PROGRESS IN BRAIN RESEARCH

VOLUME 30

CEREBRAL CIRCULATION

PROGRESS IN BRAIN RESEARCH

PROGRESS IN BRAIN RESEARCH

VOLUME 30

CEREBRAL CIRCULATION

EDITED BY

W. LUYENDIJK

Professor of Neurosurgery, Division of Neurosurgery, Academic Hospital Leyden, The Netherlands

ELSEVIER PUBLISHING COMPANY

AMSTERDAM / LONDON / NEW YORK

1968

ELSEVIER PUBLISHING COMPANY
335 JAN VAN GALENSTRAAT,
P.O. BOX 211, AMSTERDAM, THE NETHERLANDS

ELSEVIER PUBLISHING CO. LTD.
BARKING, ESSEX, ENGLAND

AMERICAN ELSEVIER PUBLISHING COMPANY, INC.
52 VANDERBILT AVENUE, NEW YORK, N.Y. 10017

LIBRARY OF CONGRESS CARD NUMBER 68–12472

STANDARD BOOK NUMBER 444–40691–3

WITH 229 ILLUSTRATIONS AND 95 TABLES

PRINTED IN THE NETHERLANDS

List of Contributors

JACOB ABRAHAM, Department of Pathology, Dartmouth Medical School, Hanover, N.H. (U.S.A.).

B. ALLIEZ, The Neuro-Surgical Clinic, Faculty of Medicine, Marseille (France).

N. O. AMELI, Department of Neurosurgery, University of Tehran, Tehran (Iran).

A. I. ARUTIUNOV, The N.N. Burdenko Research Institute of Neurosurgery, Academy of Medical Science, Moscow (U.S.S.R.).

J. J. BARCIA-GOYANES, Valencia (Spain).

J. L. BARCIA-SALORIO, Valencia (Spain).

J. BARKER, Institute of Neurological Science, Killearn Hospital, Glasgow (Great Britain).

M. BERARD, The Neuro-Surgical Clinic, Faculty of Medicine, Marseille (France).

E. BETZ, Physiological Institute, University of Marburg, Marburg/Lahn (Germany).

G. AF BJÖRKESTEN, Neurosurgical Clinic, Töölö Hospital, Helsinki (Finland).

M. BROCK, Department of Neurosurgery, University of Mainz, Mainz (Germany).

C. C. CABEZAS, Clinique Neurochirurgicale du Groupe hospitalier Pitié-Salpêtrière, Paris (France).

A. CAPON, Clinique Médicale de l'Hôpital Brugman, Université de Bruxelles, Bruxelles (Belgium).

RAUL CARREA, Centro de Investigaciones Neurológicas and Servicio de Neurocirugía, Hospital de Niños, Buenos Aires (Argentina).

ORLANDO CARVALHO, Neurologist, Lisbon Civil Hospitals, Lisbon (Portugal).

M. E. CLARK, Department of Theoretical and Applied Mechanics, College of Engineering, University of Illinois, Urbana, Ill. (U.S.A.).

H. CLEEMPOEL, Clinique Médicale de l'Hôpital Brugman, Université de Bruxelles, Bruxelles (Belgium).

A. COMBALBERT, Department of Neuroradiology, Neurobiological Research Unit, INSERM, Marseille (France).

R. COOPER, Department of Neurological Surgery, Frenchay Hospital, Bristol (Great Britain).

S. CRONQVIST, Department of Neurosurgery and Neuroradiology, University of Lund, Lund (Sweden).

MARCEL DAVID, Clinique Neurochirurgicale du Groupe hospitalier Pitié-Salpêtrière, Paris (France).

M. DE VLIEGER, Municipal Hospital Dijkzigt, Rotterdam (The Netherlands).

H. W. DICKE, Department of Surgery, Leyden University Hospital, Leyden (The Netherlands).

D. DILENGE, Clinique Neurochirurgicale de la Pitié-Salpêtrière, Paris (France).

AYKUT ERBENGI, Department of Neurosurgery, Mary Hitchcock Memorial Hospital, Hanover, N.H. (U.S.A.).

J. ESPAGNO, Neurosurgical Clinic, University Hospital Center, Toulouse (France).

J. FAURE, Department of Neuroradiology, Neurobiological Research Unit, INSERM, Marseille (France).

WILLIAM FEINDEL, Cone Laboratory for Neurosurgical Research, Montreal Neurological Institute McGill University, Montreal (Canada).

P. FIRT, Institute for Clinical and Experimental Surgery, Prague (Czechoslovakia).

H. FISCHGOLD, Clinique Neurochirurgicale de la Pitié-Salpêtrière, Paris (France).

P. FRUGONI, Via Aquileia 4, Padova (Italy).

F. J. GILLINGHAM, Royal Infirmary, Edinburgh (Great Britain).

G. GIUDICELLI, Department of Neuroradiology, Neurobiological Research Unit, INSERM, Marseille (France).

JULES C. GOVAERT, University of Ghent, Ghent (Belgium).

W. GROTE, Neurosurgical University Hospital, Bonn (Germany).

BENIAMINO GUIDETTI, Department of Neurosurgery, University of Rome Medical School, Rome (Italy).

L. HARISPE, Clinique Neurochirurgicale de la Pitié-Salpêtrière, Paris (France).

ALBERT F. HECK, Department of Neurology, University of Maryland, School of Medicine, Baltimore, Md. (U.S.A.).

L. HEJHAL, Institute for Clinical and Experimental Surgery, Prague (Czechoslovakia).

WILLIAMINA A. HIMWICH, Thudichum Psychiatric Research Laboratory, Galesburg State Research Hospital, Galesburg, Ill. (U.S.A.).

CHARLES P. HODGE, Cone Laboratory for Neurosurgical Research, Montreal Neurological Institute, McGill University, Montreal (Canada).

K. H. HOLBACH, Neurosurgical University Hospital, Bonn (Germany).

SIDNEY A. HOLLIN, Department of Neurosurgery, The Mount Sinai Hospital, New York, N.Y. (U.S.A.).

A. HULME, Department of Neurological Surgery, Frenchay Hospital, Bristol (Great Britain).

DAVID H. INGVAR, Department of Clinical Neurophysiology, University Hospital, Lund (Sweden).

JULIUS H. JACOBSON II, Department of Surgery, The Mount Sinai Hospital, New York, N.Y. (U.S.A.).

F. L. JENKNER, Department of Surgery, University of Graz, Graz (Austria).

W. BRYAN JENNETT, Institute of Neurological Sciences, Glasgow; Killearn Hospital, Glasgow (Great Britain).

A. E. KAASIK, Department of Neurology and Neurosurgery of the Tartu State University, Tartu, Estonian S.S.R. (U.S.S.R.).

VIJAY K. KAK, Department of Neurological Surgery, Royal Victoria Hospital, Belfast (N. Ireland).

P. A. KATSIOTIS, Departments of Neurosurgery and Radiology, Saint Savas Hospital, Athens (Greece).

Å. KJÄLLQUIST, Neurosurgical Research Laboratory. University Hospital, Lund (Sweden).

S. KOSTIĆ, Neurosurgical University Clinic, Belgrade (Yugoslavia).

KRISTIAN KRISTIANSEN, Ullevaal Hospital, Oslo (Norway).

ZDENĚK KUNC, Neurosurgical Clinic, Prague (Czechoslovakia).

ADAM KUNICKI, Neurosurgical Clinic, Academy of Medicine, Cracow (Poland).

E. LAINE, Clinique Neuro-Chirurgicale, Lille (France).

N. A. LASSEN, Department of Clinical Physiology, Bispebjerg Hospital, Copenhagen (Denmark).

G. LAZORTHES, Neurosurgical Clinic, University Hospital Center, Toulouse (France).

Y. LAZORTHES, Neurosurgical Clinic, University Hospital Center, Toulouse (France).

A. LENAERS, Clinique Médicale de l'Hôpital Brugman, Université de Bruxelles, Bruxelles (Belgium).

W. S. LOCKHART, JR., Department of Neurosurgery, University of Miami School of Medicine, Miami, Fla. (U.S.A.).

F. LOEW, Universitätsklinik, 665 Homburg/Saar (Germany).

N. LUNDBERG, Departments of Neurosurgery and Neuroradiology, University of Lund, Lund (Sweden).

W. C. MACCARTY, JR., Department of Radiology, Mary Hitchcock Memorial Hospital, Hanover, N.H. (U.S.A.).

D. G. McDOWALL, University Department of Anaesthesia, Western Infirmary, Glasgow (Great Britain).

GEORGE MARGOLIS, Department of Pathology, Dartmouth Medical School, Hanover, N.H. (U.S.A.).

GIOVANNI MARINI, Neurosurgical Clinic of the University of Milano, Milano (Italy).

PH. MARTIN, Clinique Médicale de l'Hôpital Brugman, Université de Bruxelles, Bruxelles (Belgium).

J. MARTIN GIRADO, Centro de Investigaciones Neurológicas and Servicio de Neurocirugía, Hospital de Niños, Buenos Aires (Argentina).

PAOLO E. MASPES, Neurosurgical Clinic of the University of Milano, Milano (Italy).

R. MESSIMY, Clinique Neurochirurgicale de la Pitié-Salpêtrière, Paris (France).

J. METZGER, Clinique Neurochirurgicale de la Pitié-Salpêtrière, Paris (France).

G. MORELLO, Istituto Neurologico di Milano, Milano (Italy).

A. MURRAY HARPER, Wellcome Surgical Research Laboratory, University of Glasgow, Glasgow (Great Britain).

G. NORLÉN, Sahlgrenska Sjukhuset, Göteborg (Sweden).

D. OECONOMOS, Athens (Greece).

JOHN O'LOUGHLIN, Department of Neurosurgery, Mary Hitchcock Memorial Hospital, Hanover, N.H. (U.S.A.).

J. E. PAILLAS, The Neuro-Surgical Clinic, Faculty of Medicine, Marseille (France).

R. M. PEARDON DONAGHY, Mary Fletcher Hospital, Burlington, Vermont (U.S.A.).

L. PERRIA, Impresa di Elettrofisiologia del C.N.R., Genova (Italy).

H. W. PIA, Neurosurgical Clinic of the University of Giessen/Lahn, Giessen/Lahn (Germany).

U. PONTÉN, Department of Neurosurgery, University of Gothenburg, Gothenburg (Sweden).

J. T. POSADA, Clinique Neurochirurgicale du Groupe hospitalier Pitié-Salpêtrière, Paris (France).

E. Raudam, Department of Neurology and Neurosurgery of the Tartu State University, Tartu, Estonian S.S.R. (U.S.S.R.).

O. M. Reinmuth, Department of Neurology, University of Miami School of Medicine, Miami, Fla. (U.S.A.).

Alan E. Richardson, Department of Neurosurgery, Atkinson Morley's Hospital, Wimbledon (Great Britain).

T. Riechert, Neurosurgical Clinic, University of Freiburg i.Br., Freiburg i.Br. (Germany).

G. Rosadini, Clinica Neurochirurgica dell'Università, Genova (Italy).

G. F. Rossi, Clinica Neurochirurgica dell'Università, Genova (Italy),

P. Röttgen, 53 Bonn-V., Heinr.-Fritsch-Str. 16 (Germany).

M. Sachs, Clinique Neurochirurgicale du Groupe Hospitalier Pitié-Salpêtrière, Paris (France).

G. Salamon, Department of Neuroradiology, Neurobiological Research Unit, INSERM, Marseille (France).

P. Scheinberg, Department of Neurology, University of Miami School of Medicine, Miami, Fla. (U.S.A.).

R. Sedan, The Neuro-Surgical Clinic Faculty of Medicine, Marseille (France).

F. A. Serbinenko, The N.N. Burdenko Research Institute of Neurosurgery, Academy of Medical Science, Moscow (U.S.S.R.).

M. N. Shalit, Department of Neurosurgery, Hadassah University Hospital, Jerusalem (Israel).

S. Shimojyo, Department of Neurology, University of Miami School of Medicine, Miami, Fla. (U.S.A.).

A. A. Shlykov, The N.N. Burdenko Research Institute of Neurosurgery, Academy of Medical Science, Moscow (U.S.S.R.).

B. K. Siesjö, Neurosurgical Clinic, University of Gothenburg, Gothenburg (Sweden).

Lucjan Stepien, 71/4 Wilcza Street, Warszawa (Poland).

Michael H. Sukoff, Department of Surgery, The Mount Sinai Hospital, New York, N.Y. (U.S.A.).

Thoralf M. Sundt, Jr., Mayo Graduate School of Medicine, University of Minnesota, Rochester, Minn. (U.S.A.).

Lindsay Symon, Department of Neurosurgical Studies, The National Hospital, Queen Square, London, W.C. 1 (Great Britain).

J. N. Taptas, Departments of Neurosurgery and Radiology, Saint Savas Hospital, Athens (Greece).

Alex R. Taylor, Department of Neurological Surgery, Royal Victoria Hospital, Belfast (N. Ireland).

M. Toga, The Neuro-Surgical Clinic, Faculty of Medicine, Marseille (France).

Eduardo Tolosa, Platón 20, Barcelona (Spain).

H. Troupp, Neurosurgical Clinic, Töölö Hospital, Helsinki (Finland).

R. Van Den Bergh, Department of Neurology and Neurosurgery, University of Louvain, Louvain (Belgium).

H. VANDER EECKEN, Department of Anatomy and Neuro-psychology, University of Ghent, Ghent (Belgium).

H. VERBIEST, Neurosurgical Clinic, University of Utrecht, Utrecht (The Netherlands).

M. VINK, Department of Surgery, Leyden University Hospital, Leyden (The Netherlands).

A. WACKENHEIM, Clinique Neurologique, Hôpital Civil, Strasbourg (France).

A. EARL WALKER, University of Ghent, Ghent (Belgium).

ARTHUR G. WALTZ, Cerebrovascular Clinical Research Center, Section of Neurology, Mayo Clinic, Rochester, Mo. (U.S.A.).

J. WAPPENSCHMIDT, Neurosurgical University Hospital, Bonn (Germany).

Y. LUCAS YAMAMOTO, Cone Laboratory for Neurosurgical Research, Montreal Neurological Institute, McGill University, Montreal (Canada).

GAZI YASARGIL, Mary Fletcher Hospital, Burlington, Vermont (U.S.A.).

PETER O. YATES, Department of Pathology, University of Manchester, Manchester (Great Britain).

J. O. ZADEH, Neurosurgical Clinic, University Hospital Center, Toulouse (France).

B. G. ZIEDSES DES PLANTES, Röntgen Laboratory, Wilhelmina Gasthuis, University of Amsterdam, Amsterdam (The Netherlands).

L. ZOLTÁN, Budapest (Hungary).

K. J. ZÜLCH, Ostmerheimer Str. 200, 5 Köln-Merheim (Germany).

R. ZUPPING, Department of Neurology and Neurosurgery of the Tartu State University, Tartu, Estonian S.S.R. (U.S.S.R.).

N. ZWETNOW, Neurosurgical Research Laboratory, University Hospital, Lund (Sweden).

x

Preface

Cerebral Circulation and its Disorders was chosen as the main subject for the IIIrd European Congress of Neurosurgery which took place in Madrid in April 1967.

The increasing interest in vascular conditions, the progress in diagnostic procedures, together with the clinical application of new methods for studying the cerebral blood flow and the development of various neurosurgical techniques for the management of these patients, led the Organization Committee of the Congress to initiate a general reassessment and discussion of certain topics in cerebral vascular pathology. For this purpose eminent European scientists and neurosurgeons were asked to write different reports as it was felt to be desirable to present a cross section of these problems in Europe today.

Very short summaries of these reports already having appeared, Professor W. Luyendijk has now edited them in full length and collected them in this volume together with a selection of free communications presented at the Congress.

I am sure that the material assembled in this book concerning fundamental anatomical and physiological studies and the more practical results obtained by diagnostic and therapeutic procedures in various vascular conditions will be of great importance for neurosurgeons and other clinicians, and specialists interested in the central nervous system.

Dr. S. Obrador
President of the IIIrd European
Congress of Neurosurgery

Contents

Section III — Neuropathology

Section IV — Neuroradiology

Section V — Other methods of investigation

Section VI — Occlusive vascular lesions

CONTENTS

Anatomy and Embryology of Cerebral Circulation

RAYMOND VAN DEN BERGH AND HENRI VANDER EECKEN

Department of Neurology and Neurosurgery and Department of Neuro-anatomy (University of Louvain, Belgium), and Department of Anatomy and Department of Neuro-psychology (University of Ghent, Belgium)

INTRODUCTION

The present report has unfortunately to be restricted to a concise and thus rather incomplete survey of recent data on cerebral arterial circulation. The topics to be discussed have been selected because of their importance in neurosurgery.

With respect to the afferent vessels, the significance of the large trunks in the establishment of cerebrovascular disturbances has recently been stressed, whereas the arteries of the basis cerebri, as a consequence of the interventions on vascular malformations, have been subject to more precise studies in relation to their frequent anatomical variants and anomalies.

The leptomeningeal arteries, spreading over the cerebral surface, have been investigated in detail, mainly from the point of view of their vascularization areas and collateral circulation.

The intracerebral circulation has been examined as to its irrigation of the cerebral parenchyma, its segmentation in vascular areas and its deep collateral circulation, which features are most important in stereotaxic surgery.

In the first chapter comments will be given on the afferent arteries culminating in the arterial circle of Willis. Upon reaching the encephalon their basal and excentric location differs from the situation in other organs, where the afferent arteries penetrate into the center by way of an hilus.

A second chapter will treat the leptomeningeal arteries, which start from the basically located main trunks and wrap around the encephalon in a dorsal direction, an organization pattern found from the telencephalon down to the medulla oblongata.

A third chapter will describe the intracerebral circulation, which is constituted by radially penetrating intraparenchymal branches of the leptomeningeal arteries.

I. AFFERENT ARTERIAL TRUNKS

The brain is supplied by four main afferent arterial trunks: the aa. carotides internae and the aa. vertebrales.

The a. carotis interna derives, together with the a. carotis externa, from the a. carotis communis at a level varying between the 3rd and 6th cervical vertebra[3,90,151,158]. Through the os petrosum it enters the cranial cavity, where its first part runs in the sinus cavernosus.

The a. vertebralis describes a delicate course through the foramina transversaria of the cervical vertebrae before reaching the foramen magnum. The aa. vertebrales fuse to an arteria basilaris at the border of pons and medulla oblongata. Anomalies are frequent. The vertebral arteries originate exceptionally from the a. carotis communis. Sometimes they persist independently without fusion. Further there are often size differences between the two arteries commonly the left being the larger.

Recently renewed attention has been given to the presence of bony rings surrounding the a. vertebralis during its course on the surface of the atlas. These rings, either external lateroglenoidal (3 to 9% according the authors) or posterior retroglenoidal (7 to 30%) consist in bony bridges covering the sulcus arteriae vertebralis[131].

Further, a venous sinus surrounding the a. vertebralis in the latters transverse course in the sulcus of the atlas has been described[90,120,191]. This "sinus atlanto-occipitalis" is found between atlas and foramen magnum and might be — not unlike the sinus cavernosus — a shock absorber and regulator of the venous circulation. In children a relatively larger sinus was observed.

Extracranially the a. carotis interna and the a. vertebralis present numerous anastomoses with the a. carotis externa, which seem to be of rather limited functional value in emergency cases.

Anastomoses between the internal and external carotid systems occur in facial structures in relation to the eye, nose and ear[24,28,38,67,85,90,111,144,145,154,156,190]. The most important connections as revealed by angiograms are end-to-end anastomoses between on one side the aa. frontales (a. ophtalmica) and on the other side the a. angularis (a. maxillaris externa) and the ramus frontalis of the a. temporalis superficialis.

Of less functional value are the connections between the aa. ethmoidales (a. ophtalmica) and the a. sphenopalatina (a. maxillaris interna), between the a. dorsalis nasi (a. ophtalmica) and the a. infraorbitalis (a. maxillaris interna), between the a. lacrimalis (a. ophtalmica) and either the a. zygomatico-orbitalis (a. temporalis superficialis) or the ramus frontalis of the a. meningea media.

In the auditory region collateral between the a. tympanica (a. carotis interna) and the a. labyrinthi (a. basilaris) on one side and branches of the a. carotis externa on the other is normally minute, devoid of any vicarious circulation possibility.

The persistence, nevertheless, of an a. stapedia primitiva might theoretically account for a significant collateral supply[183].

The frequent anastomoses between the a. occipitalis (a. carotis externa) and the rami musculares of the a. vertebralis are in general less efficient than those in the nasal and orbital regions, but they are certainly more efficient than those in the auditory region.

Intracranially the main afferent trunks anastomose under the basis cerebri, forming the circle of Willis.

Its normal structure and many variations have been thoroughly studied by numerous authors[3,11,12,31,35,37,39,41,42,46,48,51,60,66,76,77,79,83,86,90,106,112–114,118,119,133,141,150,152,185,187,188] and its morphological significance has been elucidated by B. de Vriese[41,42] and D. H. Padget[118]. The suggestion of H. A. Kaplan[80] in referring to the distal division of the a. basilaris as the aa. mesencephalicae and to the aa. communicantes posteriores as the proximal portion of the aa. cerebri posteriores should be retained. The latter terminology not only corresponds with the irrigation area but also with the morphogenesis, since B. de Vriese[42] demonstrated that the aa. cerebri posteriores phylogenetically originate from the aa. carotides internae.

With respect to the circulus arteriosus, only the usual variation types, from which most anomalies derive, will be mentioned (Fig. 1). It has been established — a fact

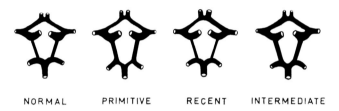

NORMAL   PRIMITIVE   RECENT   INTERMEDIATE

Fig. 1. Variation types of the circulus arteriosus cerebri.

of paramount importance to the neurosurgery of aneurysms — that the so-called normal arterial circle of Willis only occurs in a minority of cases.

Abnormal carotido-vertebro-basilar anastomoses, as the arteria trigemina primitiva, the arteria auditiva primitiva and the arteria hypoglossica primitiva, are observed[11,16,23,37,45,57,63,68,71,72,74,75,84,86,87,103,116,117,129,130,142,149,152,160]. According to literature data these persisting connections seem to be rare in adult humans (3 to 5%).

The arteria trigemina primitiva is the most important. It frequently connects the a. carotis interna with the a. basilaris. A functional consequence of this connection is a reversed, i.e. a downward circulation, in the vertebral system. This artery may cause trigeminal neuralgia and subarachnoidal hemorrhage. The latter could be due either to an embryologically incompletely formed wall, or to its frequent association with other vascular anomalies such as aneurysms. The importance of such abnormal arteries for surgery of the ponto-cerebellar area should be stressed.

II. LEPTOMENINGEAL ARTERIES

A network of leptomeningeal arteries[15,17,18,90,111,177] originating from the above mentioned basal main trunks covers the entire cerebral surface. At the basis cerebri the main trunks form an arterial circle giving rise to three cerebral arteries wrapping upward around the cerebrum. Caudally from this circle, the leptomeningeal (principally cerebellar) arteries derive from the aa. vertebrales and basilaris, embracing in an analogous circular way brain stem and cerebellum. From the leptomeningeal arteries the proper cerebral arteries perpendicularly penetrate into the cerebral parenchyma converging towards the ventricular system[165-167,169,170].

The extensive and complicated embryological development of the telencephalon as compared to that of the brain stem and cerebellum (doubling of the anterior cerebral vesicle, size increase of the gray nuclei, secondary curvature giving rise to the lateral sulcus and development of sulci and gyri) somehow obscures the annular wrapping of the neural tube at the level of the cerebrum[165]. Nevertheless, all leptomeningeal arteries can at any level be classified according to the same schema into three groups: paramedian, short circumferential and long circumferential arteries [54,90,165]. The paramedian arteries penetrate into the cerebral parenchyma after a short course (e.g. branches of the a. cerebri anterior for the infundibulum, paramedian branches of the brain stem). The short circumferential arteries run somewhat farther before ending in penetrating arteries (e.g. rami striati, aa. thalami, lateral branches of the brain stem). The long circumferential arteries are the distal ones reaching the surface of the hemispheres, the cerebellum and the dorsal surface of the brain stem.

1. Supratentorial leptomeningeal arteries

For the greater part of their course they are located in the depth of the sulci of the cerebral cortex. Throughout their course they give off fine side branches, most of which are more or less perpendicular to the direction of the sulcus and ascend on the

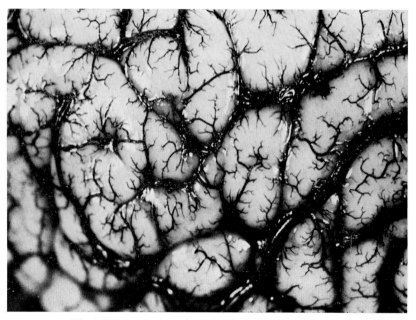

Fig. 2. Demonstration of the arterial irrigation of a gyrus.

banks of adjacent gyri to continue in close contact with the most prominent part of these gyri[173,174,177].

Our observations affirm that the ridge of the gyrus, situated between the sulci along which the arteries run, usually constitutes the border of the irrigation area of two parallel adjacent arteries which are about to overlap (Fig. 2). Occasionally an artery runs over the whole ridge of a gyrus to disappear into the sulcus on both sides, giving off side branches over its entire course. This situation expands the irrigation area of a given artery.

Although it also might suggest the existence of anastomoses between these arteries, careful dissection reveals this in most instances being rather appearance than reality.

Three sites present pronounced anatomical variations in the localization of the demarcation line between the cortical areas of the three cerebral arteries[172–174,176,177]:

(a) a displacement of 1 to 2 cm either towards the a. cerebri media or the a. cerebri posterior territory is often found in the border area of the a. parieto-occipitalis and the aa. angularis and temporalis posterior;

(b) a displacement of 1 to 1.5 cm either towards the a. cerebri anterior or the a. cerebri posterior is regularly observed on the convex surface in the border area between the a. paracentralis and the a. centralis;

(c) another variable demarcation line is located at the basal surface of the cerebral hemispheres between the a. orbitalis and the a. orbitofrontalis.

Many investigators[5,7,32–34,45,80–82,90,122,124,159,162] demonstrated that the leptomeningeal arteries are not all terminal branches and that they form numerous precapillary and capillary connections among themselves. Further, it has been established[7,8,17,25,29,36,49,55,58–62,100,101,104,146–148,176,177,181,182] that there exist fairly numerous wide anastomoses between the leptomeningeal arteries in the depth of the sulci. These anastomoses are nearly always situated in the border area of the three main cerebral arteries, forming a communication between branches originating from two different main cerebral arteries (Fig. 3, A, B, C). Anastomoses between two branches of the same cerebral artery are not common.

The leptomeningeal anastomoses, varying in size from 200 to 760 μ, constitute efficient connections. Their location at the demarcation zones may be summarized as follows:

A. Between the a. cerebri media and the a. cerebri anterior:
   (1) end-to-end anastomoses in the sulci praecentralis, centralis and parietalis anterior;
   (2) candelabra-shaped finely branched anastomoses in the sulcus frontalis superior and in or just above the sulcus interparietalis;
   (3) two or three transverse or oblique anastomoses in the region of the sulcus cruciatus.

B. Between the a. cerebri media and the a. cerebri posterior:
   (1) end-to-end anastomoses in the superior part of the sulcus parieto-occipitalis or in the inferior portion of the sulcus interparietalis;
   (2) two or three finer superficial channels in or just below the sulcus temporalis medius.

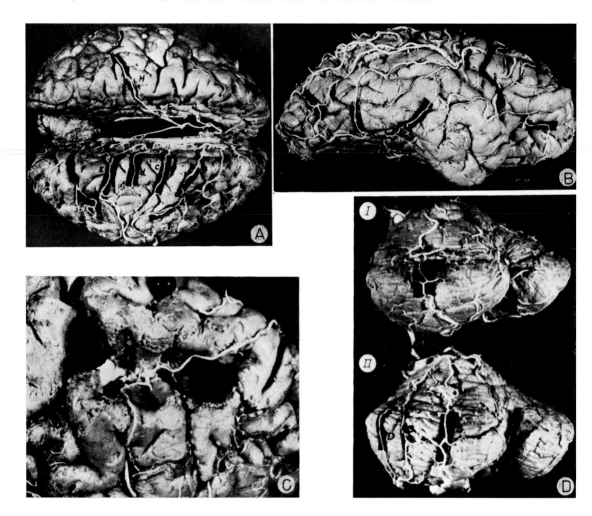

Fig. 3. *A.* Superior view of the cerebrum. Demonstration of anastomoses, on the right hemisphere, between branches of the aa. cerebri media and anterior. — *B.* Lateral view of the right hemisphere. Demonstration of anastomoses between branches of the a. cerebri media and the aa. cerebri posterior and anterior. — *C.* End-to-end anastomosis lifted from the depth of the sulcus frontalis superior dexter between a branch of the a. orbito-frontalis of a. cerebri media and the a. frontalis interna media of the a. cerebri anterior. — *D.* Demonstration of anastomoses between the a. cerebelli superior and the aa. cerebelli inferiores, ant. and post.

C. Between the a. cerebri anterior and the a. cerebri posterior: one to three end-to-end or branched anastomoses in the posterior indentation of the praecuneus at the level of the anterior tip of the sulcus parieto-occipitalis.

Recently several authors[6,9,27,30,38-40,47,50,52,68,69,88,98,107,109,110,115,132,134,138,139, 157,160,161,186] reported the presence of these peripheral anastomoses in angiographic visualisation of cerebrovascular accidents.

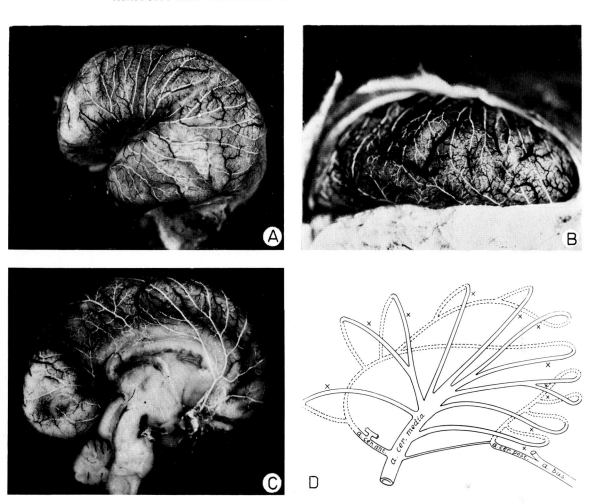

Fig. 4. *A*. Facies convexa of the left hemisphere of a foetus of about 21 weeks old. — *B*. Idem, superior view of the facies convexa of the left hemisphere. — *C*. Idem, facies interhemispherica of the left hemisphere. — *D*. Schematic representation of the main continuous arteries. The crosses indicate the place of later interruptions or anastomoses.

Number, diameter and location, however, of these leptomeningeal anastomoses show, in the human adult, large individual variations[174,176-178,180,181], which is due to a more or less pronounced regression of the more complex embryonic and foetal cerebral vascular system[172-174,176,177].

Eminent embryologists[41,42,46,78,106,118,119,140,153] have elucidated the early embryonic development of the human cerebral arterial system. It can further be observed[172-174,176,177] that in the beginning of foetal life, the cortical leptomeningeal branches form a network of wide arteries, deriving from the primordial arterial plexus, and extend as arches over the brain's surface (Fig. 4). This pattern is modified only during the last months of foetal life, when the brain sulci deepen: concommittantly the foetal loops disappear or regress to anastomoses at the sites of the future demarcation between the irrigation areas of the three cerebral arteries. Some comparative anatomical observations[26,105,172,173,176,177,189] on mammalian brains revealed the existence of arterial loops of the human foetal type in those with lissencephalon and anastomoses of the human adult type in those with gyrencephalon.

It should be stressed that the relief efficiency of these arterial collaterals with their numerous individual morphological variations entirely depends on their functional state at the "crucial" moment[192–194].

2. Infratentorial leptomeningeal arteries

The extraordinary inconstancy and variability of the infratentorial leptomeningeal arteries should always be kept in mind[13,44,64,65,89,95,121].

After branching off from the a. basilaris, a. vertebralis or a. spinalis anterior, the paramedian arteries immediately penetrate into the brain stem. They do not have particular names and are variable in number.

The short circumferential arteries end at the lateral surface of the brain stem and vary also in number. One of them is known as the lateral bulbar artery.

The long circumferential arteries are, as systematically described from below upward: the a. spinalis posterior and the a. cerebelli inferior posterior (both branches of the a. vertebralis), the a. labyrinthi, the a. cerebelli inferior anterior, and the a. cerebelli superior (all three branches of the a. basilaris).

Important variations are frequent. The a. cerebelli inferior posterior may branch off from the a. basilaris and even from the a. cerebelli inferior anterior or it may be replaced by several smaller arteries.

The a. cerebelli inferior anterior may branch off from the a. vertebralis, the a. labyrinthi or from a common branch with the a. labyrinthi of the a. basilaris.

The a. labyrinthi very often originates from the a. cerebelli inferior anterior, the latter then sometimes sinuously penetrating into the meatus acusticus internus at the level of the branching. The a. labyrinthi may provide the brain stem with recurrent branches.

The a. cerebelli superior may be double on one or both sides.

As a consequence it is often very difficult to determine the identity and the significance of an individual artery as seen isolated during a surgical intervention. For the same reason a given intraparenchymal area cannot always be allotted to a given superficial artery and it is certainly erroneous to attribute nosologically a brain stem infarct to a determined superficial artery.

Anastomoses between the infratentorial leptomeningeal arteries are relatively frequent.

Most commonly they occur between the distal branches of two different cerebellar arteries; their size varies between 180 and 550 μ (Fig. 3, D).

Anastomoses are frequently observed[172-174,176,177], between the a. cerebelli superior and the a. cerebelli inferior anterior, between the a. cerebelli superior and the a. cerebelli inferior posterior, between the a. cerebelli inferior anterior and the a. cerebelli inferior posterior.

Further, 10% of the cases present anastomoses between the aa. cerebelli superiores of both sides and between both aa. cerebelli inferiores (anteriores and posteriores).

Anastomoses between the branches of a same cerebellar artery more often occur than between the branches of a same cerebral artery.

Finally it should be mentioned that there is no pial arteriolar plexus around the brain stem as found over the cerebral and cerebellar cortex and around the spinal cord.

III. INTRAPARENCHYMAL CIRCULATION

The internal encephalic vascularization essentially concerns the irrigation of a tubular organ[165-167,170].

The excentrically and externally located afferent trunks send their branches, the leptomeningeal arteries, in an annular way round the organ, wrapping it up completely. From these branches the intraparenchymal arteries penetrate centripetally and radially towards the central lumen, i.e. the ventricle. Some penetrating arteries send secondarily centrifugal branches into the parenchyma.

This organization is found over the entire brain.

1. Cerebrum

The intracerebral arterial system[19,21,70,166,167,169,170] primarily consists of arteries of peripheral and secondarily of arteries of ventricular origin (Fig. 5, A).

A. Arteries of peripheral origin.

These arteries, branches of the leptomeningeal arteries, which cover in an annular way each hemisphere, penetrate centripetally into the cerebral parenchyma, supplying the cortex (rami corticales) and the deeper layers (rami medullares, rami striati and rami perforantes).*

The rami corticales[122-127,155,166] course parallelly and end in the cortex or immediately beneath it, where precapillary anastomoses may be found (Fig. 6).

---

* The term 'rami corticales', as mentioned by the P.N.A., is reserved for the fine intracortical arteries. The larger leptomeningeal arteries, running on the surface of the cortex, merit the name 'arteria'. On the other hand, the P.N.A. does not provide for a proper name for the arteries of the white substance. We propose the term 'rami medullares', whereas the 'rami striati' concern arteries for the gray nuclei.

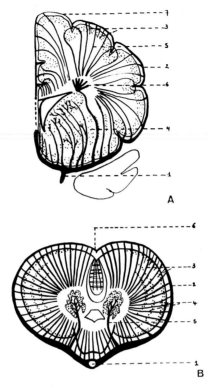

Fig. 5. *A*. Intraparenchymal circulation of the cerebrum. 1: Arteria carotis interna; 2: Leptomeningeal arteries; 3: Rami corticales; 4: Rami striati; 5: Rami medullares; 6: Ventriculofugal arteries, originating from the rami striati laterales; 7: Leptomeningeal anastomoses. — *B*. Intraparenchymal circulation of the cerebellum. 1: Arteria basilaris; 2: Leptomeningeal arteries; 3: Rami corticales; 4: Rami medullares; 5: Arteria nuclei dentati with ventriculofugal branches; 6: Leptomeningeal anastomoses.

The rami medullares[135,136,155,165–167,169,170], supplying the white substance, converge radially towards the nearest point of the ventricular wall (Fig. 6). They are rectilinear, give off but a few branches and commonly divide in two or more terminal branches in the neighbourhood of the ventricle, which they rarely reach. They exceptionally present some anastomoses, most of them smaller than 20 μ.

From an angioarchitectonic point of view[99,165–167] the rami medullares are substantially influenced by the local arrangement of nervous fibers and the glial infrastructure of the white substance[102,165–167]. At the transition zones between neighbouring nervous fascicles they frequently display deviations, dilatations, ramifications, bifurcations and sinuosities. Anastomoses, always of precapillary size, also appear at these levels (Fig. 7).

These arrangements are particularly apparent in the temporo-occipital white matter at the lateral side of the trigonum ventriculi. Here the radially oriented arteries successively penetrate through three adjacent and perpendicularly disposed fiber structures, namely the tapetum, the radiatio optica and the vertical part of the fasciculus fronto-

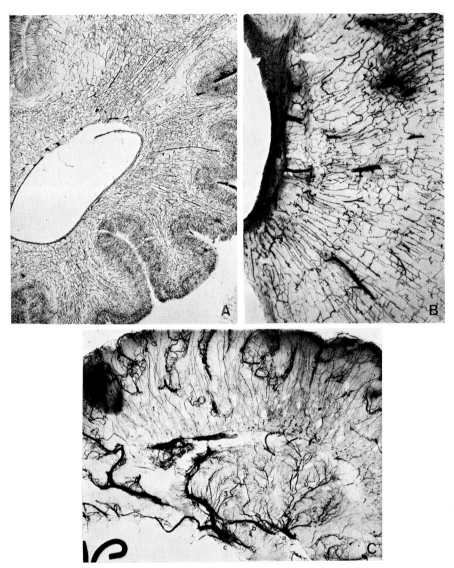

Fig. 6. *A*. Frontal section through the cornu posterius (Neonatus, Chinese ink, 200 μ × 4). Rami corticales, coursing parallelly, and rami medullares with radial and converging disposition. — *B*. Frontal section through the trigonum ventriculi lateralis (foetus 5 months old, benzidine staining, 200 μ × 12). Radial disposition of the rami medullares, influenced by the glial infrastructure of the white substance. Concentric angioarchitectonic rings. — *C*. Sagittal section (8 mm thick) through thalamus and corpus striatum (radiograph after intra-arterial injection of barium suspension). 1 : rami medullares; 2 : rami striati; 3 : rami perforantes; a : a. cerebri media; b : a. communicans posterior; c : a. cerebri posterior.

occipitalis superior. This vascular disposition probably presents a locus minoris resistentiae for intracerebral haematomes, which frequently occur in this area[162,164].

The rami striati[1,10,73,135,136,155,165–167], supplying the gray nuclei, the capsula interna

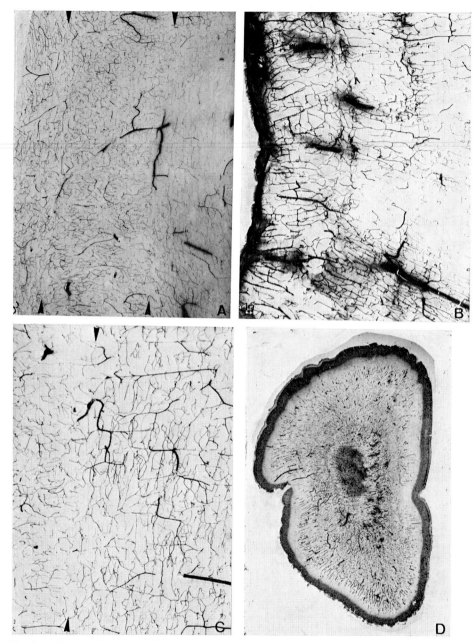

Fig. 7. *A*. Angioarchitecture of the tapetum (at the left), of the radiatio optica (in the middle) and of the fasciculus fronto-occipitalis (at the right). Deviations and ramifications in the transition zones, (frontal section of 200 μ, benzidine, $\times$ 12). — *B*. Angioarchitecture at the level of the trigonum ventriculi lateralis (at the left) in a foetus 7 months old (frontal section of 200 μ, benzidine, $\times$ 20). The rami medullares display bifurcations, sinuosities and anastomoses (precapillary size) at the transition zones between neighbouring nervous fascicles. — *C*. Angioarchitecture of the transition zone between the radiatio optica at the left and the fasciculus fronto-occipitalis at the right (frontal section of 200 μ, benzidine, $\times$ 12). — *D*. Concentric angioarchitectonic rings. Vascular deviations, sinuosities and ramifications in the transition zones (foetus of 6 months old, frontal section of lobus frontalis just in front of the cornu anterius, benzidine, $\times$ 4).

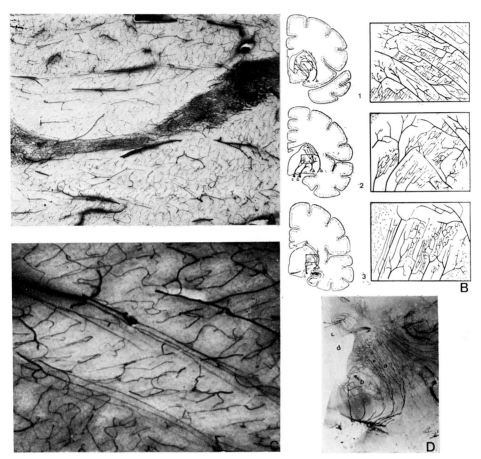

Fig. 8. *A*. Angioarchitecture of the capsula interna. Bridge of gray substance with high vascular density (frontal section of 200 μ, benzidine, $\times$ 12). — *B*. Scheme of the blood supply and of the angioarchitecture of the capsula interna. 1 = crus anterius; 2 = genu; 3 = crus posterius; a: rami striati mediales (arteria cerebri anterior); b: rami striati laterales (arteria cerebri media); c: arteria communicans posterior; d: arteria chorioidea anterior. — *C*. Angioarchitecture of the crus anterius capsulae internae. The greater part of the capillary vessels follows the direction of the nervous fibres. One finds however some very long capillary vessels, which course in a transverse way, as do the arterioles (frontal section of 200 μ, benzidine, $\times$ 40). — *D*. Blood supply of the capsula interna. Rami striati (a) and branches of the a. communicans posterior (b). Radical difference between the pattern of the same rami striati in the capsula interna and in the gray nuclei (radiograph of a frontal section after intra-arterial injection of barium suspension; c = corpus callosum, d = ventriculus lateralis).

and the laterodorsal border of the nucleus lateralis thalami, display a sinuous and arborizing course. They are larger than the rami medullares and the longest among them reach close to the ventricle (Figs. 6, C; 8, 9). The rami striati penetrate into the brain through the substantia perforata anterior. We do not agree with H. A. Kaplan and D. H. Ford[82] when they describe at this level anastomoses between medial and lateral rami striati, being respectively branches of a. cerebri anterior and of a. cerebri media. Within the gray nuclei, however, close to the ventricle and in the gray bridges of the capsula interna there are some small anastomoses reaching 50 μ.

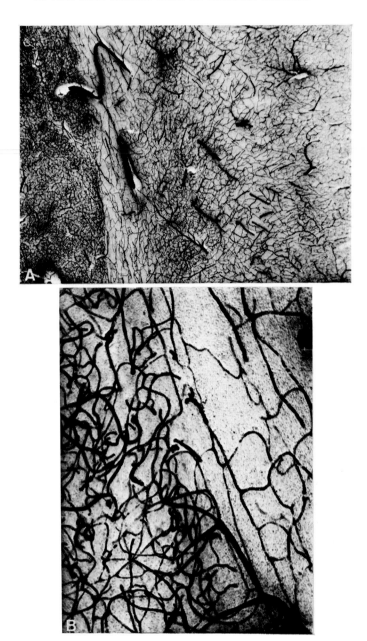

Fig. 9. Angioarchitecture of the corpus striatum and neighbourhood. *A.* From the left to the right: putamen, capsula externa, claustrum, capsula extrema, cortex insulae. (Frontal section of 200 μ, benzidine, $\times$ 12). — *B.* Putamen at the left, capsula externa at the right. (Frontal section of 200 μ, benzidine, $\times$ 60).

The angioarchitecture of the corpus striatum (Figs. 8 and 9) is highly typical[165,167,168], and, although supplied by the same arteries, there is a radical difference between the pattern in the capsula interna and in the gray nuclei[163,165,166]. The vascular density is very high, particularly in the putamen and in the medial part of the globus pallidus.

The vascular organization may play an important role in the establishment of the undesired lesions at distance during stereotaxic interventions.

The capsula interna is to a large extent supplied by arteries previously crossing the globus pallidus and putamen. In destroying one of these nuclei, a coincidental lesion of the afferent arteries will undoubtedly affect the capsula interna (Fig. 8).

The frequent occurrence of diffuse cerebral haemorrhages at the inferior external border of the putamen can to a large extent be explained by the exceptional high density of arterioles and venules in this area, where, moreover, the rami striati display a very sharp upward and inward angulation resulting in a severe cross-load.

The rami perforantes[54,90,91,97,113,128] irrigate the greater part of the thalamus and hypothalamus (Fig. 6, C).

The vessels, supplying the thalamus, can be subdivided in 5 groups: 1. rami prae-mamillarii (a. communicans posterior or a. cerebri posterior); 2. rami retromamillarii or thalamoperforantes (a. cerebri posterior); 3. rami thalamogeniculati (a. cerebri posterior); 4. rami chorioidei including lateroventral (a. chorioidea anterior), posterior and superior (a. chorioidea anterior and a. chorioidea posterior lateralis) and medial (a. chorioidea posterior medialis) vessels; 5. rami lenticulo-optici (rami striati of the a. cerebri media).

The hypothalamus is irrigated by branches, originating directly from the arteries which constitute the circulus arteriosus cerebri.

Classically rami medullares and rami corticales are considered as constituting the 'peripheral system' of the cerebral circulation, whereas the rami striati and the rami perforantes are taken to belong to the 'central system'[93,151,158]. It is questionnable if this classification is not artificial. The so-called central arteries as well as the peripheral arteries are pointed at the center of the hemisphere, i.e. the ventricle. They emanate from the same pericerebral network. The only difference resides in the fact that the central arteries branch off from the proximal portion of the large afferent arteries, whereas the peripheral arteries do this more distally. There is not any essential difference. The centripetal arteries of the gray nuclei and those of the white substance have the same peripheral origin.

The irrigation areas of the various leptomeningeal arteries may be considered as being a series of cortico-subcortical cone-shaped areas, centered around a sulcus containing the given artery. Fig. 10, 1 schematically represents the typical irrigation area of the various distal or cortical branches of the cerebral arteries over the right hemisphere (A.B.C.) and the course and irrigation area of the perforating branches of the proximal segments of the brain arteries (D.). Fig. 10, 2 represents the irrigation of the thalamus. These schemes are almost identical with those presented by Foix and coworkers[53-56]. The variations in origin of these arteries and the location of the main branches have been systematically described by numerous authors[1,4,7,22,29,36,45,53-56,58-62,90,91,104, 108,120,143,151,158,159,174,175,177].

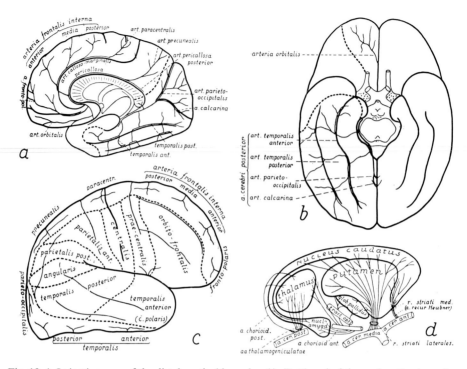

Fig. 10, 1. Irrigation area of the distal cortical branches (A, B, C) and of the perforating branches of the proximal segments (D) of the leptomeningeal arteries.

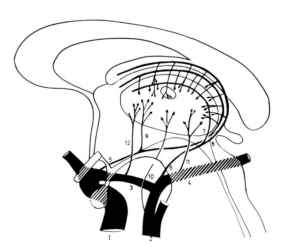

Fig. 10, 2. Irrigation of the thalamus. — 1: a. carotis interna; 2: a. basilaris; 3: a. communicans posterior; 4: a. cerebri posterior; 5: a. chorioidea anterior; 6: a. chorioidea posterior; 7: a. chorioidea posterior medialis; 8: a. chorioidea posterior lateralis; 9: rami chorioidei lateroventrales; 10: rami retromamillarii (thalamoperforantes); 11: rami thalamogeniculati; 12: rami praemamillarii.

B. Arteries of ventricular origin.

We have observed that they originate from subependymal arteries, the latter being branches of the aa. chorioideae, and from the distal branches of well-defined rami striati laterales[165–167,169–171,179]. They centri- or ventriculofugally diverge in the cerebral parenchyma. Most of them supply the periventricular white substance, some of them the paraventricular areas of the gray nuclei. They may attain a length of 1.5 cm (Fig. 11).

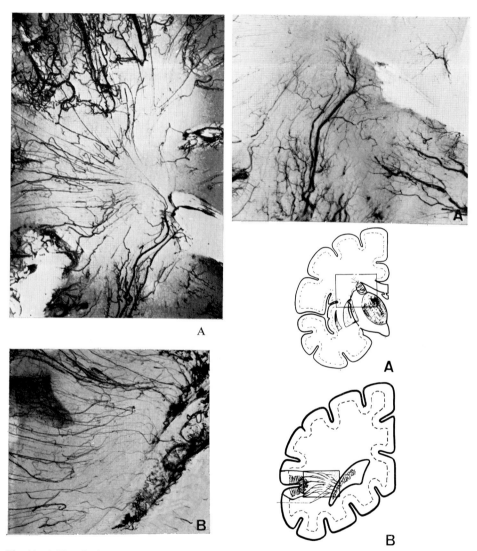

Fig. 11. *A.* Ventriculo- or centrifugal arteries at the level of the pars centralis ventriculi lateralis. They originate from the most lateral rami striati laterales. Radiograph (× 3) of a frontal section, 10 mm thick, after intra-arterial injection of Schlesinger (left picture) or Barium (right picture). — *B.* Ventriculo- or centrifugal arteries at the level of the trigonum ventriculi. They run towards the centripetal arteries, which derive from the peripheral leptomeningeal arteries, without making anastomoses.

Radiograph (× 3) of a frontal section, 10 mm thick, after intra-arterial injection of Barium.

These centrifugal arteries run towards the centripetal ones, which derive from the peripheral leptomeningeal arteries, however without making any connections or anastomoses with them. The most important and constant ones are found laterally to the external border of the pars centralis ventriculi lateralis and laterally to the trigonum and cornu posterius. Those of the pars centralis originate from the rami striati laterales; the latter ones circumscribe partially the corpus nuclei caudati, next reach the external border of the ventricle and then send their terminal branches centrifugally and divergently back into the cerebral parenchyma.

From the apparent continuity of these centrifugal arteries with those coming from the periphery some authors concluded the existence of anastomoses between medullary and striate arteries[21].

An exact knowledge of their existence is important for neurosurgical interventions in the neighbourhood of the ventricular system.

They moreover play an important role in the pathogenesis of para- and periventricular haemorrhages and infarcts and in the safeguarding of these areas in case of infarcts in the neighbourhood[171].

This means that an occlusion of some rami striati laterales can cause a selective infarct of the paraventricular white matter whereas the latter can escape a cone-shaped infarct affecting the white substance from the periphery.

The periventricular leukomalacia in the newborn is considered by most authors as an anoxemic lesion preferentially affecting these areas because of their terminal location with respect to the vascular irrigation from the periphery and of their location on the border of several cortico-subcortical vascular areas[2,14,43]. In our opinion, however, these leukomalacia areas perfectly coincide with the demarcation zone between the centrifugal and centripetal vascular systems[166,167,170,171].

Except the border areas and the 'Letzte Wiesen'[192-194], determined by the depth

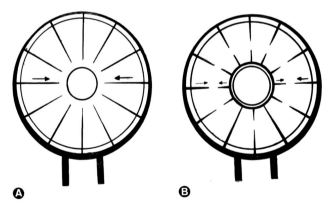

Ⓐ   Ⓑ

Fig. 12. *A*. Scheme of the classic conception of the cerebral blood supply. The brain is envelopped by a network of leptomeningeal arteries, coming from afferent trunks, which remain basally and outside the brain. From this network the intracerebral arteries converge towards the ventricle (represented by a circle). — *B*. Ventriculofugal arteries, originating from deep penetrating vessels. They run towards the ventriculopetal vessels, without making anastomoses. Between the two systems there exists a periventricular demarcation line.

projection of the cortical cerebral arteries, there also exists in the deep blood supply of the brain a three-dimensional periventricular border area (Fig. 12) between a centripetal network surging from the periphery and a centrifugal network, dependent from well-defined branches[171].

2. Cerebellum

The same pattern of centripetal and centrifugal arteries, as described in the cerebrum, applies to the cerebellum and the pons, when considered as a whole with the fourth ventricle as its center (Fig. 5, B).

The important development, dorsally of the fourth ventricle, of the cerebellum as a separate organ entails a new feature. The three cerebellar peduncles deeply penetrate into the cerebellum and form some kind of a hilus, directed towards the cerebellar nuclei, the latter being centrally located close to the fourth ventricle. As a consequence the cerebellar centrifugal intraparenchymal circulation is more extensive than that in the telencephalon.

The centripetal arteries are branches of the leptomeningeal vascular plexus, which spread over the cerebellar surface. They are directed to the cerebellar nuclei and the fourth ventricle[20,94,95,121]. Most of these arteries terminate in the white substance without reaching the former structures. They irrigate the cortex and the white substance, whereas some of them do reach the external border of the nucleus dentatus[95,96].

The centrifugal arteries branch off from the proximal segments of the various cerebellar arteries and course with the cerebellar peduncles directly to the center of the cerebellum by-passing the cortex. The most typical one, the a. nuclei dentati, a branch of the a. cerebelli inferior anterior[29] or of the a. cerebelli superior ([95,96,184]) follows the pedunculus cerebellaris superior and directly reaches the cerebellar center close to the fourth ventricle. Its branches radiate centrifugally towards the concavity of the nucleus dentatus, while some side-branches supply the other gray nuclei.

3. Brain Stem

The intraparenchymal vascularization of the brain stem, already thoroughly studied from an anatomoclinical point of view, was the object of important recent research[64,65,92]. A crown of radial arteries, converging towards the aqueduct and fourth ventricle, can be divided in a median or anterior, a paramedian or anterolateral, a lateral and a posterior area.

These vascular territories differ by the size and the length of the arteries and by their vascular density.

REFERENCES

1 ABBIE, A. (1934) The morphology of the fore-brain arteries, with special reference to the evolution of the basal ganglia. *J. Anat.*, **68**, 433–470.

2 ABRAMOWICZ, A. (1964) The pathogenesis of experimental periventricular cerebral necrosis and its possible relation to the periventricular leucomalacia of birth trauma. *J. Neurol. Neurosurg. Psychiat.*, **27**, 85–95.

3 ADACHI, B. (1928) *Das Arteriensystem der Japaner.* Bd.l, Kyoto.

4 ADAMS, R. D. AND VANDER EECKEN, H. (1953) Vascular diseases of the brain. *Ann. Rev. Med.*, **4**, 213–252.

5 ALAJOUANINE, TH., CASTAIGNE, P. AND LHERMITTE, F. (1958) A new technical approach to the study of the cerebral circulation in cases of arterial occlusion. *Circulation*, **1**, 341–351.

6 ALAJOUANINE, TH., CASTAIGNE, P., LHERMITTE, F. ET CLAY, R. (1957) Aspects artériographiques des thromboses artérielles et de la circulation de suppléance. *Sem. hôp. Paris*, **33**, 2135–2150.

7 ALAJOUANINE, TH., CASTAIGNE, P., LHERMITTE, F. ET GAUTIER, J. C. (1959) Nouvelle méthode d'exploration des artères cérébrales. *Sem. hôp. Paris*, **35**, 171–173.

8 ALAJOUANINE, TH. ET THUREL, R. (1936) La pathologie de la circulation cérébrale. *Rev. Neurol.*, **68**, 1276–1458.

9 ALEMA, G. E. E CASTORINA, G. (1953) Il quadro clinico e angiografico dell' occlusione dell' arteria silviana. *Rev. Neurol.*, **23**, 625–660.

10 ALEXANDER, L. (1947) The vascular supply of the strio-pallidum. *Ass. Res. Nerv. Dis. Proc.*, **21**, 77–132.

11 ALTMANN, F. (1947) Anomalies of the internal carotid artery and its branches: their embryological and comparative anatomical significance. *Laryngoscope*, **57**, 313–316.

12 ALPERS, B., BERRY, G. P. AND PADDISON, R. M. (1959) Anatomical studies of the circle of Willis in normal brains. *Arch. Neurol. Psych.*, **81**, 409–418.

13 ATKINSON, N. J. (1949) The anterior-inferior cerebellar artery. *J. Neurol.*, **12**, 137–146.

14 BANKER, B. Q. AND LARROCHE, J. C. (1962) Periventricular leukomalacia of infancy. *Arch. Neurol.*, **7**, 386–410.

15 BAPTISTA, A. G. (1964) Studies on the arteries of the brain. *Acta Neurol. Scand.*, **26**, 1–18.

16 BATUJEFF, N. (1889) Eine seltene Arterienanomalie. *Anat. Anz.*, **4**, 282–285.

17 BEEVOR, C. E. (1907) The cerebral arterial supply. *Brain*, **30**, 403–425.

18 — (1909) On the distribution of the different arteries supplying the human brain. *Philos. Trans. (B)*, **200**, 1–56.

19 BERKOL, M., MOUCHET, A., ZEREN, Z. ET OYA, K. (1939) Distribution intracérébrale des artères provenant du réseau pie-mérien. *Ann. Anat. Pat.*, **16**, 861–865.

20 BIEMOND, A. (1949) *Anatomie du cervelet.* Traité de Médecine. Tome XV. Masson. Paris.

21 BOLONYI, F. (1951) Étude sur la vascularisation du lobe frontal au point de vue phylogénétique. *Acta Anat.*, **12**, 110–116.

22 BRAUS, H. (1940) *Anatomie des Menschen.* Bd. IV.

23 BREA, J. B. (1956) Sulla persistenza della anastomosi carotido-basilare. *Sistema nerv.*, **8**, 17–23.

24 BREGEAT, P., DAVID, M., FISCHGOLD, H. ET TALAIRACH, J. (1952) Opacification des vaisseaux orbitaires et de la choroïde par l'angiographie carotidienne. *Rev. Neurol.*, **87**, 549–551.

25 CADIAT, P. (1881) Bulletins et mémoires de la Société de Biologie 1876. *Traité d'Anatomie générale.*

26 CAMPBELL, A. C. (1937) The vascular architecture of the cat's brain. *Res. Nerv. Ment. Dis.*, **17**, 719–725.

27 CASTORINA, G. E FRANCESCONI, G. (1956) I rapporti tra sintomatologia clinica e circolo collaterale di compenso nell'occlusione dell' arteria cerebrale media. *Il. Lav. Neuropsichiat.*, **19**, 23–82.

28 CHARACHON, R. ET LATARJET, M. (1952) Les injections de matières plastiques appliquées à l' étude de l' artère auditive interne. *C. R. Assoc. anat.*, **3**, 436–441.

29 CHARPY, A. (1902) *Traité d'Anatomie humaine.* Poirier-Charpy, **3**.

30 CHAVANY, J., MESSIMY, R., DJINDJIAN, R. ET MAMO, H. (1955) Considérations sur l'artériographie au cours des oblitérations thrombosiques et emboliques des artères cérébrales. *Sem. hôp. Paris*, **31**, 1661–1668.

31 CAVATORTI, P. (1908) Il Tipo norma e le variazioni delle arterie della base dell'encefalo nell' uomo. *Monit. zool. ital.*, **19**, 248–257.

32 COBB, S. (1931) The question of endarteries in the brain and the mechanism of endarteries. *Arch. Neurol. Psych.*, **25**, 273–281.

33 —, (1937) Cerebral circulation. A critical discussion of the symposion. *Assoc. Res. nerv. ment. dis.*, **17**, 719–726.

34 COBB, S. AND TALBOTT, J. (1937) Studies on cerebral circulation. II. Quantitative study of cerebral capillaries. *Trans. Assoc. Am. Phys.*, **42**, 255–272.

35 CONGDON, E. D. (1922) Transformation of the aortic arch system during the development of the human embryo. *Carnegie Inst. Work Publ., contrib. Embryol.*, **14**, 47–110.

36 CRITCHLEY, MC. D. (1930) The anterior cerebral artery and its syndromes. *Brain*, **53**, 120–165.

37 DECKER, F. (1886) *Über eine seltene Varietät der Arterien der Hirnbasis*. Bd. 5 Phys. Med. Ges., Würzburg.

38 DECKER, K. (1955) Die Arteria ophtalmica im Karotisangiogramm. *Fortschr. Röntgenstr.*, **82**, 667–673.

39 DECKER, K. UND HIPP, E. (1958) Der basale Gefäszkranz. Morphologie und Angiographie. *Anat. Anz.*, **105**, 100–116.

40 DECKER, K. UND HOLZER, E. (1954) Gefäszverschlüsse im Carotis- und Vertebralisangiogramm. *Fortschr. Röntgenstr.*, **80**, 565–575.

41 DE VRIESE, B. (1904) Sur la recherche morphologique des artères cérébrales. *Arch. Biol.*, **21**, 357–457.

42 —, (1905) *Recherches sur la morphologie de l'artère basilaire*. Thèse, Gand.

43 DINSDALE, H. (1962) Quoted by Abramowicz.

44 DONEGANI, G. (1965) *Anatomia vascolare del rombencefalo e mesencefalo*. Tipografia Toso, Torino.

45 DURET, H. (1874) Recherches anatomiques sur la circulation de l'Encéphale. *Arch. Phys. norm. path.*, sér. **2**, 60–91, 316–354; 664–693; 919–957.

46 EVANS, H. M. (1911) Handbuch der Entwicklungsgeschichte des Menschen. *Keibel u. Mall.*, **11**, 551–688.

47 FASANO, V. A., MASPES, P. E. AND BROGGI, G. (1953) Remarks on the adjustment of the cerebral circulation in some cases of internal carotid and middle cerebral artery occlusion. *5e Congr. Neurol. Intern., Lisbonne*.

48 FAWZETT, E. AND BLACKFORD, J. V. (1906) The circle of Willis: an examination of 700 specimen. *J. Anat. Physiol.*, **40**, 63–73.

49 FAY, T. (1925) The cerebral vasculature. *J. Am. Med. Ass.*, **84**, 1729–1731.

50 FEIRING, E. H. AND SUSSMAN, H. (1956) Spontaneous occlusion of the middle cerebral artery. *Neurol.*, **6**, 529–546.

51 FETTERMAN, G. H. AND MORAN, T. J. (1932) Anomalies of the circle of Willis in relation to cerebral softening. *Arch. Path.*, 251–257.

52 FLETCHER, T. M., TAVERAS, J. M. AND POOL, J. L. (1959) Cerebral vasospasm in angiography for intracranial aneurysms. *Arch. Neurol.*, **1**, 38–44.

53 FOIX, C. ET HILLEMAND, P. (1925) Le syndrome de l'artère cérébrale antérieure. *Encéphale*, **4**, 209–232.

54 —, (1925) Les artères de l'axe encéphalique jusqu'au diencéphale inclusivement. *Rev. Neurol.*, **32**, 705–739.

55 FOIX, C. ET LEVY, M. (1927) Les ramollissements sylviens. *Rev. Neurol.*, **2**, 1–51.

56 FOIX, C. ET MASSON, A. (1923) Le syndrome de l'artère cérébrale postérieure. *Presse Méd.*, **32**, 361–365.

57 FRUGONI, P. (1952) Persistenza della anastomosi carotido basilare. *Chirurgia*, **7**, 327–335.

58 GABRIELLE, H., LATARJET, M. ET DUROUX, P. E. (1949) Contribution à l'étude du tronc de l'artère sylvienne et de la vascularisation artérielle du lobe de l'insula chez l'homme. *C. R. Ass. Anat.*, **36**, 291–325.

59 GABRIELLE, H., LATARJET, M., LECUIRE, J. ET EICHOLZ, L. (1949) Contribution à l'étude de l'anatomie macroscopique de l'artère cérébrale postérieure et de la vascularisation artérielle du lobe occipital chez l'homme. *C. R. Ass. Anat.*, **36**, 326–338.

60 GABRIELLE, H., LATARJET, M., LECUIRE, J. ET MEUNIER, M. (1949) Anatomie macroscopique des artères de l'écorce cérébrale humaine. *C. R. Ass. Anat.*, **36**, 230–276.

61 GABRIELLE, H., LATARJET, M., LECUIRE, J. ET MILLERET, P. (1949) Contribution à l'étude macroscopique de la vascularisation du lobe temporal chez l'homme. *C. R. Ass. Anat.*, **36**, 339–352.

62 GABRIELLE, H., LATARJET, M., LECUIRE, J., SANTOT, J. ET CHARPIN, M. (1949) Contribution à l'étude microscopique de l'artère cérébrale antérieure et de la vascularisation artérielle du lobe frontal chez l'homme. *C. R. Ass. Anat.*, **36**, 277–290.

63 GESSURI, L. E FRUGONI, P. (1954) Considerazioni sulla persistenza della anastomosi carotido basilare. *Rev. di Neurol.*, **24**, 338–348.

64 GILLILAN, L. A. (1955) Angioarchitecture of the human brainstem. *Anat. Rec.*, **121**, 299–312.

65 —, (1964) The correlation of the blood supply to the human brainstem with clinical brainstem lesions. *J. Neuropath. Exptl. Neurol.*, **23**, 78–108.

66 GODINOV, V. M. (1929) The arterial system of the brain. *Am. J. Phys. Anthropol.*, **13**, 359–388.
67 GRINO, A. AND BILLET, E. (1949) The diagnosis of orbital tumors by angiography. *Am. J. Ophthal.*, **32**, 897–911.
68 GROS, CL., MINVEILLE, J. ET VLAHOVITCH, B. (1956) Anastomoses artérielles intracraniennes. Etude artériographique et clinique. *Neurochir.*, **2**, 281–302.
69 GUIOT, G. ET LESBESNERAIS, J. (1955) Oblitération de l'artère cérébrale moyenne sans sequelles neurologiques. *Neurochir.*, **1**, 287–291.
70 HALE, R. AND REED, F. (1963) Studies in cerebral circulation. Methods for the qualitative and quantitative study of human cerebral b'ood vessels. *Am. Heart. J.*, **2**, 226–242.
71 HARRISON, C. E LUTTRELL, J. (1953) Persistent carotid basilar anastomosis. *J. Neurol.*, **10**, 205–215.
72 HASENJÄGER, TH. (1937) Ein Beitrag zu den Abnormitäten des circulus arteriosus Willisi. *Neurochir.*, **2**, 34–39.
73 HEUBNER, D. (1874) *Die luetische Erkrankung der Hirnarterien.* Leipzig.
74 HINCK, (1964) Persistent primitive trigeminal artery. *Radiology*, **83**, 41–45.
75 HOCHSTETTER, F. (1885) Über zwei Fälle einer seltenen Varietät der Art. Carotis interna. *Arch. Anat. Physiol.*, **1**, 396–400.
76 HODES, PH. J., CAMPOY, F., RIGGS, H. E. AND BLY, P. (1953) Cerebral angiography. *Am. J. Röntgen.*, **70**, 61–82.
77 HODES, PH. J., PERREYMAN, C. R. AND CHAMBERLIN, R. H. (1947) Cerebral angiography. *Am. J. Röntgen.*, **58**, 543–582.
78 HIS, W. (1885) *Anatomie menschlicher Embryonen*, **3**, 185–199, Leipzig.
79 HUTCHINSON, E. C. (1965) *The circle of Willis today. The modern trends in Neurology.* Williams, London.
80 KAPLAN, H. A. (1956) Arteries of the brain. *Acta Radiologica*, **46**, 364–370.
81 —, (1961) Collateral circulation of the brain. *Neurol.*, **2**, 9–15.
82 KAPLAN, H. A. AND FORD, D. H. (1966) *The brain vascular system.* Elsevier, Amsterdam.
83 KLEISS, E. (1942) Die verschiedenen Formen des circulus arteriosus cerebri Willisi (Eine statistische Untersuchung von 325 menschlichen Gehirnen). *Anat. Anz.*, **92**, 216–230.
84 KLOSS, K. (1953) Persistierende Carotis-Basilaris Anastomose als Ursache einer Subarachnoidalblutung. *Neurochir.*, **13**, 166–171.
85 KRAYENBÜHL, H. (1958) Diagnostic value of orbital angiography. *Brit. J. Ophtal.*, **42**, 180–190.
86 KRAYENBÜHL, H. UND YASARGIL, M. G. (1957) *Die vaskulären Erkrankungen im Gebiet der Arteria vertebralis und Arteria basilaris.* G. Thieme Verl., Stuttgart.
87 —, (1958) Der cerebrale kollaterale Blutkreislauf im angiographischen Bild. *Acta Neurochir.*, **6**, 30–80.
88 LAFON, R., GROS, CL., BETOULIERES, P., MINVIEILLE, J., PALEIRAC, R. ET VLAHOVITCH, B., (1956) La circulation collatérale dans les thromboses carotidiennes: étude artériographique. *J. Radiol.*, **37**, 12–16.
89 LANDOLT, F. (1949) Zur Topografie der Kleinhirnarterien. Abnorme Verlaufsformen der Arteria cerebellaris inferior posterior. *Schweiz. Arch. Neurol.*, **64**, 329–335.
90 LAZORTHES, G. (1961) *Vascularisation et circulation cérébrales.* Masson. Paris.
91 LAZORTHES, G., GAUBERT, J. ET POULHÈS, J. (1956) La distribution centrale et corticale de l'artère cérébrale antérieure. Etude anatomique et incidences neurochirurgicales. *Neurochir.*, **2**, 237–253.
92 LAZORTHES, G., POULHÈS, J., BASTIDE, G., ET ROULLEAU, J. (1958) Les territoires artériels du tronc cérébral. Recherches anatomiques et syndromes vasculaires. *Presse Médicale*, **91**, 2048–2051.
93 LAZORTHES, G., POULHÈS, J., BASTIDE, G., ROULLEAU, J. ET AMARAL-GOMES, F. (1960) Les grands courants artériels du cerveau. *Presse Médicale*, **68**, 137–140.
94 LAZORTHES, G., POULHÈS, J. ET ESPAGNO, J. (1967) Les territoires vasculaires du cortex cérébelleux. *C.R. Ass. Anat.*
95 —, (1967) Les artères du cervelet. *C.R. Ass. Anat.*
96 —, (1951) La vascularisation artérielle des noyaux du cervelet. *C.R. Ass. Anat.*, **68**, 649–653.
97 LAZORTHES, G., POULHÈS, J. ET GAUBERT, J. (1956) Les artères et les territoires vasculaires de l'Hypothalamus. Applications neurochirurgicales. *Presse Médicale*, **64**, 1701–1703.
98 LEHRER, G. M. (1958) Arteriographic demonstration of collateral circulation in cerebro-vascular disease. *Neurol.*, **8**, 27–32.
99 LEPHENE, G. (1919) Zerfall der roten Blutkörperchen beim Ikterus infectiosus. *Beitr. path. Anat. allgem. Path.*, **65**, 163–174.
100 LEY, G. (1931) Oblitération embolique totale de l'artère sylvienne sans ramollissement en aval. Les "artères terminales du cerveau". *J.B. Neur. Psych.*, **8**, 497–509.

101 —, (1932) Contribution à l'étude du ramollissement cérébral envisagé au point de vue de la pathogénie de l'ictus apoplectique. *J.B. Neur. Psych.*, **11**, 785–875; **12**, 895–970.

102 LIERSE, W. (1963) Über die Beeinflussung der Hirnangioarchitektur durch die Morphogenese. *Acta Anat.*, **53**, 1–54.

103 LINDGREN, E. (1950) Percutaneous angiography of the vertebral artery. *Acta Radiol.*, **33**, 389–404.

104 LOOTEN, R. (1906) *Recherches anatomiques sur la circulation artérielle du cerveau.* Thèse, Lille.

105 LORENTE DE NÓ, R. (1927) Ein Beitrag zur Kenntnis der Gefässverteilung in der Hirnrinde. *J. Psych. Neur.*, **35**, 19–24.

106 MALL, F. P. (1905) On the development of the bloodvessels of the brain in the human embryo. *Am. J. Anat.*, **4**, 1–18.

107 MASPES, P., FASANO, V. ET BROGGI, G. (1955) Aspect angiographique de la circulation collatérale dans les cas de thrombose de la carotide interne. *Neurochir.*, **1**, 273–278.

108 METTLER, F. R. (1948) *Neuro-anatomy.* 2nd Edit. Mosby, St. Louis.

109 MINVIELLE, J. ET VLAHOVITCH, B. (1959) *Les hémiplégies vasculaires.* Masson, Paris.

110 MOFFAT, D. B. (1962) The embryology of the arteries of the brain. *Ann. Roy. Coll. Surg. Engl.*, **30**, 368–382.

111 MONIZ, E. (1940) *Die cerebrale Arteriographie und Phlebographie.* "Handbuch der Neurologie". II. Springer, Berlin.

112 MOREL, F. ET WILDI, E. (1953) Examen anatomique du polygone de Willis et ses anomalies. Etude statistique. *Neurochir.*, **13**, 174–175.

113 MOUCHET, A. (1911) *Étude radiographique des artères du cerveau.* Thèse, Toulouse.

114 —, (1933) Note sur les artères du cerveau. *Ann. Anat. path.*, **10**, 669–675.

115 MOUNT, L. A. AND TAVERAS, J. M. (1957) Angiographic demonstration of the collateral circulation of the cerebral hemispheres. *Arch. Neurol. Psych.*, **78**, 235–253.

116 MURTACH, F., STAUFFER, H. AND HARLEY, A., (1955) A case of persistent carotid-basilar anastomosis. *J. Neurosurg.*, **12**, 46–49.

117 OERTEL, P. (1922) Über die Persistenz embryonaler Verbindungen zwischen der A. carotis interna und der A. vertebralis. *Anat. Anz.*, **55**, 281–295.

118 PADGET, D. H. (1945) *The circle of Willis. Its Embryology and Anatomy in intracranial arterial aneurysms.* W. E. Dandy and Co., New York.

119 —, (1948) The development of the cranial arteries in the human embryo. *Carnegie Inst. Washington*, **32**, 205–261.

120 PATURET, G. (1964) *Traité d'Anatomie humaine. Tome IV: Système nerveux.* Masson, Paris.

121 PERRIA, L. (1941) La vascolarizzazione del cerveletto dell'uomo. *Rev. Pat. Nerv.*, **58**, 1–11.

122 PFEIFER, R. A. (1928) *Die Angioarchitektonik der Grosshirnrinde.* Springer, Berlin.

123 —, (1930) *Grundlegende Untersuchungen für die Angioarchitektonik des menschlichen Gehirns.* Springer Berlin.

124 —, (1931) Anastomosen der Hirngefässe. *J. Psych. Neurol.*, **42**, 1–173.

125 —, (1936) Neue Ergbnisse über die Morphologie der Hirngefäsze. *Klin. Wschr.*, **15**, 469–483.

126 —, (1940) *Die Angioarchitektonische areale Gliederung der Groszhirnrinde.* Thieme, Leipzig.

127 PICKWORTH, F. A. (1934) A new method of study of the braincapillaries and its application to the regional localization of mental disorder. *J. Anat.*, **69**, 62–68.

128 PLETS, C. (1966) Vascularisation topographique du thalamus humain. *Acta Neurol. Psych. Belg.*, **66**, 752–770.

129 POBLETE, R. E ASENJO, A. (1955) Anastomosis carotido-basilar por persistenzia de la arteria trigeminial. *Neurocir.*, **11**, 1–5.

130 QUAIN, R. (1844) *The anatomy of the arteries of the human body and its application to pathology and operative surgery with a series of lithographic drawings.* Taylor and Walton, London.

131 RADOJEVIC, S. ET NEGOVANOVIC, B. (1963) La gouttière et les anneaux osseux de l'artère vertébrale de l'atlas. *Acta Anat.*, **55**, 186–194.

132 RANEY, R., RANEY, A. AND SAUCHEZ-PEREZ, J. J. (1949) The role of complete cerebral angiography in neurosurgery. *J. Neurosurg.*, **6**, 222–237.

133 RIGGS, H. E. (1937) Anomalies of circle of Willis. *Trans. Philad. Neurol. Soc.*

134 ROSEGAY, H. AND WELCH, K. (1954) Peripheral collateral circulation between cerebral arteries. A demonstration by angiography of the meningeal anastomoses. *J. Neurosurg.*, **11**, 363–377.

135 ROWBOTHAM, G. F. AND LITTLE, E. (1965) Circulations of the Cerebral Hemispheres. *Brit. J. Surg.*, **1**, 8–20.

136 —, (1965) A new concept of the circulation and the circulations of the brain. *Brit. J. Surg.*, **7**, 539–542.

137 SCHARRER, E. (1938) Über cerebrale Endarterien. *Z. ges. Neurol. Psychiat.*, **162**, 401–406.

138 SCHIEFER, W. (1956) Der diagnostiche Wert einer funktionellen Serieangiographie bei intrakraniellen Prozessen. *Acta Radiol.*, **46**, 299–309.

139 SCHIEFER, W. UND STRUCK, G. (1957) Serienangiographische Untersuchungen bei diffusen cerebralen Gefässerkrankungen. *Dtsch. Z. Nervenheilk.*, **176**, 595–616.

140 SABIN, F. R. (1917) Origin and development of the primitive vessels of the Chick and the Pig. *Contr. Embryol., Carnegie Inst., Washington*, **6**, 61–124.

141 SAPHIR, O. (1935) Anomalies of the circle of Willis with resulting encephalomalacia and cerebal hemorrhage. *Am. J. Path.*, **11**, 775–787.

142 SCHAERER, J. P. (1955) A case of carotid-basilar anastomosis with multiple associated cerebro-vascular anomalies. *J. Neurosurg.*, **12**, 62–65.

143 SCHIFF-WERTHEIMER, S. (1926) *Le syndrome hémianopsique dans le ramollissement cérébral.* Thèse, Paris.

144 SCHURR, PH. (1951) Angiography of normal ophtalmic artery and choroidal plexus of eye. *Brit. J. Ophthal.*, **35**, 473–478.

145 SCHURR, PH. AND WICKBORN, I. (1952) Rapid serial angiography. *J. Neurol.*, **15**, 110–118.

146 SEZE, S. DE (1931) *Pression artérielle et ramollissement cérébral.* Thèse, Paris.

147 SHELLSHEAR, J. L. (1920) The basal arteries of the forebrain. *J. Anat.*, **55**, 33–37.

148 —, (1930) Arterial supply of cerebral cortex in chimpanzee. *J. Anat.*, **45**, 65–69.

149 SICCURO, A. ET BAGGIORE, P. (1953) *Le tronc anastomique carotido-basilaire. 5e Congr. Int. Neurol.*, Lisbonne.

150 SLANY, A. (1938) Anomalien der Circulus arteriosus Willisi in ihrer Beziehung zur Aneurysmenbildung an der Hirnbasis. *Virchow Arch. Path. Anat.*, **301**, 62–69.

151 SOBOTTA, J. (1958) *Deskriptive Anatomie.* 3. Teil. Lehmanns Verl., München.

152 STENVERS, H. W., BANNENBERG, P. M. ET LENSHÖCH, C. H. (1953) Anastomose carotido-basilaire persistante. *Rev. Neurol.*, **6**, 575–577.

153 STREETER, G. L. (1918) The developmental alterations in the vascular system of the brain of the human embryo. *Contr. Embryol. Carnegie Inst. Washington*, **8**, 5–38.

154 SZAPIRO, J. AND PAKULA, H. (1963) Anatomical studies of the collateral blood supply to the brain and the retina. *J. Neurol. Neurosurg. Psychiat.*, **26**, 414–417.

155 SZIKLA, G. UND ZOLNAI, G. (1956) Der Nachweis der Gehirnangioarchitektur mittels mit Kunstharz verfertigten Korrosion-präparaten. *Anat. Anz.*, **103**, 386–393.

156 TARTIRINI, E. E GUIGNI, L. (1955) Studio arteriografico del sifone carotideo in condizioni normalie patologiche. *Sist. Nerv.*, **3**, 3–31.

157 TAVERAS, J. M. (1961) Angiographic observation in occlusive cerebrovascular disease. *Neurol.*, **1**, 86–90.

158 TESTUT, J. L. (1948) *Traité d'Anatomie humaine.* Anatomie descriptive, histologie, développement. Paris.

159 TIXIER, J. (1922) *Artère sylvienne, branches collatérales et réseau de la pie-mère.* Thèse, Paris.

160 TÖNNIS, W. UND SCHIEFER, W. (1959) *Zirkulationsstörungen des Gehirns im Serienangiogramm* Springer Verl., Berlin.

161 TORKILDSEN, A. AND KOPPANG, H. (1953) Notes on the collateral cerebral circulation as demonstrated by carotid angiography. *J. Neurosurg.*, **8**, 269–278.

162 VAN DEN BERGH, R. (1959) L'angioarchitecture des radiations optiques. Son rôle éventuel dans la pathogénie de l'hématome intracérébral spontané. *Acta Neurochir.*, **7**, 178–189.

163 —, (1959) L'angioarchitecture de la capsule interne. *C.R. Ass. Anat.*, **104**, 749–753.

164 —, (1960) Contribution à l'étude de la pathogénie de l'hématome intracérébral spontané. *Acta Neurol. Belg.*, **3**, 312–319.

165 —, (1961) *De subcorticale angioarchitectuur van het menselijk telencephalon.* Thesis, Leuven, 1960. Arscia, Brussel.

166 —, (1961) La vascularisation artérielle intracérébrale. *Acta Neurol. Psych. Belg.*, **61**, 1013–1023.

167 —, (1962) Les caractères fondamentaux de l'angioarchitecture sous-corticale du télencéphalon humain. *World Neurology*, **7**, 546–560.

168 —, (1963) Blood supply and angioarchitecture of the corpus striatum. Neurological and neurosurgical aspects. *Exc. Med., Intern. Congr. Ser.*, **60**, 125–127.

169 —, (1964) Bijzonderheden over de anatomie van de hersenbloedvaten. *Belg. Tijdschr. Geneesk.*, **17**, 891–898.

170 —, (1965) Einige Besonderheiten der intrazerebralen Gefässanordnung. *Zentr. Neuroch.*, **4/5**, 180–197.

171 —, (1967) *The periventricular intracerebral blood supply*. IIIrd Symposium of the "International study group on brain circulation", Salzburg oct. '66. Charles C. Thomas, Springfield, in press.

172 VANDER EECKEN, H. (1953) *Les anastomoses des artères cérébrales et leur signification morphologique*. Ve. Congr. Neurol. Intern., Lisbonne, **2**, 8–9.

173 —, (1954) Signification morphologique des anastomoses leptoméningées aux confins du territoire des artères cérébrales. *Acta Neurol. Psych. Belg.*, **7**, 525–532.

174 —, (1955) *De anastomosen tussen de leptomeningiale slagaders van het encephalon*. Thesis, Erasmus, Gent.

175 —, (1957) De arteria cerebri anterior bij de mens. *Verhl. Kon. Vl. Akad. Gen. Belg.*, **19**, 149–174.

176 —, (1958) Les anastomoses des artères leptoméningées. *C.R. Ass. Anat.*, **3**, 1–39.

177 —, (1959) *Anastomoses between the leptomeningeal arteries of the brain. Their morphological, pathological and clinical significance*. Charles C. Thomas, Springfield.

178 —, (1961) Discussion of "collateral circulation of the brain". *Neurol.*, **11**, 16–19.

179 —, (1967) *Arterial topography and architecture at the level of the intracerebral arterial demarcation zones in human adult and foetus brains*. IIIrd Symposium of the "International study group on brain circulation", Salzburg, oct. '66. Charles C. Thomas, Springfield, in press.

180 VANDER EECKEN, H. AND ADAMS, R. D. (1953) The anatomy and functional significance of the meningeal arterial anastomoses of the human brain. *J. Neurol. exp. Neurol.*, **12**, 132–157.

181 VANDER EECKEN, H., FISCHER, C. M. AND ADAMS, R. D. (1952) The arterial anastomoses of the human brain and their importance in the delimitation of infarcts. *J. Neurol. exp. Neurol.*, **2**, 91–94.

182 VANDER EECKEN, H., HOFFMANN, G. ET DE HAENE, A. (1956) Hémisphérectomie pour hémiplégie infantile. Etude des anastomoses leptoméningées. *Neurochir.*, **2**, 436–440.

183 VANDER EECKEN, H. AND KLUYSKENS, P. (1958) *A study of the stapedial artery in the course of stapes mobilization operation in 485 adults*. (to be published).

184 VERRESEN, H. (1961) *De subcorticale angioarchitectuur van het menselijke cerebellum*. Reisbeurzenwedstrijd 1961. (Thesis Leuven).

185 WATT, J. AND MAC KILLOP (1935) The arteries on the base of the brain. *Arch. Surg.*, **12**, 330–348.

186 WELCH, K., STEPHENS, J., HUBER, W. AND INGERSOLL, C. (1955) The collateral circulation following middle cerebral branch occlusion. *J. Neurosurg.*, **12**, 360–368.

187 WILLIS, TH. (1664) *Cerebri anatomia nevrorumque descriptio et usus*. J. Flesher. London.

188 WINDLE, B. C. (1887) On the arteries forming the circle of Willis. *J. Anat. Phys.*, **1**, 22–26.

189 WISLOCKI, G. B. AND CAMPBELL, A. C. (1937) The unusual manner of vascularization of the brain of the Opossum. *Anat. Rec.*, **67**, 177–183.

190 YASARGIL, G. (1957) *Die Röntgendiagnostik des Exophtalmus unilateralis*. S. Karger, Basel.

191 ZÜLCH, J. K. (1955) Gedanken zur Enstehung und Behandlung der "Schlaganfälle." *Wien. Med. Wschr.*, **50**, 1035–1041.

192 —, (1961) Über die Entstehung und Lokalisation der Hirninfarkte. *Zentralblatt Neurochir.*, **1**, 158–177.

193 —, (1963) Conceptions nouvelles concernant la pathogénie de l'ischémie cérébrale. *Ann. Radiol.*, **6**, 7–14.

The Vascular Architecture of the Cortex and the Cortical Blood Flow

G. LAZORTHES, J. ESPAGNO, Y. LAZORTHES AND J. O. ZADEH

Neurosurgical Clinic, University Hospital Center, Toulouse (France)

The writers have been investigating the cortical angioarchitecture over a number of years by means of angiographic techniques and by diaphanisation.

Our initial findings were published[4] in 1961. We are now in a position to confirm that the main cortical areas differ in the organization of their respective vascular beds (Fig. 1).

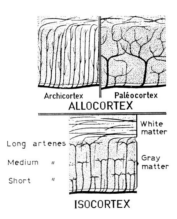

Fig. 1. The vascular patterns of the cortex (schematic representation).

The archicortex (hippocampus) shows a simple vascular bed corresponding to its primitive structure; the arteries, of approximately the same length, are parallel and thin.

The paleocortex (olfactory area) shows typical arterial ramifications 'en calice' (goblet-like) or 'en chandelier' (chandelier-like). Amygdaloid nucleus is very abundantly supplied by branching arteries.

The neocortex (isocortex), on the other hand, is supplied by arteries of variable length, which seem to terminate in different cellular layers. The short arteries give off very few collateral branches and terminate 'en bouquet', probably in layers 2 and 3. The medium length arteries give off a few branches at right angles and also end 'en bouquet', probably in layers 4 and 5.

The long arteries are often difficult to distinguish from the medium ones and end in the deeper layers of the cortex near the boundary between the grey matter and the white matter.

This pattern repeats itself throughout the homotypical isocortex. So far, we have been unable to demonstrate any variation of the pattern which could be considered characteristic of any particular area of the vast expanse of the cortex of the cyto-architectural type in question.

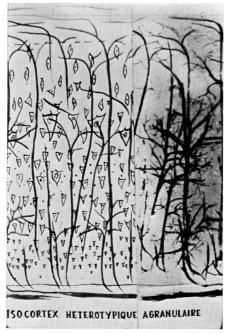

Fig. 2. The vascular pattern of heterotypical agranulous isocortex (angiographic technique).

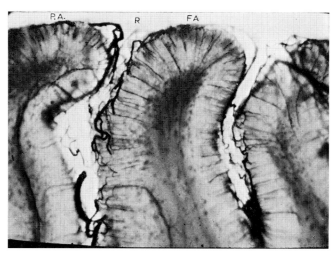

Fig. 3. The vascular pattern of the precentral and postcentral gyri (an example of section treated by diaphanisation technique).

The heterotypical agranulous isocortex (area 4) shows a very rich and dense vascular tree. Its medium and long arteries are more numerous and branch more freely than elsewhere and their endings are found in the great pyramidal (Betz) cells (Figs. 2, 3).

The heterotypical granulous isocortex (coniocortex) seems relatively poorly supplied. The first temporal convolution, and mainly its upper surface corresponding to Heschl's convolutions (auditosensory), shows a poorer blood supply than that of other temporal convolutions (homotypical isocortex). The contrast is quite definite. The 5th and 6th occipital convolutions seem superficially very vascular while the cortex of the depth of the calcarine sulcus does not show a particularly rich arterial tree (Fig. 4).

Finally, the cerebellar cortex presents an entirely different pattern. The arteries are relatively thicker than those of the cerebral cortex, they are all of the same type and they divide dichotomously.

Are the differences of cyto- and angio-architecture of the cerebral cortex reflected in the blood flow?

Measurements of blood flow by local intraparenchymatous injections of radioactive inert gas (Xenon 133) enabled us first to confirm the great difference between the blood flow in the white matter (constant and poor) and that in the grey matter (variable and abundant) [1,2,3].

The following points must be stressed, however:

Our measurements were not made under physiological conditions. The blood flow was usually determined during operations inside the skull. The patients were anesthetized and were usually in a sitting position. In each case there was some intracranial lesion which was, of course, the object of the intervention. On the other hand the blood pressure was maintained at the preoperative level and there was never any evidence of respiratory depression, pO_2 and pCO_2 having been determined in each case simultaneously with blood flow measurement, the latter always being carried out as far from the lesion as possible (Fig. 5).

The variability noticeable in our results is essentially attributable to the different values given to the coefficient of diffusion of Xenon. In our calculations we currently accept the figure of 0.8 for the grey matter, as suggested recently by Mallet and Veall. These workers were able to use techniques inapplicable to our studies.

With these reservations, our results seem to lead to two important conclusions [3,5].

1. *The cerebral cortex, which is not a homogeneous structure* as far as its cyto-architecture and angio-architecture are concerned, is also not homogeneous from the point of view of its hemodynamics.

The majority of our measurements of the cortical blood flow produced a bi-exponential clearance curve. The injection was, however, of very small volume (1 to 5 μl) and given into the cortex; the fact that the gas did not diffuse beyond the cortex was confirmed by experimental cortical biopsies and microscopic examination of the fragments. The mean half value for the quick component was 0.65 ± 0.1/min, which gives a calculated blood flow of the order of 85 ml/100 g/min. For the slow component the half value was 4.5 ± 0.5/min, which gives a calculated blood flow of the order of 12.5 ml/100 g/min.

The relative importance of the two components in the conditions in question seemed

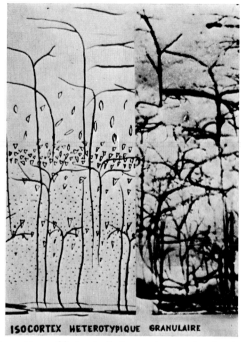

Fig. 4. The vascular pattern of heterotypical granulous cortex (angiographic technique).

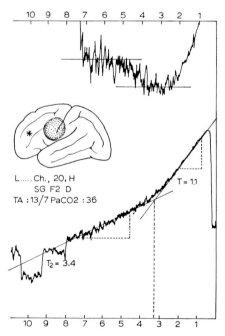

Fig. 5. A typical elimination curve following an injection of Xenon 133 into cerebral cortex.

to depend on the depth at which the injection was made. A very superficial injection of a very small volume usually produced a monoexponential curve analogous to the slow component of the bi-exponential curve produced by the injection of the cortical type.

In the pathologically altered areas (peritumoral edema, and especially after trauma) the blood flow characteristically showed not only an absolute reduction, but also a much greater degree of uniformity between the different zones due to reduction of the quick component (Fig. 6).

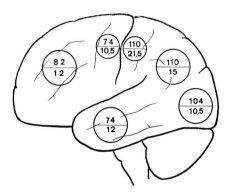

Fig. 6. Blood flow of the principal cortical regions (two components quoted).

2. *Different areas of the cortex seem to show topographic variations of the blood flow.* The blood flow calculated for different zones seems to show significant variations. So far, 110 measurements have been obtained by means of intraparenchymatous injections, but we are not yet in a position to offer actual firm figures for each area of every functional or cyto-angio-architectural region of the cortex. The mean results can however be listed.

The lowest values were obtained for the frontal lobe (82 ml/100 g/min), precentral gyrus (74 ml/100 g/min) and temporal lobe (74 ml/100 g/min), while the parietal (110 ml/100 g/min) and occipital lobes (104 ml/100 g/min) produced the highest figures.

One obvious difficulty is to know the exact location, particularly at the level of the precentral gyrus.

Finally, we obtained a number of values for the blood flow of the cerebellar cortex. The gradient of the mono-exponential clearance curve for 2.4 corresponds to a relatively slow flow, but as no coefficient is available for blood-cortex diffusion of Xenon in the cerebellum, no absolute figures could be calculated.

Our results therefore indicate that the blood flow of the cerebral cortex is not uniform, and considerable differences exist between the individual functional zones. We do not believe, however, that one should talk in terms of proper blood flow values for each of the cortical areas.

REFERENCES

1. ESPAGNO, J. AND LAZORTHES, Y. (1965) Determination of local cerebral blood flow values by intracerebral injection of Xenon 133. Comparative flow values in various regions and formations. *Proc. Third Intern. Congr. Neurol. Surg., Copenhagen, August 1965.* pp. 612–618.

2. ESPAGNO, J. AND LAZORTHES, Y. (1965) Measurement of regional cerebral blood flow in man by local injections of Xenon 133. Symposium on R.C.B.F., Lund, March 1965. *Acta Neurol. Scand., Suppl.* **14**, 58–63.

3. ESPAGNO, J. AND LAZORTHES, Y. (1966) The measurement of the local cerebral blood flow in man by intraparenchymatous injections of Xenon 133. *Presse Médicale*, **74**, (37) 1881–1887.

4. LAZORTHES, G. AND AMARAL-GOMES, F. (1961) Arterial angio-architecture of cerebral cortex. Attempted systematization by personal studies. *Bull. Acad. Natl. Méd.*, **145**, (33-34) 698–703.

5. LAZORTHES, Y. (1967) *A study of local cerebral blood flow.* The technique and clinical applications. The technique of intraparenchymatous injections of Xenon 133. Volume 214 pp., 18 figs., 26 tables.

Microradiographic Study of the Arterial Circulation of the Brain

G. SALAMON*, A. COMBALBERT, J. FAURE AND G. GIUDICELLI

Department of Neuroradiology, Neurobiological Research Unit, INSERM, and Neurosurgical Clinic, Marseilles (France)

INTRODUCTION

The recent development of carotid and vertebral arteriography, the use of photographic techniques such as subtraction or logetron now enable us to study blood vessels of under 0.5 mm in diameter.

By these means, we have the possibility of examining on the angiogram the area of the lenticulo-striate or thalamic arteries, the meningeal blood vessels and the branches of the ophthalmic artery.

These concepts of vascular anatomy can only be developed if our arteriographic data are compared with opaque injections or any other method of studying cerebral arteries where the results can be used for normal reference purposes (Fischgold *et al.*, 1965).

Among these methods, radiopaque injections with the possibility of microradiography hold an important place.

In 1898, Heycock and Neville presented for the first time a method enabling enlargements to be made of an object photographed by X-ray.

In 1913, Goby reported to the Academy of Sciences in Paris on: "the new method of using X-rays which I have the honour to introduce under the name of Microradiography, the object of which is to render easily and completely observable the internal structure of objects which by their very minutenes necessitate the use of the microscope but which escape observation owing to their opacity".

This method, based on the use of very fine grain film, capable of considerable enlargement and of tubes with sometimes microscopic lenses, could hardly fail to arouse great enthusiasm.

Among others, Lamarque (1936) and Collette (1955) carried out work on the radiography of tissues or microlymphography.

At the same time as this method was being perfected, it was undergoing technical modifications which included the use of an X-ray microscope (Cosslett and Nixon, 1952).

Thus an opaque object examined by fine focus X-ray on an extremely sensitive

---

* Electro-radiologiste des Hôpitaux, Professeur Agrégé à la Faculté, Hôpital de la Timone, 13 Marseille.

References p. 40–41

plate can yield a radiographic picture which, when enlarged photographically, reveals details of micron size.

In 1960, a Symposium was held in Stockholm on Microscopy by X-rays attended by Engström, Cosslett and Pattee (Saunders 1960) at which more than 75 contributions concerning this method and its developments were received. Six of them were exclusively concerned with the study of blood vessels.

Among the techniques at our disposal for the study of cerebral blood vessels, as indeed those of any other area, microradiography represents a method of selective opacification of arteries or veins which permits the study of very fine details (20 to 30 μ).

However, many other procedures also remain available to us.

We will rapidly summarize them. They can be classed in several groups according to whether they require: (1) Dye injections; (2) Histological dyes; (3) Use of plastic materials; (4) Use of fluorescent products; (5) Injections with decolourization of the brain (diaphanization); (6) Use of opaque substances with X-rays.

1. Dye injections

The injection of dyes is the simplest and longest-standing method.

Heubner (1872) described the recurrent branches of the anterior cerebral artery after injecting Prussian blue.

Duret (1874) used injections of carmine or Prussian blue to observe the arterial system of the brain stem, the central grey nuclei and the cortex.

These injections were perfected by Beevor (1907) and taken up by Shellshear (1920) who perfused each cerebral artery simultaneously with a mixture of gelatine and different dyes in order to observe the various regions of cerebral vascularization at one and the same time on a single specimen.

The use of Indian ink by Pfeiffer (1928) permitted a very detailed analysis of cerebral circulation. Unfortunately these preparations show the opacification both of the arterial and venous systems.

Thin sections may be photographed or analysed by microscope.

On the other hand, these different methods do not allow the complete analysis of an arterial system since such analysis depends exclusivley on the study of sections.

2. Histological dyes

The use of products which dye haemoglobin has resulted in a series of histological dyes of which the best known are Pickworth's (1934), later taken up by Schlesinger (1939) — a method employing benzidine.

Eros (1941) modified the procedure by using the action of fuchsin.

In this way it is possible to dye the arterial and venous systems and to carry out microscopic examination of a fine series of sections (of micron size).

3. Plastic injections with corrosion

The ease of utilizing synthetic resins has made possible the use of intravascular njections of plastic materials.

When it is extracted in its entirety, the brain is plunged into an alkaline or acid solution which destroys the parenchyma in order to leave only a moulding of the injected blood vessels.

Preparations in space are thus obtained (Tompsett, 1956) which, if the resins are mixed with an opaque product, make it possible to take radiographs.

The disadvantage of this method lies in the fact that any study of the related nervous substance is impossible, since the latter must be dissolved in order to render the moulding visible.

4. Fluorescent injections

Recent publications by Castaing and Gouaze (1963), Delarue *et al.* (1965, 1966) have shown the value of the information which can be derived from the injection of biological fluorescents. Sections are examined and photographed by ultra-violet light. It is then possible to discern real areas of vascularization. These areas are functional since this is the only technique of injection *in vivo* which does not modify the haemodynamics of the area under examination.

For this reason, this method is, of course, inapplicable to human pathology.

5. Injections with decolourization of the brain and plastic filling: "diaphanization".

Duret (1874) was apparently one of the first to propose decolouring cerebral substance where the blood vessels had been previously injected.

Thus, through a brain cross-section, a picture may be obtained of arterial or venous pedicles, seen in isolation, since the path of the vessels appears clearly visible in the thickness of the segment subjected to decolourization.

This method was perfected by Lazorthes (1961), and Poulhes and Galy (1962) in particular.

Such diaphanization offers the very great advantage in the case of sections of less than one centimetre in thickness of seeing in isolation vessel and nerve relationships because the diaphanized segment, although transparent, still leaves the most visible structures clearly discernible (cortex, nucleus and white matter).

6. Opaque injections with X-ray

The injection of opaque products enables very detailed pictures to be obtained from several angles.

The method appears to have been applied for the first time by Mouchet (1911) and enabled him to study the pattern of brain arteries from coronal or sagittal sections.

Foix and Hillemand (1925) in their work on the arteries of the brain stem and of the thalamus also used a mixture of collargol in albuminous solution.

This has since become a routine method and has been the basis for most of the work undertaken on cerebral vascularization. The use of aluminum or barium in oil or gelatinous solution was thus widely used by Lazorthes (1955, 1961), Kaplan and Ford (1966), and the Scandinavian School of Neuroradiology.

References p. 40–41

The use of finer opaque products making it possible to achieve injections even in capillary regions and photography by microradiographic techniques have enabled Saunders (1960), Hassler (1966), Delarue *et al.* (1965, 1966) and ourselves to secure very detailed pictures of more limited vascular areas.

It appears that the analysis of the major arteries should be carried out, especially in the case of a more selective injection, on the basis of normal opaque injections, while more detailed analysis of a given area should make use of micro-radiographic techniques.

TECHNIQUE AND RESULTS

Brains for examination should be extracted soon after death (between 6 and 12 h). Any subject whose death is the result of cerebral disease of vascular or tumoural type is unsuitable.

The extraction is carried out very carefully to avoid any injury to the cerebral cortex.

As far as possible the brain is removed with the dura mater. A very slow perfusion of the brain (4 to 6 h) is made with a 10% dilute solution of micropaque. This perfusion is normally made through a vertebral artery, the other vertebral together with the two carotids being tied. When this perfusion, which must always be made at low pressure, is completed, a seal of micropaque in gelatinous solution is injected to prevent leakage of the product.

The brain is fixed in a 10% saline formol solution. Maximum precaution must be taken to avoid any deformation either during injection or during the fixing process. One month later, usually after a median sagittal section, the anterior and posterior commissures are marked; these thereafter serve as reference points for determining the cross-section planes. All sections are in fact made either coronally, sagitally or horizontally in order to be strictly perpendicular or parallel to the bicommissural line.

Each section is one centimetre thick.

The sections are numbered according to their location in relation to the bicommissural plane, like the Atlas sections of Schaltenbrand and Bailey (1959).

In some particular cases (study of the posterior fossa or a given structure) the sections are made differently.

Each section is radiographed on metallographic film (KODAK M) with micro-radiographic apparatus (TUBIX). Colour photos of each section are also made in such a way that it is possible to compare on life-size prints the appearance of blood vessels which have been radiographed and their relation to the cerebral structures which they irrigate.

From each radiographic image obtained, the most interesting areas are optically enlarged (Durst): standard enlargements are of the order of 4 to 20. When greater enlargements are necessary, other, thinner sections of 200 to 500 μ are made with the freezer microtome and photos are taken on finer grain plates (M.R. plates).

Thus details may be obtained of blood vessels with diameters varying between 5 and 20 μ.

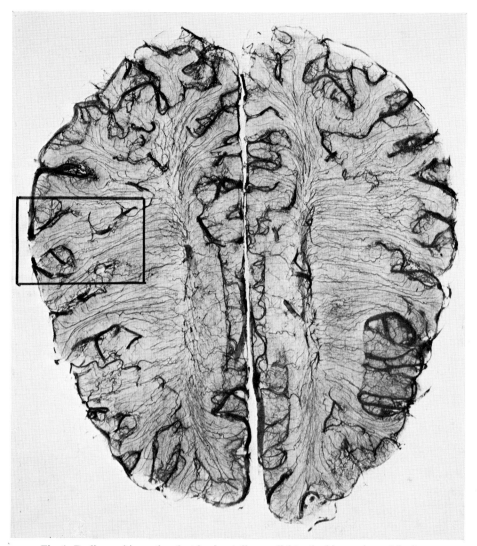

Fig. 1. Radiographic section (cut horizontally parallel to the bicommissural line).

We should like to illustrate this technique by three examples concerning the vascularization of white matter from the parietal region, the optic radiations and the corpus callosum.

Fig. 1 shows a radiographic section, cut horizontally parallel to the bicommissural line (on an area located 3 centimetres above this line). The outline of the cortical arteries may be clearly seen as well as the transverse arborizations of the medullary long arteries of the white matter at this level.

Fig. 2, enlargement of the area indicated by a rectangle on Fig. 1, makes it possible to see more clearly the medullary long branches. These vessels arise from the cortical arteries and have a very long path of 2 to 3 cm. Their calibre is much greater than that of the fine perforating cortical arteries (100 to 300 microns). Some vessels first

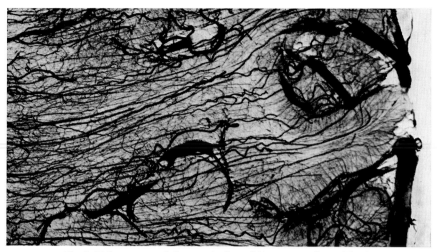

Fig. 2. Enlargement of the area indicated by a rectangle on Fig. 1.

follow a perpendicular path to the cortex they are about to traverse, then turn off at right angles towards the centre line; others rising in the depths of a fold follow an almost straight path. The first intra-axial segment of these vessels is indicated by the almost constant existence of vascular sinuosity in spirals. Vascular density at this level is considerable.

Besides these larger branches, there is a system of very fine vessels of lesser diameter comparable to the arteries of the cerebral cortex.

Fig. 3 shows an entirely different arrangement of the white matter arteries. It consists of a median parasagittal section one centimeter in thickness (5 cm from the bicommissural area) including the optic radiations. Here the path of the long arteries is entirely different, following the optic radiations themselves. There is a sort of fanwise spread of the vessels whose diameter is comparable to those of the arteries in the two previous sections but without apparent anastomosis. The considerable vascular density of an area ordinarily regarded as a poorly irrigated borderline territory is noteworthy.

Fig. 4 is also a sagittal paramedian section showing the vascularization of the whole of the corpus callosum.

This is very slightly different type of vascularization made up of parallel terminal type branches arising from the pericallosal artery.

The very considerable vascularization of the corpus callosum almost certainly explains the frequent propagation of infiltrating malignant tumours at this level.

In this presentation may also be seen the thalamic perforating branches of the posterior communicant and of the posterior cerebral artery.

SUMMARY

The authors report on the results obtained by use of a microradiographic technique in the examination of brain arteries.

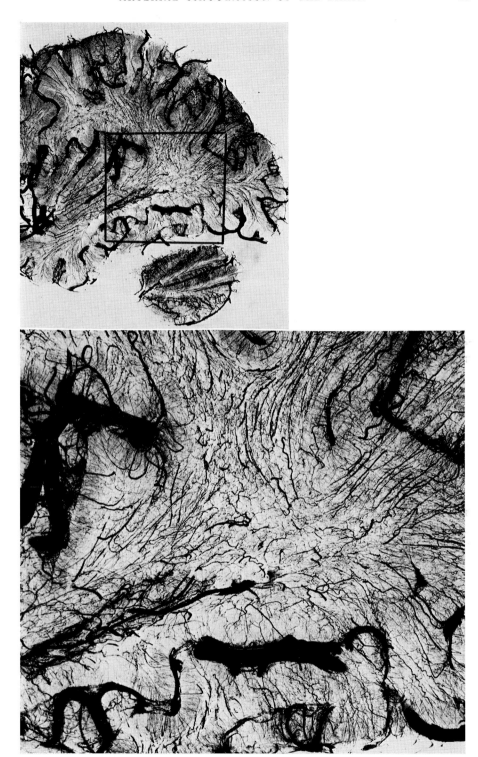

Fig. 3. Arrangement of the white matter arteries. (Median parasagittal section.)

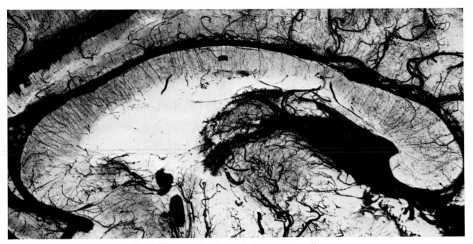

Fig. 4. Vascularization of the corpus callosum.

They illustrate their report with some examples relating to vascularization of the white matter in the frontal lobe, optic radiations and the corpus callosum.

This technique is compared with other methods of morphological study of the cerebral circulation.

REFERENCES

BEEVOR, C. E., (1907); The cerebral arterial supply. *Brain*, **30**, 403–425.

CASTAING, J., ET GOUAZE, A., (1963); Les fluorescents biologiques. Nouvelle possibilité de marquage du courant sanguin. *Presse Médicale*, **55**, 2723–2726.

COLLETTE, J. M., (1955); La Microradiographie. Bases et principes de la technique. *J. Belge Radiol.*, **36**, 293–312.

COSSLETT, V. E., ET NIXON, W. C., (1952); An experimental X Ray shadow microscope. *Proc. Roy. Soc. Med., London*, **53**, 422–431.

DELARUE, J., ABELANET, R., ET VEDRENNE, C., (1966); Etude de la vascularisation des tumeurs cérébrales malignes. *Ann. Anat. Pathol.*, 151–168.

—, MIGNOT, J., CAULET, T., DIEBOLD, J., ET DADDI, G., (1965); Les microunités vasculaires (angions). *Ann. Anat. Pathol.*, 5–20.

DURST, H., (1874); Recherches anatomiques sur la circulation de l'encéphale. *Arch. Physiol.*, 60–91, 316–353.

EROS, G., (1941); Method for fuchsin staining of the network of cerebral blood vessels. *Arch. Pathol.*, 215–219.

FISCHGOLD, H., GRISOLI, J., SALAMON, G., GUERINEL, G., ET LOUIS, R., (1965); Radio-Anatomie et Neuroradiologie. *Presse Médicale*, **73**, 3223–3228.

FOIX, C., ET HILLEMAND, P. L., (1925); Les artères de l'arc encéphalique jusqu'au diencéphale inclusivement. *Rev. Neurol.*, **6**, 705–739.

GOBY, P., (1913); Une nouvelle méthode d'application des Rayons X : la Microradiographie. *C. R. Acad. Sci.*, **156**, 686–688.

HASSLER, O., (1966); Deep cerebral venous system in man. A microangiographic study on its area of drainage and its anastomoses with superficial cerebral veins. *Neurology (Minneap.)*, **16**, 504–511.

HEUBNER, (1872); Zur topographie der Ernährungsgebiete der einzelnen Hirnarterien. *Centrbl. med. Wiss.*, **7**, 817–821.

HEYCOK, C. T., ET NEVILLE, F. H., (1898); Roentgen rays photography applied to alloys. *Trans. Chem. Soc. Lond.*, **73**, 714–723.

KAPLAN, H. A., ET FORD, D. H., (1966); *The brain vascular system.* Elsevier, Amsterdam.

LAMARQUE, P., (1936); Historadiographie. *C.R. Acad. Sci.*, pp. 684–685.

LAZORTHES, G., (1955); *Neuroanatomie*. Viguier, Toulouse.

—, (1961); *Vascularisation et circulation cérébrales*. Masson, Paris.

MOUCHET, A., (1911); *Etude radiographique des artères du cerveau*. (Thèse Médecine) Toulouse.

PFEIFFER, R. A., (1928); *Die Angioarchitektonik der Grosshirnrinde*. Mitt. 130, Springer (Berlin 1928).

PICKWORTH, F. A., (1934); A new method of study of the brain capillaries and its application to the regional localisation of mental disorder. *J. Anat.*, **35**, 62–70.

POULHES, J., ET GALY, E., (1962); Présentation de pièces anatomiques traitées par diaphanisation inclusion. *C.R. Ass. Anat. (Toulouse)*.

SALAMON, G., BOUDOURESQUES, J., COMBALBERT, A., KHALIL, R., FAURE, J., ET GIUDICELLI, G., Les artères lenticulo-striées. *Rev. Neurol.*, **114**, 361–373.

SAUNDERS, R. L., (1960); Microangiography of the brain and spinal cord. In: *X Ray microscopy and microanalysis*, A. Engström, V. F. Cosslett et H. H. Pattee (Eds.), Elsevier, Amsterdam, pp. 244–256.

SCHALTENBRAND, G., AND BAILEY, P., (1959); *Introduction to stereotaxis with an atlas of the human brain*. Thieme, Stuttgart.

SHELSHEAR, J. L., (1920); The basal arteries of the forebrain and their functional significance. *J. Anat.*, **55**, 27–35.

SCHLESINGER, B., (1939); The venous drainage of the brain with special reference to the galenic system. *Brain*, **62**, 274–291.

TOMPSETT, D. H., (1956); *Anatomical techniques*. Livingstone, London.

Methodology of cerebral blood flow measurement

A. CAPON, H. CLEEMPOEL, A. LENAERS* AND PH. MARTIN

Hôpital Saint-Pierre, Université de Bruxelles (Belgium)

The ideal method for measuring cerebral blood flow should be highly sensitive, accurate and perfectly quantitative. It should allow for continuous recording and indicate even transient hemodynamic variations. Moreover, it should not disturb brain function and ought to be utilizable in man as well as in laboratory animals in the absence of anesthesia. None of the methods described so far meet all of these requirements simultaneously.

METHODS FOR MEASUREMENT OF CEREBRAL BLOOD FLOW IN ANIMALS

Among the methods used primarily in animals, direct inspection of pial vessels (Riser, 1936) and plethysmography obtained by measuring CSF pressure can supply only qualitative values (Ryder *et al.*, 1952; Schmitt, 1956).

Measuring blood flow in the arteries of the neck necessitates complete isolation of the arteries specifically supplying the brain. In most laboratory animals, this isolation is impossible in practice because of the numerous anastomoses between branches of the internal and external carotid arteries (Schmidt, 1944). In the cat, the internal carotid artery is virtually replaced by a 'rete mirabile' (Batson, 1944). Techniques which have been described in the dog are laborious (Bouckaert and Heymans, 1935; Green and Denison, 1956; Sagawa, and Guyton, 1961) and must be undertaken under deep anesthesia. In the rabbit (Schmidt and Hendrix, 1934) and the monkey (Dumke and Schmidt, 1942), however, the territory of the internal carotid artery can be more easily distinguished from the external carotid artery. In general, prolonged surgical preparation disturbs brain function; deep anesthesia abolishes vasomotor reactions and dilates cerebral vessels (Lubsen, 1941).

Measuring the venous outflow — as well as measuring the arterial inflow — allows continuous recording of quantitative data values, but also meets with surgical difficulties. Ingvar and Soderberg (1956) have developed a technique for measuring flow in the superior longitudinal sinus of anesthetized cats. Anastomoses between the sinus and the veins of the skull are interrupted by the craniotomy, and the intracranial pressure is later restored by artificially reconstituting the skull vault (1958). A few anastomoses with the skull veins remain intact, however, and the physiological venous pressure is abolished. The blood flow actually measured is the outflow from the rostral and parietal regions of the brain.

---

* *Chargé de recherches au Fond National de la Recherche Scientifique.*

References p. 49–52

The method used by Meyer *et al.* (1964) in the monkey consists of measuring the flow in both the internal jugular veins by means of electromagnetic flowmeters. Numerous ligatures suppress most of the anastomoses but leave both vertebral veins intact.

The thermodilution technique of Gibbs (1933) consists of introducing into the brain a thermocouple heated by an electric current and cooled by the local blood flow. Recording of potentials from the thermocouple gives continuous information on local blood flow. All variations, even when transient, are recorded but the values obtained are by no means quantitative.

The technique can be used without anesthesia and has been applied in the cat (Schmidt, 1934; Schmidt and Pierson, 1934), in the rabbit (Field *et al.*, 1951) and even in man (Betz and Wüllenweber, 1962). In its more recent applications, the thermocouple has been replaced by a thermistor, which has smaller inertia together with greater sensitivity (Fumagalli *et al.*, 1957; Molnar and Csanaky, 1961; Capon, 1962; Suzuki and Tukahara, 1963).

Grayson (1952) thought the method could be quantitated and that the square of the intensity of the heating current necessary to maintain a constant temperature difference (1°C) between the thermocouple and the tissue was at all times directly related to local blood flow. Linzell (1953), however, showed that this relationship held true only for the smallest flows.

Despite its qualitative nature, Gibbs' method meets with many of the requirements of an ideal method for measuring cerebral blood flow. Fig. 1 shows its application to the rabbit's brain.

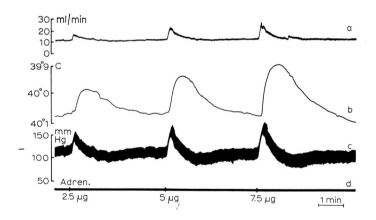

Fig. 1. Thermistor flowmeter recording of transient increase of brain blood flow in response to intravenous injection of adrenalin. Rabbit under neuroleptanalgesia. From above downwards: (a) Arterial blood flow measured by a Wilson rotameter in both carotid arteries, with external carotid and vertebral arteries ligated; (b) Blood flow at rest in the depth of the right hemisphere measured with a thermistor flowmeter heated to 2°C above cerebral temperature; (c) Femoral blood pressure; (d) Signal indicating injection into the inferior vena cava.

METHODS FOR MEASUREMENT OF CEREBRAL BLOOD FLOW IN MAN

Methods employed to measure cerebral blood flow in man furnish information either about the total blood flow in the brain or about the blood flow in the various parts of the brain.

1. Total cerebral blood flow

Methods developed for measurement of total cerebral blood flow have been based on the Fick principle (1870) or on the Stewart-Hamilton principle (Stewart, 1921; Moore et al., 1929). More recently Sapirstein (1958) proposed measurement of cerebral blood flow by use of the indicator fractionation technique.

(a) Methods based on the Fick principle

Kety and Schmidt (1945), described the earliest method wherein the subject was required to inhale a mixture of air and nitrous oxide for ten minutes. By taking blood samples from a peripheral artery and from the internal jugular vein throughout the duration of the test, it was possible to plot the concentration of nitrous oxide in the arterial and venous blood of the brain. Fig. 2 shows the blood concentration curves

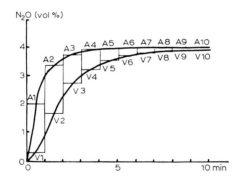

Fig. 2. Nitrous oxide methode. Saturation curves (Kety and Schmidt). Blood flow/min/100g tissue =

$$\frac{V_{10} \times K \times 100}{S_0 \int^{10} (A - V)dt}$$

derived and how cerebral blood flow value is obtained. Cerebral blood flow is expressed in terms of ml/100 g brain tissue perfused per minute, calculated on the basis of the concentration in the venous blood, the coefficient of distribution between the blood and the brain tissue and the integrated difference between venous and arterial concentrations. This method has been modified several times. In 1955 Lassen and Munck proposed replacing nitrous oxide with krypton 85. Krypton beta radiation was measured by means of a Geiger counter. The inhalation period was lengthened to 15 minutes. It was shown that after the eighth minute, the venous curve tended to monoexponentially approximate the arterial curve, which by then had stabilized; thus it was possible to extrapolate arterial/venous differences to infinity. This correction is especially important when cerebral blood flow is reduced. If the development of the arterial/venous difference is observed during the desaturation period, i.e. from the moment when krypton 85 inhalation is ended, inverse curves are obtained (Mc Henry, 1964; Lassen and Klee, 1965). This modification seems to give more regular curves. The inhalation period before blood samples are taken must be sufficiently long, i.e. from 20 to 30 minutes. Other variations on this method concern the manner of sampling (Scheinberg and Stead, 1949) or the manner of assay disposal (Albert *et al.*, 1960).

This method, or one of its variations, has been widely used in humans and enables one to obtain accurate quantitative information about cerebral blood flow and cerebral metabolism (Lassen *et al.*, 1960; Geraud *et al.*, 1963; Alexander *et al.*, 1964). It is not possible, however, to follow rapid variations in these parameters by this method and one can obtain cerebral blood flow only in terms of the quantity of brain perfused.

Lewis *et al.* (1960) have perfected a similar method whereby the quantity of gas in the brain is no longer calculated on the basis of sampled blood concentration, but is measured directly by counting externally over the skull. For this purpose, a gamma-emitting substance, krypton 79 is administered by inhalation while radioactivity of the blood is measured every minute. With this technique it is possible to follow rapid variations in the cerebral blood flow, but larger blood flows are obtained with this method than with other methods. Unfortunately, the detector is sensitive to radioactivity in tissues outside the brain and is more influenced by radioactivity in the brain cortex than by that in deeper layers. Reinmuth *et al.* (1965) replaced krypton 79 with another gamma-emitting substance, [^{131}I]labelled iodoantipyrine. Summing up regarding methods based on the Fick principle, it should be remembered that certain authors consider the arterial/venous difference to be a very good indication of the brain blood flow. The method is dependent on the remarkably steady rate of oxygen consumption by the brain.

(b) Methods based on the Stewart-Hamilton principle

Various authors have used the method of indicator dilution graphs to attempt to measure total cerebral blood flow. According to this principle, cerebral blood flow is equal to the quantity of tracer injected into the brain arterial system divided by the surface of the concentration curve during the initial circulation of the tracer.

Gibbs *et al.* (1947) used Evans Blue injected into the carotid artery and collected from the internal jugular vein. The method was improved by Sheakin and colleagues. Hellinger (1962), using indocyanine green, took samples of venous blood from the two internal jugular veins and obtained results very similar to those obtained by the Fick principle employing the gaseous indicators. Nylin *et al.* (1961) injected red cells labelled with various radioisotopes. Finally, many authors have used injection of non-diffusible radioactive tracers the distribution of which is detected at one or more points in the cranium by external counting methods. It is not possible by these methods to measure the actual cerebral blood flow quantitatively. Indices of blood flow and the time taken to flow through various parts can be measured.

(c) Methods based on the indicator fractionation technique

The method developed by Sapirstein (1962) studies the distribution of an indicator introduced into the general circulatory system. An indicator, spreading rapidly in the tissues, is distributed in the various organs of a human being in proportion to that fraction of the total blood flow to each organ. This is true only for a brief time after a single injection of the indicator. Thus it is possible to determine the cranial blood flow measuring the radioactivity of the cranium by means of a scintillation detector after injection of a tracer which diffuses rapidly into all cranial tissues. Similarly, it is possible to determine the cranial blood flow outside the brain by repeating the test with a tracer which diffuses rapidly into extra-cerebral tissue. The difference between the two determinations represents the cerebral blood flow. With this method Sapirstein measured cerebral blood flow by injecting iodoantipyrine labelled with Iodine 131 and with Potassium 42.

2. Regional cerebral blood flow in man — intact skull methods

(a) Qualitative methods

Rheoencephalography measures the impedance of cranial tissue to an alternating current applied through external electrodes. This method records variation in blood volume rather than variation in blood flow. It is not quantitative. Moreover it monitors variations in external as well as internal carotid distribution (Jenkner, 1962; Perez-Borja and Meyer, 1964).

(b) Tracer methods — non-diffusible tracers

Cerebral angiography

Rapid serial angiography provides fairly precise information on the circulation time in either carotid or vertebral areas, as well as on the size of the main draining vessels (subtraction). But it measures cerebral blood flow inaccurately because no definite measurement of the cerebral blood volume in the explored area is obtained (Tönnis and Schiefer, 1959; Dilenge and David, 1964).

Radiorheography — non-diffusible radioactive tracers

The method consists of injecting [131I]- or [125I]labelled paraaminohippuric acid or human serum albumin either into the carotid artery or intravenously and recording externally the variations in radioactivity over the skull and neck vessels. The relationship between variation in blood flow and the rate of radioactivity recorded, however, is not linear and, as in serial angiography, only the circulation time can be measured accurately (Fazio *et al.*, 1963; Agnoli *et al.*, 1964; Oldendorf, 1963).

(c) Quantitative methods — non-gaseous diffusible tracers

Injection of non-metabolizable, diffusible radioactive tracers, [125I]- or [131I]labelled antipyrine, via intravenous or intra-arterial routes with recording of radioactivity over the skull shows regional differences in activity, but generally does not permit

References p. 49–52

precise measurement of the regional blood flow. External counting is contaminated by the circulation of the scalp.

The Fick principle may be applied and analysis of the clearance curve of the tracer may be made to give a precise measurement of the regional cerebral blood flow provided the following conditions are met:

(1) the partition coefficient of the tracer between blood and brain is known; (2) an immediate equilibrium is established by diffusion of the tracer between capillaries and the brain; (3) the intra-arterial injection is rapid; (4) the error due to recirculation of the tracer is corrected.

(d) Intra-arterial injection of a radioactive gas in saline

The method used experimentally in animals by Lassen and Ingvar (1961) consists of injecting ^{85}Kr in saline into the internal carotid artery and recording the radioactivity by means of a counter placed in direct contact with the cortex. The beta-emission of ^{85}Kr explores cortical blood flow. The authors later applied their method to man (1963). The clearance curve of ^{85}Kr, used as a gamma-radiation emitter was recorded by means of one or more scintillation detectors placed over the skull. Later ^{133}Xe, a more easily detectable gamma-radiation emitter, was utilized (Glass and Harper, 1963; Lassen and Ingvar, 1963; Bes and Espagno, 1965; Géraud *et al.*, 1965). Injection into the internal carotid artery is made in the course of angiography. Inert gases have the advantage of low solubility and the error due to recirculation is very much reduced by their elimination through the lungs. Diffusion of the gas is rapid and since its partition coefficient between blood and brain is known, the Fick principle and the Kety-Schmidt formula:

$$\text{mean } \gamma \text{ CB}^{\text{F}} = \frac{\text{H}_{\max} - \text{H}^t}{\text{A}^t corr} \lambda \text{ ml/g/min*}$$

permits calculation of blood flow in the region seen by the scintillation detector. Figures are corrected taking into account pCO_2 and hematocrit. Analysis of the curve resolves it into two uniexponential components (Fig. 3), a rapid and a slow component, which seem to correspond under normal conditions to the blood flow in the gray matter and in the white matter respectively. By analysis of clearance curves of ^{85}Kr or ^{133}Xe injected into the cortex of animals and man, Nilson, Espagno and Lazorthes confirmed the values obtained by Lassen and, by successive excision of the injected area, also confirmed his interpretation of the curve. Furthermore, they demonstrated the existence of a third type of blood flow in the subcortical white matter.

Recently, Ingvar and Lassen have applied the gamma camera to a two dimensional analysis of regional cerebral blood flow.

---

* $\text{H}_{\max}$ = Radioactivity recorded at the start of desaturation.
H^t = Radioactivity at time *t*.
$\text{A}^t corr$ = Area under the curve corrected for background and recirculation.
γ = blood: tissue partition coefficient.

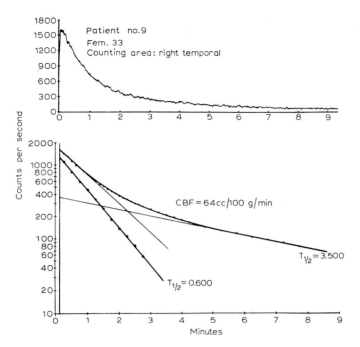

Fig. 3. Upper diagram shows clearance curve of krypton 85 obtained over the right temporal region, in a 33-year-old female patient. The isotope was dissolved in about 10 ml of saline and injected into the right internal carotid artery. Lower diagram shows semilogarithmic plot of the same clearance curve. Note final rectilinear part of the curve indicating a slow perfusion phase (T $\frac{1}{2}$ = 3.5 minutes). Graphical analysis yielded a fast component with a T $\frac{1}{2}$ of 0.6 minutes. The average flow (f = 64 cc/100 gm/min) was obtained by calculating a weighted average of the two flow rates according to the following equations for krypton 85:

$$f = L_1 f_1 + L_2 f_2 \; \text{ml/gm/min}$$

where $f_1 = 0.95 \dfrac{0.693}{\text{T}\frac{1}{2}\,(\text{fast component})}$; $f_2 = 1.30 \dfrac{0.693}{\text{T}\frac{1}{2}\,(\text{slow component})}$; $L_1 = \dfrac{I_1}{I_1 + I_2(f_1/f_2)}$;

$L_2 = \dfrac{I_2(f_1 f_2)}{I_1 + I_2(f_1/f_2)}$; I_1 = zero time intercept of fast component;
I_2 = zero time intercept of slow component.

With ^{133}Xe the solubility coefficients used to calculate f_1 and f_2 from their time constants are 0.83 and 1.57 (instead of 0.95 and 1.30 for ^{85}Kr); otherwise the calculations are identical with those shown above.

Inhalation of a radioactive gas

Veal and Mallet proposed giving a gaseous tracer (^{133}Xe) through inhalation. This entirely atraumatic method is attractive. Unfortunately, measurements are contaminated by the activity of extra-cerebral tissues; recirculation is great and the method is influenced by pulmonary conditions (Espagno and Lazorthes, 1965).

REFERENCES

AGNOLI, A., BONAMINI, F. ET FIESCHI, C. (1964) Etude de la circulation cérébrale dans les syndromes obstructifs des artères encéphaliques au moyen de l'injection intracarotidienne de radioisotopes. *Neurochir.*, **10**, 339–360.

ALBERT, S. N., ALBERT, C. A. AND FAZEKAS, J. F. (1960) Rapid and simple method for measuring rate of cerebral blood flow in humans with krypton. *J. Lab. Clin. Med.*, **56**, 473–482.

ALEXANDER, S. C. *et al.* (1964) Krypton-85 and nitrous oxide uptake of human brain during anesthesia. *Anesthesiol.*, **25**, 37–42.

BATSON, O. V. (1944) Anatomical problems concerned in the study of cerebral blood flow. *Fed. Proc.*, **3**, 139–144.

BES, A. ET ESPAGNO, J. (1965) Les méthodes d'exploration de la circulation cérébrale. Le débit cérébral. *Symp. Intern. circul. cérébrale. Paris.*

BETZ, E. UND WÜLLENWEBER, R. (1962) Fortlaufende Registrierung der lokalen Gehirndurchblutung mit Wärmeleitsonde am Menschen. *Klin. Wschr.*, **40**, 1056–1058.

BOUCKAERT, J. J. AND HEYMANS, C. (1935) On the reflex regulation of the cerebral blood flow and the cerebral vasomotor tone. *J. Physiol.*, **84**, 367–380.

CAPON, A. (1962) Discussion du rapport de Zülch sur la physiopathologie des troubles vasculaires médullaires. *Rev. Neurol.*, **106**, 659–663.

DILENGE, D. ET DAVID, M. (1964) Place de l'angiographie dans l'étude de l'hémodynamique cérébrale. *Neurochir.*, **10**, 567–586.

DUMKE, P. R. AND SCHMIDT, C. F. (1942) Quantitative measurements of blood flow in the macaque monkey. *Amer. J. Physiol.*, **138**, 421–431.

ESPAGNO, J. ET LAZORTHES, Y. (1965) Etude du débit sanguin cérébral par injection locale intra-parenchymateuse de Xénon 133. Premiers résultats. *Neurochir.*, **11**, 199–202.

FAZIO, C., FIESCHI, C. AND AGNOLI, A. (1963) Direct common carotid injection in cerebral circulatory disturbances in man. *Neurol.*, **13**, 561–574.

FICK, A. (1870) Ueber die Messung des Blutquantums in den Herzventrikel. *Sitzungsb. Phys-Med. Ges. Würzburg*, **36**.

FIELD, E. J., GRAYSON, J. AND ROGERS, A. F. (1951) Observations on the blood flow in the spinal cord of the rabbit. *J. Physiol.*, **114**, 56–70.

FIESCHI, C. (1963) Clinical evaluation of radioisotope rheoencephalography. Dynamic clinical studies with radioisotopes. *U.S. Atomic Energy Commission. Oak Ridge 1963*, 171–188.

FUMAGALLI, B., CASELLA, C. ET NOLI, S. (1957) Il comportamento del circolo cerebrale nel gatto e nel coniglio studiato con metodo termoelettrico. *Boll. Soc. Med. Chir. Pavia*, **71**, 3–27.

GERAUD, J., BES, A., RASCOL, A., DELPLA, M. ET MARC-VERGNES, J. P. (1963) Mesure du débit sanguin cérébral au krypton 85. Quelques applications physiopathologiques et cliniques. *Rev. Neurol.*, **108**, 542–557.

—, —, —, —, — ET LAZORTHES, Y. (1965) Le débit sanguin cérébral régional par injection intracarotidienne de Xénon-133. *Rev. Med. (Toulouse)*, **1**, 357–368.

GIBBS, F. A. (1933) A thermoelectric blood flow recorder in the form of a needle. *Proc. Soc. Exper. Biol. Med.*, **31**, 141–146.

—, MAXWELL, H. AND GIBBS, E. L. (1947) Volume flow of blood through human brain. *Arch. Neurol. Psychiat.*, **57**, 137–144.

GLASS, H. I. AND HARPER, A. M. (1963) Measurement of regional blood flow in cerebral cortex of man through intact skull. *Brit. Med. J.*, **2**, 593.

GRAYSON, J. (1952) Internal calorimetry in the determination of thermal conductivity and blood flow. *J. Physiol.*, **118**, 54–72.

GREEN, H. D. AND DENISON, A. B. (1956) Absence of vasomotor response to epinephrine and arterenol in an isolated intracranial circulation. *Circ. Res.*, **4**, 565–573.

HELLINGER, F. R., BLOOR, B. M. AND McCUTCHEN, J. J. (1962) Total cerebral blood flow and oxygen consumption using dye-dilution method: study of occlusive arterial disease and cerebral infarction. *J. Neurosurg.*, **19**, 964–970.

INGVAR, D. H. AND SODERBERG, U. (1956) A new method for measuring cerebral blood flow in relation to the electroencephalogram. *E.E.G. Clin. Neurophysiol.*, **8**, 403–412.

— AND — (1958) Cortical blood flow related to EEG patterns evoked by stimulation of the brain stem. *Acta Physiol. Scand.*, **42**, 130–143.

JENKNER, F. L. (1962) *Rheoencephalography*. Charles C. Thomas, Publisher, Springfield, Ill.

KETY, S. S. AND SCHMIDT, C. F. (1945) Determination of the cerebral blood flow in man by use of nitrous oxide in low concentrations. *Amer. J. Physiol.*, **143**, 53–66.

LASSEN, A., FEINBERG, I. AND LANE M. H. (1960) Bilateral studies of cerebral oxygen uptake in young and aged normal subjects and in patients with organic dementia. *J. Clin. Invest.*, **39**, 491–500.

— AND INGVAR, D. H. (1963) Regional cerebral blood flow in man. *Arch. Neurol.*, **9**, 615–622.

— AND MUNCK, O. (1955) Cerebral blood flow in man determined by use of radioactive krypton. *Acta Physiol. Scand.*, **33**, 30–49.

— AND INGVAR, D. H. (1961) The blood flow of the cerebral cortex determined by radioactive Krypton 85. *Experientia*, **17**, 42–45.

— *et al.* (1963) Regional cerebral blood flow in man determined by Krypton 85. *Neurology*, **13**, 719–727.

— AND KLEE, A. (1965) Cerebral blood flow determination by saturation and desaturation with krypton-85: evaluation of validity of inert gas method of Kety and Schmidt. *Circ. Res.*, **16**, 26–32.

LEWIS, B. M., SOKOLOFF, L., WECHSLER, R. L., WENTZ, W. B. AND KETY, S. S. (1960) Method for continuous measurement of cerebral blood flow in man by means of radioactive krypton (Kr79). *J. Clin. Invest.*, **39**, 707–716.

LINZELL, J. L. (1953) Internal calorimetry in the measurement of blood flow with heated thermocouples. *J. Physiol.*, **121**, 390–402.

LUBSEN, N. (1941) Experimental studies on the cerebral circulation of the unanaesthetized rabbit. *Arch. Neerl. de Physiol.*, **25**, 287–305.

MEYER, J. S., ISHIKAWA, S. AND LEE, T. K. (1964) Electromagnetic measurement of internal jugular venous flow in the monkey. *J. Neurosurg.*, **21**, 524–539.

MCHENRY, L. C., JR. (1964) Quantitative cerebral blood flow determination, application of krypton-85 desaturation technique in man. *Neurology*, **14**, 785–793.

MOLNAR, L. ET CSANAKY, A. (1961) Méthode pour l'enregistrement synchrone du débit du sang et de l'activité électrique du cerveau. *C.R. Soc. Biol.*, **155**, 2269–2272.

MOORE, J. W., KINSMAN, J. M., HAMILTON, W. F. AND SPURLING, G. (1929) Studies on the circulation. II. Cardiac output determination; comparison of the injection method with the direct Fick procedure. *Amer. J. Physiol.*, **89**, 331.

NYLIN, G., HEDLUND, S. AND RENGSTROM, O. (1961) Studies of the cerebral circulation with labeled erythrocytes in healthy man. *Circulat. Res.*, **9**, 664–674.

OLDENDORF, W. H. (1962) Measurement of mean transit time of cerebral circulation by external detection of intravenously injected radioisotope. *J. Nuclear Med.*, **3**, 382–398.

— (1963) Monitoring certain aspects of the cranial blood pool. *Proceedings of the San Diego Symposium for Biomedical Engineering*, 65–72.

PEREZ-BORJA, G. AND MEYER, J. S. (1964) A critical evaluation of rheo-encephalography in control subject and proven cases of cerebrovascular disease. *J. Neurol. Neurosurg. Psychiat.*, **27**, 66–72.

REINMUTH, O. M., SCHEINBERG, P. AND BOURNE, B. (1965) Total cerebral blood flow and metabolism: new method for repeated serial measurement of total cerebral blood flow using iodoantipyrine (I^{131}) with report of determination in normal human beings of blood flow, oxygen consumption, glucose utilization and respiratory quotient of whole brain. *Arch. Neurol.*, **12**, 49–66.

RISER, M. (1936) La circulation cérébrale. *Rev. Neurol.*, **65**, 1061–1173.

RYDER, H. W. *et al.* (1952) Influence of changes in cerebral blood flow on the cerebrospinal fluid pressure. *Arch. Neurol. Psychiat.*, **68**, 165–169.

SAGAWA, K. AND GUYTON, A. C. (1961) Pressure-flow relationship in isolated canine cerebral circulation. *Amer. J. Physiol.*, **200**, 711–714.

SAPIRSTEIN, L. A. (1958) Regional blood flow by fractional distribution of indicators. *Amer. J. Physiol.*, **193**, 161–168.

— (1962) Measurement of the cephalic and cerebral blood flow fractions of the cardiac output in man. *J. Clin. Invest.*, **41**, 1429–1435.

SCHEINBERG, P. (1961) Applications of blood flow measurements to future Investigations. In *Cerebral vascular diseases.* C. H. Millikan, R. G. Siekert et J. P. Whisnant (Eds.), Grune and Stratton, New York.

— AND STEAD, E. A., JR. (1949) Cerebral blood flow in male subjects as measured by nitrous oxide technique: normal values for blood flow, oxygen utilization, glucose utilization, and peripheral resistance with observations on effect of tilting and anxiety. *J. Clin. Invest.*, **28**, 1163–1171.

SCHMIDT, C. F. (1934) The intrinsic regulation of the circulation in the hypothalamus of the cat. *Amer. J. Physiol.*, **110**, 137–152.

— (1944) The present status of knowledge concerning the intrinsic control of the cerebral circulation and the effects of functional derangements in it. *Fed. Proc.*, **3**, 131–139.

— AND HENDRIX, J. P. (1934) The action of chemical substances on cerebral blood vessels. *Res. Pub. Ass. Nerv. Ment. Dis.*, **18**, 241.

— AND PIERSON, J. C. (1934) The intrinsic regulation of the blood vessels of the medulla oblongata. *Amer. J. Physiol.*, **108**, 241–263.

SCHMITT, H. (1956) Inversion de l'action de l'adrénaline et de la noradrénaline sur les vaisseaux cérébraux du chien. *J. Physiol. (Paris)*, **48**, 1035–1043.

STEWART, G. N. (1921) The pulmonary circulation time, the quantity of blood in the lungs and the output of the heart. *Amer. J. Physiol.*, **58**, 20.

SUZUKI, H. AND TUKAHARA, Y. (1963) A heated thermistor method for measuring local blood flow in the brain. *Tohoku J. Exper. Med.*, **81**, 238–245.

TÖNNIS, W. UND SCHIEFER, W. (1959) *Zirkulationsstörungen des Gehirns im Serienangiogramm.* Springer, Göttingen-Heidelberg.

Blood Flow Measurements in Clinical Neurosurgery

W. BRYAN JENNETT AND A. MURRAY HARPER

Institute of Neurological Sciences, Glasgow, and the Wellcome Surgical Research Laboratory, University of Glasgow

The question which must be in the minds of many neurosurgeons is, what is the possible clinical use of the blood flow techniques currently being developed? Are they likely to help the surgeon to make decisions about individual patients, or will they be limited to providing information about the physiopathology of simulated situations in the laboratory, with only secondary deductive applications in hospital?

CEREBRAL BLOOD FLOW MEASUREMENTS IN NEUROSURGERY

Cerebral ischaemia after carotid ligation
Carotid stenosis and endarterectomy
Recovery from circulatory insults (SAH, HI)

Effect of non-surgical treatment — OHP / anaesthesia / anti-spasmodics

Fig. 1. Some possible applications of blood flow measurements in neurosurgery

There seem at present to be four possible fields of application for blood flow measurements in neurosurgery (Fig. 1). One is *carotid ligation* and this will be described later. Another is *carotid endarterectomy* for atheromatous stenosis; this aims primarily to remove a source of emboli and to prevent complete occlusion, but claims are also made that it improves blood flow. Only by measurement can we discover whether this claim is well founded: if so it would be important to know in which patients this was likely to be of benefit. We have carried out measurements during the course of endarterectomy and demonstrated the feasibility of this manoeuvre.

Aneurysm surgery is still bedevilled by the problem of vasospasm, and of choosing the optimum time for operation. Repeated angiography is unacceptable as a means of assessing the resolution of spasm, because it may by itself aggravate it as well as adding other risks; serial blood flow measurements might give just the information which the surgeon wishes (Kak and Taylor, 1967). Similar measurements have also been used to study the post-concussional syndrome (Taylor and Bell, 1966) and this method might prove even more useful in the earlier stages after head injury, particularly in predicting the likelihood of recovery from severe injuries.

The effect of various drugs on cerebral blood flow can also be monitored both to indicate the side effects on the cerebral circulation as well as the extent of the desired effects. *Anti-spasmodics* are being marketed now and the claim that they improve the cerebral circulation clearly cannot be substantiated on the grounds of clinical improvement alone. The effect of *anaesthetics* on cerebral blood flow has interested us and Dr. McDowall will deal with this in a later paper. Then again there is the effect of *hyperbaric oxygen* which is being proposed as a method of increasing the availability of oxygen to the brain in certain situations. We have now measured the effect on cerebral blood flow of oxygen at two atmospheres on a number of patients undergoing surgery in the pressure chamber.

TABLE 1

CEREBRAL BLOOD FLOW MEASUREMENTS IN MAN

Technique	Procedure required						
	No needles	Arm vein puncture	Jugular vein puncture	Artery puncture	Carotid puncture	Neck oper- ation	IC oper- ation
Inhalation	×						
Impedence pulsation	×						
Mode circulation time		×					
Heat clearance (Hermann)			×				
Kety-Schmidt			×	×			
Inert gas clearance (gamma)					×		
Rapid serial angiography					×		
Flowmeter						×	
Heat clearance (Betz)							×
Hydrogen polography							×
Inert gas clearance (beta)					×		×
Dyes					×		×

	TYPE OF DATA		
Total	qualitative	Repeatable	Slow
Regional	quantitative	Once only	Rapid

Fig. 2. Type of data yielded by different blood flow methods

Having indicated the possible fields of useful application the methods available must be considered. The familiar clinical dilemma confronts us — that the most scientifically satisfying methods are apt to demand the most elaborate interventions on our patients. Some aspects of this equation are explored in Table 1 in which the complexity of the procedure is plotted against the method available. In Fig. 2 the different types of data yielded by various methods are set out; there is still some controversy in a growing subject as to exactly which methods yield which type of data and no attempt is made to indicate this correlation. It is, however, obvious that electro-magnetic flow meters or heat clearance techniques can give information about rapid changes in cerebral blood flow, whereas the clearance methods give the average flow over ten or fifteen minutes. On the other hand, the mean circulation time method and xenon inhalation are methods which can be repeated whereas those involving intracarotid injection or surgical operation clearly cannot. Much theoretical work remains to be done before we can say with confidence just what quantitative validity we can attach to the various methods. In the Institute of Neurological Sciences, Glasgow, we are mainly concerned at present with comparing the value of beta counting from the cortex with gamma counting with external detectors, and in comparing the mean circulation time with the xenon clearance; and with comparing internal and common carotid injections of isotope for clearance measurements.

There is no answer to the question which is the best method? The clinician interested in this field must have more than one method in his repertoire and let the special circumstances of the problem facing him at the time dictate which method he uses. For example, we might be able to assess quantitatively the changes in cerebral circulation after subarachnoid haemorrhage by undertaking, at the time of the diagnostic angiogram, xenon clearance simultaneously with a mean circulation time, whereby the latter simple and repeatable method could be calibrated for that patient. We could then repeat the mean circulation time in the ward on successive days and get useful information about flow changes.

I wish briefly now to recount the use we have made of the xenon clearance method during the course of carotid ligation, as a means of predicting the risk of cerebral ischaemia and of comparing the risks of internal and common carotid ligation (Jennett et al., 1966). Methods employed hitherto to predict the likelihood of hemiplegia after therapeutic carotid ligation have proved unreliable (Wilkinson et al., 1965). Because of the efficiency of the circle of Willis assessments of flow in neck vessels may bear little relation to cerebral blood flow and a more direct method is required. This paper describes the adaptation of the radio-active inert gas clearance technique of measuring rCBF for use in the operating theatre during carotid ligation. The clearance rate of ^{133}Xe from the brain after internal carotid injection is measured by counting the gamma emissions through the intact skull using a collimated scintillation crystal. Clearance rates are estimated before and after temporary clamping of the common and the internal carotid arteries in turn.

The degree of reduction in rCBF during internal carotid clamping was related to the development of immediate or delayed hemiparesis. Of the ten studies during internal carotid clamping four patients showed more than 25% reduction in rCBF and every one of them developed immediate or delayed hemiparesis; no patient with less than 25% reduction developed any neurological complication.

A comparison of the reduction in rCBF during common and internal carotid clamping in eight patients suggested a steal from internal to external in four because clearance was much slower during clamping of the common carotid than when the internal carotid was clamped. Because of the amount of isotope in the external carotid circulation under these circumstances it is not possible at present to calculate rCBF quantitatively during a steal. In four other patients the reduction in rCBF was similar during common and internal clamping, and in only two was the external apparently serving as a useful collateral. This technique gives the surgeon an immediate guide in the operating theatre. Comparison of the flow before and after temporary clamping of the internal and common carotid arteries in turn gives an indication of the risk to the cerebral circulation of permanent ligation of either artery.

ACKNOWLEDGEMENTS

This work was supported by The Medical Research Council, The Wellcome Trust and The Scottish Hospital Endowment Research Trust.

REFERENCES

JENNETT, W. B., HARPER, A. M. AND GILLESPIE, F. C. (1966) *Lancet*, **ii**, 1162.
KAK, V. K. AND TAYLOR, A. R. (1967) *Lancet*, **i**, 875
TAYLOR, A. R. AND BELL, T. K. (1966) *Lancet*, **ii**, 178.
WILKINSON, H. A., WRIGHT, R. L. AND SWEET, W. H. (1965) *J. Neurosurg.*, **22**, 241.

Regional Cerebral Blood Flow in Cerebrovascular Disorders *

DAVID H. INGVAR

Department of Clinical Neurophysiology, University Hospital, Lund, Sweden

INTRODUCTION

The majority of cerebrovascular disorders are *regional* in character. A cerebral thrombosis, an embolus, or a cerebral hemorrhage does not as a rule involve the whole of the brain but only a circumscribed part of it. In order to study the pathophysiology of these disorders it is therefore a prerequisite that methods for the measurement of *regional* cerebral blood flow (rCBF) are available (Lassen *et al.*, 1963; Høedt-Rasmussen *et al.*, 1966; Ingvar *et al.*, 1965).

This is a review of some principal findings concerning rCBF in focal cerebrovascular disorders.

TECHNICAL ASPECTS

Very early in the development of isotope clearance techniques for measurement of rCBF, it became evident that the resolution of such measurements could be augmented by the use of multiple detectors. At present, we are regularly using 8, or 16 detectors which are mounted at right angle to the side of the skull. By suitable collimation the overlap between the individual detector fields is kept at a minimum. For a simple analysis of the large number of clearance curves obtained with 16 detectors, it has recently been suggested to use the initial slope of the clearance curve as an expression of the flow (Høedt-Rasmussen *et al.*, 1967). However, for the calculation of absolute flow values, and of differential flows in the grey and white matter, including the relative weights of these two components, the earlier proposed computer analyses of the curves are still being used routinely (Høedt-Rasmussen *et al.*, 1966).

We have also recently added various dynamic procedures in order to study the rCBF during different functional conditions. Thus, *mental activity* has been found to produce regional patterns of rCBF changes. These patterns may be altered by focal brain lesions (Ingvar and Risberg, 1967). *Alterations of the arterial pressure* and *inhalation of carbon dioxide* have also been used in order to establish whether a given brain region demonstrates autoregulation of the blood flow which is normal, or whether this regulation is absent (Høedt-Rasmussen *et al.*, 1967).

* Several investigations summarized in this paper were sponsored by the Swedish Medical Research Council (projects nr 21X-84-01 and 21X-84-02) and by the Wallenberg Foundation.

References p. 61

CLINICAL RESULTS

From an unselected group of patients studied at the University Hospital of Lund and at the Bispebjerg Hospital in Copenhagen, comprising about 70 cases of acute cerebrovascular disorder, the following main results have been obtained (*cf.* Ingvar, 1967; Ingvar and Risberg, 1967).

In the acute phase of an occlusive cerebrovascular lesion, when angiography only shows subtle changes, often in the form of a local contrast "blush" or a few early filling veins (Cronqvist, 1966; Cronqvist and Laroche, 1967), multiple rCBF measurements may demonstrate a region with *fast flow* corresponding to the angiographic abnormality. Cerebral infarcts pertaining to this group, may be of the transient type, and the rCBF may be normal in clinically and angiographically normal parts of the hemisphere studied. Hence, the fast flow within the focal lesion might represent an absolute hyperemia. The clearance curves over such lesions often show an initial peak which indicates the presence of abnormal rapidly perfused tissue compartments (Cronqvist and Laroche, 1967). With the 16-detector unit, at present used in Copenhagen, it has clearly been demonstrated that with this number of detectors one can outline similar *hyperemic infarct* in substantial detail (Høedt-Rasmussen *et al.*, 1967).

As shown recently by Høedt-Rasmussen *et al.* (1967), the flow within hyperemic infarcts follows passively variations in the arterial pressure. This demonstrates that there is a regional lack of autoregulation.

A general cerebral vasodilatation, on the other hand, induced by e.g. carbon dioxide inhalation, may diminish the flow within the hyperemic region (Høedt-Rasmussen *et al.*, 1967; Symon, 1967; Shalit *et al.*, 1967). When carbon dioxide dilates the normal part of the cerebral vascular bed, the perfusion pressure within collaterals to the hyperemic infarct drops. Since the vessels around the lesion lack autoregulation the drop of pressure leads to a decrease in perfusion (Fig. 1). For this phenomenon the term '*intracerebral steal*' has been used. It seems likely that such a mechanism may have direct therapeutic implications. Vasodilatory drugs may not benefit the flow in an infarcted area, but, instead, set up a deleterious reduction of the flow, when (not only the

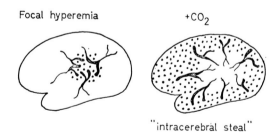

Fig. 1. The 'intracerebral steal' phenomenon. Hypothetical diagram of a possible mechanism behind the observations that the blood flow and perfusion pressure inside the collateral flow to an infarcted area may decrease following carbon dioxide inhalation. The dilatation induced by carbon dioxide affects only the intact part of the cerebral vascular bed. In the perifocal collaterals this leads to a fall in perfusion pressure and — since there is a lack of autoregulation — also to a fall in the perfusion.

systemic pressure may decrease, but also) the perfusion pressure drops in collaterals leading to the hyperemic region.

In larger cerebrovascular lesions, we have observed a second type of rCBF change. Here an *ischemic area* can be outlined which corresponds to the angiographic abnormality (occlusion of a large vessel, or signs of an expansive mass). The clinical symptoms in such cases are usually very severe and the EEG demonstrates a marked general disturbance (Ingvar, 1966). The rCBF in parts of the hemisphere which are not primarily involved by the large lesion is usually also substantially reduced.

While the two types described thus show *focal* abnormalities of the rCBF, a third type has been encountered in which neither focal ischemia nor hyperemia could be detected. These patients often still demonstrated definite focal neurological deficits, but they were often investigated late in the course of the disease. In most of them there was a general reduction of the rCBF to a uniform low level in all areas measured.

An analysis of the EEG in the patients mentioned showed that the EEG abnormalities only to a limited extent reflected the size and the location of the vascular lesion. This is probably due to the limited covering of the brain by external electrodes, and, also, to the fact that deep lesions may create "remote" EEG changes when structures regulating the cortical rhythms are affected. A detailed account of the EEG findings in relation to rCBF measurements has been presented elsewhere recently (Ingvar, 1966). The radiological findings in the Lund material of cerebrovascular patients, studied simultaneously with cerebral angiography and rCBF measurements, have recently been summarized by Cronqvist (1966) and Cronqvist and Laroche (1967).

DISCUSSION

It appears likely that the three types presented above of different rCBF patterns in focal cerebrovascular lesions, may in fact represent important stages in the pathogenesis of such lesions (Fig. 2).

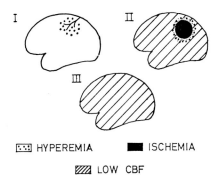

Fig. 2. Schematic diagram of the three main types of occlusive cerebrovascular lesions discussed in this paper. These principal (sometimes overlapping) types have emerged from studies of patients with occlusive cerebrovascular lesions which were examined with cerebral angiography and multiple simultaneous measurements of regional cerebral blood flow. There is some evidence that these three types may represent subsequent phases in the pathogenesis of certain occlusive lesions.

References p. 61

The *focal hyperemic type* was usually found in the acute stage of an occlusive lesion and could disappear later. The hyperemia and the concomitant 'shunt' picture in the angiogram with early filling veins and/or contrast 'blush', most likely represents a regional "luxury perfusion syndrome" (See Lassen, 1966). The hyperemia is probably caused by a regional post-anoxic dilatation of the vascular bed due to anaerobic (acid) metabolites. Smaller such lesions may apparently disappear completely and within a few days a normal angiogram and rCBF pattern may then be seen (Cronqvist and Laroche, 1967).

The ischemic type would represent a larger cerebrovascular lesion with a central core which may not be perfused at all. This non-perfused part is of course not measured by the rCBF technique, but only the periphery in which an insufficient collateral flow gives rise to the very low rCBF values measured over such lesions. The size of the lesion and secondary edema often gives rise to an increase of the intracranial pressure which to some extent may be responsible for the severity of the clinical symptoms and the general EEG abnormalities.

Finally, the last mentioned type, the *non-focal low rCBF type*, seems to represent the "chronic brain syndrome" following a focal vascular lesion. It is well known that such patients when studied with the KETY technique often show a reduced mean cerebral oxygen uptake and blood flow. The original focus may have passed through its hyperemic and/or ischemic stage and the rCBF detectors do not see any focal deviations from the generally low rCBF level. This level is set by the general depression of the cerebral functional activity caused by the focal lesion.

However, it should be pointed out that the three types outlined above often may overlap and that they are not always seen in clean forms. At present, serial studies with detailed clinical analyses, as well as repeated angiographic studies and rCBF measurements, are under way. Such studies will reveal whether the above interpretation of the rCBF patterns seen in cerebrovascular lesions is a correct one.

CONCLUDING REMARKS

Multiple simultaneous measurements of regional cerebral blood flow in patients with focal cerebrovascular lesions have revealed new details in the pathophysiology of such disorders. An acute focal occlusive lesion sets up a regional vasodilatation in the surrounding, which can both be seen in the acute phase directly on the angiogram, and measured by means of isotope clearance as a regional hyperemia. In larger lesions an ischemic region with low flow can be actually found, corresponding to an expansive mass shown on the angiogram. In the chronic phase the over-all reduction of the cerebral blood flow gives a measure of the general functional sequelae of the primary focal lesion.

These findings would seem to have a general bearing on the problem of focal cerebral ischemia encountered in neurosurgical disorders of traumatic, neoplastic or vascular origin.

REFERENCES

CRONQVIST, S. (1966) Transitory hyperaemia in focal cerebral ischemic lesions. *3rd Intern. Symp. Cerebral Circulation, Salzburg.*

CRONQVIST, S. AND LAROCHE, F. (1967) Transitory "hyperemia" in focal cerebral vascular lesions studied by angiography and regional cerebral blood flow measurement. *Brit. J. Radiol.,* 40, 270.

HØEDT-RASMUSSEN, K., SKINHØJ, E. AND LASSEN, N. A. (1966) Regional cerebral blood flow in man determined by intra-arterial injection of radioactive inert gas. *Circ. Res.,* **18,** 237.

HØEDT-RASMUSSEN, K., SKINHØJ, E., PAULSON, O., EWALD, J., BJERROM, J. K., FAHRENKROG, A. AND LASSEN, N. A. (1967) Regional cerebral blood flow in acute apoplexy with a demonstration of local hyperemia ("the luxury perfusion syndrome") of the brain tissue. *Arch. Neurol. (Chicago),* in press.

INGVAR, D. H. (1966) The pathophysiology of the stroke related to findings in EEG and to measurements of regional cerebral blood flow. *Thule International Symposia, Stroke,* p. 105.

—, (1967) The pathophysiology of occlusive cerebrovascular disorders, related to neuroradiological findings, EEG, and measurements of regional cerebral blood flow. *Contr. 18th Scand. Congr. Neurol., Helsinki,* June 19-22, 1967.

INGVAR, D. H., CRONQVIST, S., EKBERG, R., RISBERG, J. AND HØEDT-RASMUSSEN, K. (1965) Normal values of regional cerebral blood flow in man, including flow and weight estimates of gray and white matter. *Acta Neurol. Scand.,* Suppl. **14,** 72.

INGVAR, D. H. AND RISBERG, J. (1967) Increase of regional cerebral blood flow during mental effort in normals and in patients with focal brain disorders. *Exptl. Brain Res.,* **3,** 195.

LASSEN, N. A. (1966) The luxury-perfusion syndrome and its possible relation to acute metabolic acidosis localised within the brain. *Lancet,* 1113.

LASSEN, N. A., HØEDT-RASMUSSEN, K., SØRENSEN, S. C., SKINHØJ, E., CRONQVIST, S., BODFORSS, B., ENG, E. AND INGVAR, D. H. (1963) Regional cerebral blood flow in man determined by Krypton[85]. *Neurology,* **13,** 719.

SHALIT, M. N., SHIMOYO, S., REINMUTH, D. M., LOCKHART, W. S. JR. AND SCHEINBERG, P. (1967) The mechanism of action of carbon dioxide in the regulation of cerebral blood flow. Abstr. *III. Europ. Congr. Neurosurg., Madrid,* April.

SYMON, L. (1967) Experimental study of cerebral arterial spasm. *Abstr. III. Europ. Congr. Neurosurg., Madrid,* April.

A Method for the Study of Experimental Cerebral Vasospasm

LINDSAY SYMON

The Department of Neurosurgical Studies, The National Hospital, Queen Square, London

Narrowing of cerebral arteries is seen in the area of intracranial aneurysms after sub-arachnoid haemorrhage. It has been regarded as arterial spasm and associated by some surgeons with the narrowing of cerebral vessels which can be produced at operation by traumatic stimuli (Pool, 1958; Gillingham, 1958; Johnson *et al.*, 1958). Experimentally produced traumatic arterial spasm has been much studied therefore, since spasm has been thought to be important in the production of ischaemic symptoms after sub-arachnoid haemorrhage. Most of this experimental work has confined itself to visual description of spasm without quantitation and the concept has remained scientifically vague as a result. The present work attempts to study experimental spasm in a form in which numerical analysis is possible so that its character and its variability may be analysed. There is no proof that experimental and clinical spasm are the same, but angiographically they are indistinguishable (Symon, 1967).

The method of production and recording of spasm has been fully described elsewhere (Symon, 1963, 1967). A small catheter is introduced into a leptomeningeal branch of the middle cerebral artery, and the pulse pressure and intravascular pressure in the middle cerebral field continuously measured. The main middle cerebral artery is bared of arachnoid within the first 5 mm of its course and stimulated by light repetitive occlusions using a stopped non-toothed dissecting forceps to produce approximately the same pressure at each occlusion. The resulting spasm produces the appearance shown in Fig. 1.

Shortly after the stimulus there is a reduction in intravascular pressure and pulse pressure increasing to a maximum and then slowly decreasing. This gives three measurements, the total duration of spasm, the time it takes to reach its maximum and the intensity of the spasm measured as a percentage reduction in pulse pressure. Other recordings essential from the control point of view are endtidal CO_2 monitored continuously, arterial pCO_2 quantitatively from time to time, and systemic blood pressure continuously. A further recording shown is a superficial thermistor recording from a small pial artery of similar size to that catheterised indicating that blood flow is reduced during the period of spasm. The mean values obtained from these three measurements in a group of 15 animals are shown in Table 1. The variation from one animal to the next is not inconsiderable. Mean duration varies from 12 to 29 min, the time of development from nearly 2 min to over 7 min, and the intensity from a pulse pressure reduc-

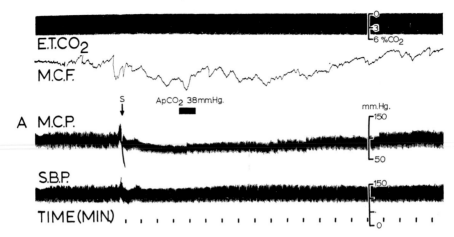

Fig. 1. Records of systemic blood pressure (S.B.P.), endtidal CO_2 tension ($ETCO_2$) and middle cerebral pressure and flow (M.C.P., M.C.F.) from a parietal branch of the middle cerebral artery, in a baboon under chloralose anaesthesia. Traumatic stimulus at S.

tion of 24% to one of over 50%. The mean and standard errors for the group as a whole are shown.

In a group of five animals which formed the first in Table I, the control observations were the only ones made, and a series of spasms were produced over a prolonged period of time. The analysis of this group in which five control episodes were made in each case is shown in Table II. There is appreciable variation from maximum to minimum, both in the duration of spasm, in the time of the development of the spasm, and in the intensity of the spasm. In most cases there is a narrow standard error for the

TABLE I

Experiment number	Number of observations	Mean duration (min)	Mean time to maximum (min)	Mean % reduction in pulse pressure
11	5	22.6	3.9	41.6
12	5	12.6	3.8	44.5
13	5	15.1	3.3	29.4
16	5	15.3	4.1	33.4
17	5	20.7	3.9	53.2
18	3	13.3	2.7	53
19	3	14.4	3.3	37
20	3	20.3	3.3	41.5
21	3	20.3	3.4	47
22	3	19.0	1.8	46
24	3	16.2	1.9	49
26	3	28.0	6.0	54
27	3	28.6	6.5	30
29	3	22.4	3.4	45
30	3	18.5	4.4	40
Mean		19.2	3.7	43.6
S.D.		±4.9	±0.4	±8.1

TABLE II

Experiment number	Number of observations	Duration of spasm (min)			Time to maximum (min)			Reduction in pial pulse pressure (%)		
		Max.	Min.	Mean ± S.D.	Max.	Min.	Mean ± S.D.	Max.	Min.	Mean ± S.D.
11	5	34.5	14.0	22.6 ± 10.8	8.4	2.6	3.9 ± 2.6	50	38	41.6 ± 8.5
12	5	19.3	10.6	12.6 ± 3.8	4.0	3.6	3.8 ± 0.6	66	20	44.5 ± 18.6
13	5	16.6	12.2	15.1 ± 3.0	4.9	1.8	3.3 ± 1.2	33	20	29.4 ± 5.4
16	5	18.3	11.9	15.3 ± 2.5	5.0	3.5	4.1 ± 0.6	56	20	33.4 ± 13.7
17	5	26.2	14.8	20.7 ± 5.3	5.0	3.2	3.9 ± 2.7	61	30	53.2 ± 10.9

References p. 67

duration of spasm. The variability of the time of development of spasm is rather large and the variability in the intensity of the spasm is also seen to be considerable. Electrical and more complicated mechanical methods of applying the stimulus did not prove satisfactory. Electrical stimuli in particular applied in the region of the base of the brain considerably altered the animal's systemic blood pressure during the passage of the current.

Thus, descriptive experiments which do not provide adequate objective and statistical evidence of the standards of variation to be expected in a particular preparation, are unlikely to be of scientific value. The range of random variation in the experimental preparation used must be stated.

Using this method I have analysed the reproducibilityof arterial spasm at high and low levels of arterial pCO_2. The normocapnic controls were artificially ventilated to maintain an arterial pCO_2 between 35 and 45 mm Hg. Hypocapnic animals were hyperventilated to reduce the arterial pCO_2 to less than 20 mm Hg. Hypercapnic animals had CO_2 added to the respiratory inlet to raise the arterial pCO_2 to more than 50 mm Hg. The three parameters of spasm were not significantly different in any case.

A troublesome complicating factor was the production of clear emboli from the area of artery traumatised. This may be associated with the appearance of whiteness and narrowness of the main trunk indistinguishable photographically from severe arterial spasm. The picture is different on the end arterial recording, however, as is shown in Fig. 2 where a traumatic stimulus results in the appearance of severe spasm which appears to be resolving. Suddenly it progresses to obliteration of the pulse and instead of resolving in about 20 min intravascular pressure remains very low until 30 min when it suddenly recovers, unlike the gradual recovery of arterial spasm. Repeated trauma again abolished the pulse for a prolonged period of time. Each sudden reappearance of the pulse in this instance was associated with a shower of clear bodies in the peripheral circulation similar to those described by Denny Brown after carotid

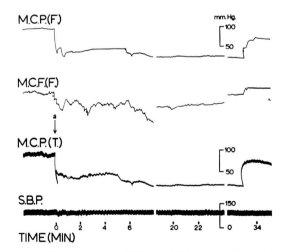

Fig. 2. Records of systemic blood pressure (S.B.P.), middle cerebral arterial pressure (M.C.P.) and middle cerebral flow (M.C.F.) in a baboon under chloralose anaesthesia. Traumatic stimulus at A.

trauma. I believe them to be platelet emboli from the area of damage to the artery.

Histological examination of the traumatised area of artery shows that the intima is damaged and the internal elastic lamina broken up into spirals which project into the lumen and contain small aggregates of structureless granular material suggesting that these may be aggregates of platelets. The histological appearances are independent of the production of spasm since spasm has been produced in animals which subsequently show no histological changes. Animals who have proceeded to apparent complete obliteration of the artery which has subsequently resolved do not show thrombosis of the vessel but they show the histological damage to the intima.

Using this preparation also, various agents have been applied to the middle cerebral artery in an attempt to produce or encourage traumatic arterial spasm. These have included fresh and stored blood, serum, CSF from subarachnoid cases, haemolysed blood, concentrations of catecholamine up to 100 μg/ml, of 5-HT up to 100 μg/ml and of bradykinin and histamine. None of these produced the appearances of reduced peripheral blood flow, or of reduced pulse and intravascular pressures such as are associated with traumatic arterial spasm. The appearances of the wave of spasm coming on and slowly relaxing is very suggestive of focal liberation of some pharmacologically active material, as yet uncertain in nature. It may be that although vaso-active material externally applied does not produce significant spasm in this preparation, the liberation of some vaso-active compound intra-murally from the area of damaged arterial wall may yet be effective in producing spasm.

REFERENCES

GILLINGHAM, F. J. (1958) The management of ruptured intracranial aneurysm. *Ann. Roy. Coll. Surg. Eng.*, **23**, 89–117.

JOHNSON, R. J., POTTER, J. M. AND REID, R. C. (1958) Arterial spasm in subarachnoid haemorrhage: mechanical considerations. *J. Neurol. Neurosurg. Psychiat.*, **21**, 68.

POOL, J. L. (1958) Cerebral vasospasm. *New Engl. J. Med.*, **259**, 1259–1264.

SYMON, L. (1963) Cerebral arterial pressure recording in dogs and macacus rhesus. *J. Physiol.*, **165**, 62P.

—, (1967) Vascular spasm in the cerebral circulation. *Proc. First Migraine Symposium* (in press).

—, (1967) A comparative study of middle cerebral arterial pressure in dogs and macaques. *J. Physiol.* (in press).

Clinical Investigations on Interrelations Between Intracranial Pressure and Intracranial Hemodynamics

N. LUNDBERG, S. CRONQVIST AND Å. KJÄLLQUIST

Departments of Neurosurgery and Neuroradiology, University and Hospital of Lund, Sweden

Studies of the ventricular fluid pressure (VFP) by continuous recording have shown that, in patients with intracranial hypertension the VFP has a marked tendency to rapid variations and that these variations often follow certain well defined patterns. It has been possible to distinguish three main forms of variations. Two are of a rhythmic nature and related to periodic breathing of the Cheyne-Stokes' type and to Traube-Hering-Mayer waves of the systemic blood pressure (frequency: $\frac{1}{2}$–2/min and 6/min respectively). They are probably related to an intrinsic rhythmic acitivity of medullary centers, released from influence of higher centra in the upper brain stem (Kjällquist *et al.*, 1964) and may serve as examples of variations of the VFP caused by variations of the blood pressure within the cerebral vascular bed.

The third type of pressure variations is of an entirely different character (Fig. 1). They occur with varying intervals and often with considerable amplitude (60–100 mm Hg) and duration (5–20 min). In accordance with their form we have called them "plateau waves" (Lundberg *et al.*, 1959; Lundberg, 1960; Ingvar and Lundberg, 1961). These waves are frequently accompanied by transient, sometimes paroxysmal symptoms, such as headache, nausea, vomiting, facial flush, impairment of consciousness,

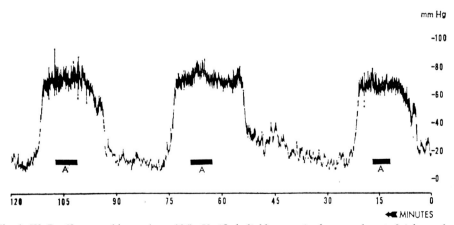

Fig. 1. W. P., 60-years old man (case 136). *Verified glioblastoma in the central part of right cerebral hemisphere.* Spontaneous plateau waves. Horizontal lines marked A = attacks of headache, restlessness, impaired consciousness and increased rigidity of the limbs.

confusion, forced breathing as well as by various motor phenomena such as clonic movements and tonic rigidity of the limbs. The plateau waves may be regarded as a pathophysiological basis of acute disorders of the brain stem in patients with increased intracranial pressure. Hence their origin is of considerable interest to the neurosurgeons.

The following observations may serve to elucidate this problem.

(1) Plateau waves occur during a fairly advanced stage of intracranial hypertension (roughly corresponding to the second and third stage of Kocher) and only if the mean intracranial pressure is substantially elevated (> 20 mm Hg). By decreasing the intracranial pressure (and/or brain volume) by drainage of CSF or administration of hypertonic solutions the plateau waves can always be temporarily abolished.

(2) Plateau waves have not been observed in hydrocephalic infants with open fontanels and increased intracranial pressure. They have been found to diminish or disappear after subtemporal decompression in spite of the mean pressure remaining at about the same level as before the operation.

(3) Plateau waves may occur without any appreciable change of the systemic arterial blood pressure. When that is the case the arterio-venous pressure difference may be heavily reduced (Fig. 2). However, a rise of the arterial systemic blood pressure concomitant with plateau waves in many cases aids in preserving a sufficient perfusion pressure.

(4) Simultaneous recording of the VFP, respiration and alveolar pCO_2 during plateau waves show that respiratory irregularities causing hypercapnia may precede the rise in pressure. On the other hand, forced breathing with hypocapnia may precede the fall in pressure. In some cases the VFP is markedly resistant to hypocapnia during a plateau wave, in others a prompt fall in pressure can be induced by voluntary hyperventilation. Furthermore, plateau waves may occur during artificial respiration at a constant ventilation rate, a constant alveolar pCO_2, and a constant mean intrathoracic pressure.

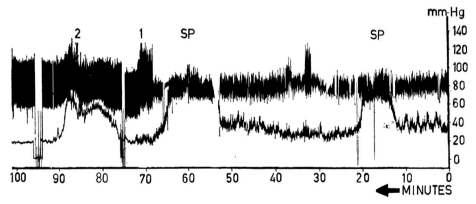

Fig. 2. M. N., 26-years old woman (case 579). *Verified glioblastoma in left frontal lobe.* Preoperative recording of VFP (lower curve) and blood pressure in left femoral artery (upper curve). Common reference level: anterior axillary line. S P = spontaneous plateau waves; Arrow 1 = induction of general anesthesia; Arrow 2 = intubation.

(5) In patients with spontaneous plateau waves similar pressure waves can be provoked a) by inducing a relatively small rise in intracranial pressue (e.g. 20 mm Hg in 5") by instillation of gas or fluid into the ventricles or by pressing upon a cranial defect (Fig. 3), b) by inducing hypercapnia or by intravenous injection of histamine.

(6) Spontaneous plateau waves often occur without visible cause. However, it is sometimes obvious that the initial rise in pressure coincides with bodily activity, emotional upset, painful stimuli or arousal from sleep.

(7) Angiograms made during spontaneous plateau waves show wider vessels in the arterial phase as compared with angiograms taken during the interval between two waves (Fig. 4). The venograms show the large parasagittal veins to be about equally contrast filled during as between the waves.

(8) Measurements of the CBF by the isotope clearance technique (Lassen *et al.*, 1963) during plateau waves show a decrease in CBF as compared with measurements made during the intervals of low pressure (Fig. 4).

DISCUSSION

Plateau waves occur during a state of intracranial hypertension when the mechanisms for intracranial spatial compensation can be assumed to be markedly impaired (observation 1). Furthermore plateau waves disappear or diminish if the distensibility of the walls of the cranial cavity is increased or the brain volume decreased (observations 1 and 2). These facts indicate that plateau waves occur when the interrelations between pressure and volume are represented on the steep part of the intracranial pressure/volume curve (Langfitt *et al.*, 1965a), i.e. where a relatively small increase in volume of the intracranial content gives rise to a relatively great increase of the intracranial pressure.

The necessary net increase of the intracranial content can theoretically occur within any of the three intracranial compartments: vascular bed, CSF pathways or brain tissue. The rapidity and the prompt reversibility of the pressure variations suggest that

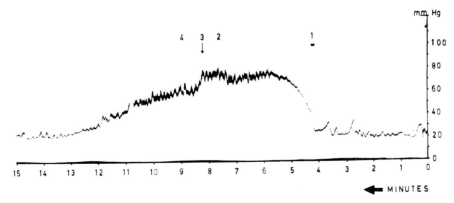

Fig. 3. E. N., 41-years old man (case 503). *Verified glioblastoma in right cerebral hemisphere.* Spontaneous plateau waves before operation. Recording of the VFP 2 weeks after subtemporal decompression. Blood pressure cuff fixed around the head with the rubber bag over the bone defect. 1 = inflation of cuff to 100 mm Hg in 8"; 2 = patient drowsy; 3 = deflation of cuff; 4 = patient alert.

they are caused by dilatation (or constriction) of resistance-determining blood vessels permitting a greater (or lesser) part of the systemic blood pressure to be transmitted to the cerebral vascular bed. This view is supported by the dilatation of cerebral arteries which can be seen in angiograms taken during plateau waves (observation 7). However, variations of the volume of the two other compartments cannot be excluded as a possible parameters involved in the mechanism.

From the fact that plateau waves may occur irrespectively of any variations of the systemic blood pressure and the respiration (observation 3 and 4) it can be inferred that they may be exclusively due to changes of the cerebral vascular resistance. However, changes of the systemic blood pressure and respiration, including reactions secondary to the elevation of the intracranial pressure (e.g. rise in blood pressure, hyperpnea, irregular breathing) may act as modifying factors (Langfitt *et al.*, 1965a and b, observation 4).

Dilatation of pial arteries as a response to an acute increase of the intracranial pressure was observed in animals by Wolff and Forbes (1929) and Fog (1933). Noell and Schneider (1948) found that a substantial reduction of the CBF provoked by increasing the CSF pressure was compensated for by cerebral vasodilatation, due to the influence of hypoxia and followed by a "reactive hyperemia" when the CSF pressure was lowered

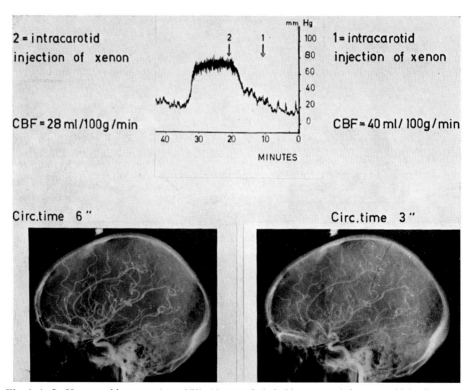

Fig. 4. A. J., 58-years old woman (case 378). *Non verified glioblastoma in left temporal lobe.* Spontaneous plateau waves. Repeated angiography and CBF measurements. Arrows 1 and 2 = first and second injection of xenon[133]. Left angiogram taken during the plateau wave. Right angiogram taken between 2 plateau waves.

again. Similar phenomena were observed by Häggendal *et al.* (1967). By filling an intracranial balloon in monkeys Langfitt *et al.* (1965a) could demonstrate a secondary rise of the intracranial pressure and present evidence suggesting that this rise was due to cerebral vasodilatation. It seems reasonable to assume that a similar vasomotor response to an increase of the intracranial pressure is responsible for the secondary rise in pressure, demonstrated in Fig. 3, and also for the ascending shank of the spontaneous plateau waves.

Not least from a clinical point of view it would be of interest to know which stimuli may be capable of initiating plateau waves in patients with intracranial hypertension. In our clinical experiments, besides by raising the intracranial pressure mechanically, pressure waves similar to spontaneous plateau waves have been provoked by agents known to cause dilatation of cerebral vessels such as CO_2 and histamine (observation 5). The most common cause related to neurosurgical measures has surely been incautious injection of gas into the ventricles or the subarachnoidal space for pneumography (Cronqvist *et al.*, 1963) and hypercapnia due to inadequate anesthesiological technique. Valsalva mechanisms may also be responsible for an initiating rise of the intracranial pressure.

A less known cause of increase in intracranial pressure is augmentation of the functional activity of the brain. By continuous recording via a lumbar needle Haug (1932) found that mental stimuli and pain provoked elevations of the CSF pressure. In one case of status epilepticus without permanent intracranial hypertension we have been able to record the VFP when the patient was curarized and ventilated with a respirator. In spite of the absence of any motor activity the VFP rose 15–20 mm Hg at the same time as the EEG indicated seizure (Cronqvist *et al.*, 1967). Cooper and Hulme (1966) found that during sleep, plateau waves were most frequent during states of "paradoxical" sleep characterized by electroencephalographic signs of increased functional activity of the brain. Our observations (6) suggest that also changes of cerebral functional activity caused e.g. by emotional upset, painful stimuli, bodily or mental activity and arousal might be capable of initiating plateau waves by causing cerebral vasodilatation (Ingvar and Lundberg, 1961). This could explain the apparently arbitrary and unpredictable occurrence of plateau waves which is typical in many cases of intracranial hypertension as well as the beneficial effect of bedrest in such cases. It could perhaps also explain why tracheal intubation so often is accompanied by acute rise in intracranial pressure even if the arterial pCO_2 is kept at a normal level.

A decrease in CBF during spontaneous plateau waves has been shown by the isotope clearance technique (Lassen *et al.*, 1963) (observation 8) and by the thermo-electric technique of Hensel and Betz (Betz, 1965; Wüllenweber, 1965). This observation suggests a paradoxical change of the cerebrovascular resistance on dilatation of cerebral arteries. It seems reasonable to assume that this paradoxical reaction is a consequence of the normal facilities for spatial compensation being absent in patients with intracranial hypertension and rigid cranial walls. Wright (1938) and Greenfield and Tindall (1965) observed filled convexity and parasagittal veins during induced intracranial hypertension. We have made the same observation (8) in angiograms taken during plateau waves. As pointed out by Greenfield and Tindall this signifies that the pressure in the parasagittal veins is at least as high as the intracranial pressure and that the locus for the main pressure drop has shifted from the arterioli to the entrance of the cerebral veins into the venous sinuses.

From Fig. 2 it is evident that the perfusion pressure may be heavily reduced during plateau waves. A consequent reduction in CBF giving rise to hypoxia in the brain tissue may certainly be the cause of signs of cerebral dysfunction which often accompany plateau waves (Figs. 1 and 3). Another possible explanation is increased mechanical stress on the brain stem produced by increased herniation or distortion.

The nature of the reaction by which an increase of the intracranial pressure causes vasodilatation is not known. One possible explanation would be that an intracranial pressure-sensitive "baro-receptor" transmits pressure stimuli into impulses in vasomotor nerves. Another that the rise in intra-cranial pressure causes a decrease in CBF followed by hypoxia and that the vasodilatation is due to the local action of hypoxic metabolites. The latter explanation would be in accordance with the increasing evidence that the autoregulation of the CBF is mainly governed by the cerebral metabolism (see also papers by Ingvar, Lassen, Siesjö and Zwetnow in this volume).

REFERENCES

BETZ, E. (1965) Local heat clearance from the brain as a measure of blood flow in acute and chronic experiments. In: *Regional Cerebral Blood Flow*. Ed. by D. H. Ingvar and N. A. Lassen. Copenhagen, Munksgaard. 29–37.

COOPER, RAY AND HULME, A. (1966) Intracranial pressure and related phenomena during sleep. *J. Neurol. Neurosurg. Psychiat.*, **29**, 564–570.

CRONQVIST, S., LUNDBERG, N. AND PONTÉN, U. (1963) Cerebral pneumography with continuous control of ventricular fluid pressure. *Acta Radiol.*, **1**, 558–564.

CRONQVIST, S., INGVAR, D. H., KJÄLLQUIST, Å., LUNDBERG, N. AND PONTÉN, U. (1967) Intrakranieller Druck, EEG und Hirndurchblutung bei einem Fall von Status epilepticus. *Acta Neurochirurg.*, **16**, 167–168.

FOG, M. (1933) Influence of intracranial hypertension upon the cerebral circulation. *Acta Psychiat. Neurol.*, **8**, 191–198.

GREENFIELD, J. C., JR. AND TINDALL, G. T. (1965) Effect of acute increase in intracranial pressure on blood flow in the internal carotid artery of man. *J. Clin. Invest.*, **44**, 1343–1351.

INGVAR, D. H. AND LUNDBERG, N. (1961) Paroxysmal symptoms in intracranial hypertension, studied with ventricular fluid pressure recording and electroencephalography. *Brain*, **84**, 446–459.

HAUG, K. (1932) Klinische und pharmakodynamische Untersuchungen des Liquordrucks vermittelst Dauerdruckmessungen bei Geisteskranken. *Arch. Psychiat. Nervenkrankh.*, **97**, 185–206.

HÄGGENDAL, E., LÖFGREN, L., NILSSON, N. J. AND ZWETNOW, N. (1967) Die Gehirndurchblutung bei experimentellen Liquordruckänderungen. *Acta Neurochirurg.*, **16**, 163.

KJÄLLQUIST, Å., LUNDBERG, N. AND PONTÉN, U. (1964) Respiratory and cardiovascular changes during rapid spontaneous variations of ventricular fluid pressure in patients with intracranial hypertension. *Acta Neurol. Scand.*, **40**, 291–317.

LANGFITT, T. W., WEINSTEIN, J. D. AND KASSELL, J. F. (1965a) Cerebral vasomotor paralysis produced by intracranial hypertension. *Neurology*, **15**, 622–641.

LANGFITT, T. W., KASSELL, N. F. AND WEINSTEIN, J. D. (1965b) Cerebral blood flow with intracranial hypertension. *Neurology*, **15**, 761–773.

LASSEN, N. A., HØEDT-RASMUSSEN, K., SØRENSEN, S. C., SKINHÖJ, E., CRONQVIST, S., BODFORSS, B. AND INGVAR, D. H. (1963) Regional cerebral blood flow in man determined by Krypton[85]. *Neurology*, **13**, 719–727.

LUNDBERG, N. (1960) Continuous recording and control of ventricular fluid pressure in neurosurgical practice. *Acta Psych. Neurol. Scand.*, **36**, suppl. 149.

LUNDBERG, N., KJÄLLQUIST, Å. AND BIEN, CH. (1959) Reduction of increased intracranial pressure by hyperventilation. *Acta Psych. Neurol. Scand.*, **34**, suppl. 139.

NOELL, W. AND SCHNEIDER, M. (1948) Zur Hämodynamik der Gehirndurchblutung bei Liquordruck-steigerung. *Arch. Psychiat.*, **180**, 713–730.

WOLFF, H. G. AND FORBES, H. S. (1929) The cerebral circulation. Observations of the pial circulation during changes in intracranial pressure. In: The Intracranial Pressure in Health and Disease. A. *Res. Nerv. Ment.*, **8**, 91–103.

WRIGHT, R. D. (1938) Experimental observations on increased intracranial pressure. *Austr. N.Z. J. Surg.*, **7**, 215.

WÜLLENWEBER, R. (1965) Schwankungen der Hirndurchblutung unter physiologischen und patho-physiologischen Bedingungen. *Acta Neurochir.*, **13**, 64–76.

Cerebral Blood Flow During Sleep in Patients with Raised Intracranial Pressure

A. HULME AND R. COOPER

Department of Neurological Surgery, Frenchay Hospital, Bristol, England

Several investigations have demonstrated reduction in total cerebral blood flow (CBF) when intracranial pressure (ICP) is raised above a critical level, lying between 350 and 550 mm. of water. Key, Shenkin and Schmidt (1948) using the nitrous oxide technique in thirteen patients found that flow was significantly diminsihed at pressures in excess of 450 mm of water. Greenfield and Tindall (1965) using an electro-magnetic flowmeter to estimate carotid artery blood flow in thirteen human subjects reported that flow was not significantly reduced until ICP reached a level approximately 1.8 times the control value. The mean results in the cases studied indicated a critical level of 380 mm of water. At a cerebrospinal fluid (CSF) pressure of 920 mm of H_2O, carotid blood flow averaged 25% less than the control value. No associated rise in systemic blood pressure was observed.

A technique for long term monitoring of ICP variations by means of a very small pressure transducer inserted in the skull, together with changes in cortical available oxygen, electrical impedance and blood flow, by means of thin gold electrodes and thermistors in the subdural space has been described in detail elsewhere (Cooper and Hulme, 1966; Hulme and Cooper, 1966). The electrical impedance (electroplethysmograph, EPG) of two electrodes in the subdural space is primarily determined by the thickness of the layer of CSF which is of low impedance compared with blood and other tissues (Porter *et al.*, 1964; Robinson and Tompkins, 1964). The impedance rises if brain volume increases as in generalised cerebral vasodilatation (Moskalenko *et al.*, 1964). Electroencephalogram (EEG), heart rate and respiration were also recorded simultaneously.

Protracted continuous monitoring of ICP in patients with intracranial hypertension due to a variety of causes has demonstrated large spontaneous increases of the order of 500–1000 mm of H_2O superimposed on the mean resting level. Peak pressure approaching or exceeding the diastolic blood pressure commonly occurs. Our records closely resemble those of Lundberg and his colleagues (Lundberg, 1960; Ingvar and Lundberg, 1961). These workers have identified several types of ventricular fluid pressure wave, the most significant being the large high pressure 'plateau' waves. Our polygraphic studies show that an episode of considerably increased cerebral hypoxia occurs during each of these waves and we postulate that these have a cumulative effect on neurons. They are believed to be initiated by swelling of the brain (shown by an increase in the electrical impedance) caused by vasodilatation in response to accumulation of CO_2 in the brain when ICP is high enough to cause some impairment of blood flow. In support of this hypothesis is the observation that the spontaneous fluctuations in available oxygen, which are believed to be caused by local variations in vascular tone also diminish in amplitude or disappear completely as the pressue wave builds up. They are known to cease if cortical pCO_2 is increased (Clark *et al.*, 1958; Cooper *et al.*, 1966). In these conditions the additional rise in ICP reduces the effective perfusion pressure and results, paradoxically, in a further fall rather than an increase in CBF. A typical record shows a marked fall in local blood flow and available oxygen during two successive pressure waves. (Fig. 1).

The increase in the amplitude of the transmitted arterial pulse wave during periods of higher pressure also provides evidence of relaxation of the arteriolar walls which allows an increasing fraction of the systemic blood pressure to be transmitted to the intracranial contents. In many instances a pressure wave is seen to terminate abruptly, suggesting the intervention of some compensatory mechanism (Fig. 2). An increase in heart rate and sometimes in depth or rate of respiration usually commences a few seconds before the pressure begins to fall. This may represent a reflex response mediated through the medullary centres which breaks the vicious circle by improving CBF and reducing CO_2. Greenfield and Tindall (1965) have shown that at high ICP levels the CBF is largely dependent on the pulsatile component accompanying each systole. Thus an increased heart rate would produce a rise in flow even if the systemic blood pressure remained unchanged. Further compensation might occur as a result of a rise in blood pressure, although in these studies we have found no close correlation between

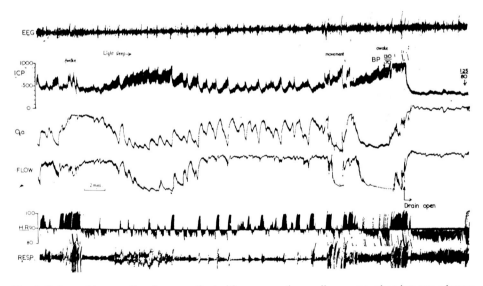

Fig. 1. Polygraphic recording from a patient with an acoustic neurilemmoma, showing two plateau waves with peak pressures rising to 1000 mm H_2O. During each of these there was a marked fall in local blood flow and available oxygen and increased depth of respiration. The second plateau wave was terminated by opening a ventricular drain. Sharp one per minute waves accompanied by fluctuations in heart rate, cortical oxygen and EEG occurred during the intervening period.

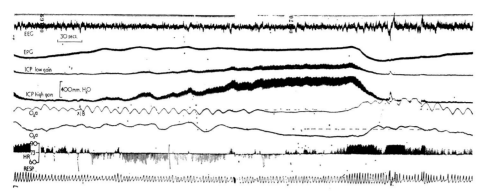

Fig. 2. Polygraphic recording of plateau wave from a patient with an infiltrating glioma. Intracranial pressure, shown in channels 3 and 4 at low and high gains respectively, rose gradually over a period of about five minutes to a peak level some 600 mm of water above the mean resting pressure of 400 mm, and fell abruptly in less than one minute to the previous level. The amplitude of the transmitted cardiac pulse wave increased fourfold as the pressure rose. The increase of pressure was preceded by an increase of impedance (channel 2), indicating an increase of brain volume. There was a fall in the level of available oxygen and the spontaneous low frequency oscillations disappeared (channels 5 and 6). An increase in heart rate and depth of respiration commenced about 30 seconds before the end of the pressure wave and continued for about two minutes (channels 7 and 8). As the pressure fell there was a marked increase in the level of available oxygen and the oscillations returned. There was a rapid fall of impedance. The EEG throughout this pressure wave showed low-amplitude fast activity.

this and the ICP. In patients whose mean resting pressure was in the moderately increased range, i.e. 400–500 mm of H_2O, pressure waves were found to have a marked association with certain stages of sleep as determined by the EEG. Thus they were rarely observed in these subjects during the waking state or during periods of deep sleep characterised by high amplitude low frequency activity (stage 4 sleep). They occurred most frequently on transition from a period of deep to 'paradoxical' sleep as shown by desynchronisation of the EEG and the appearance of rapid eye movements (Fig. 3). It is suggested that this increased incidence is a reflection of enhanced cerebral metabolic activity and therefore of CO_2 production during this phase.

Experimental work on animals indicates that cerebral metabolic rate during the paradoxical (rapid eye movement, REM) stage of sleep may exceed that of the normal alert state (Kanzow, 1965; Kawamura and Sawyer, 1965; Kety, 1965; Rechtschaffen et al., 1966).

Brebbia and Altshuler (1965) reported significant differences in oxygen consumption during different stages of sleep as defined by the EEG in human subjects. They found that oxygen consumption was highest during the REM (dreaming) stage, least in stages 3 and 4 (deep sleep) and intermediate in stage 2 (light sleep). Since cerebral circulation is seriously compromised during each high pressure wave, it is probable that the repeated episodes of relative ischaemia and hypoxia have a cumulative effect on the brain. The increased frequency of pressure waves during some stages of sleep offers a possible explanation for the familiar observation that clinical deterioration and accentuation of symptoms of raised intracranial pressure commonly occur during the night.

References p. 81

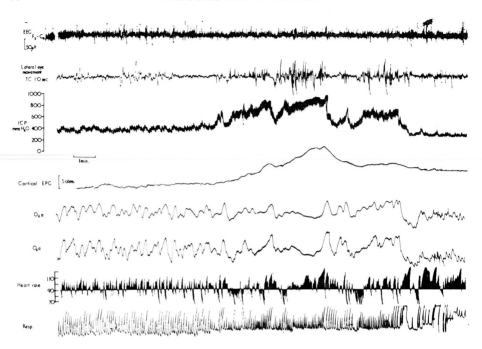

Fig. 3. Plateau wave accompanied by rapid eye movements and change in pattern of EEG. There was a rise of impedance (EPG) and the low frequency fluctuations of available oxygen (O₂a) disappeared at the height of the pressure wave. During the periods of high pressure there were sustained increases of heart rate and a doubling of the respiration rate. This patient had a tumour obstructing the third ventricle.

The importance of measures to lower the mean level of ICP, especially during the night, is obvious. Osmotically active agents such as hypertonic sucrose, urea or Mannitol appear to be of limited value since their effects last for only a few hours at the most and may be followed by a rebound rise of pressure. In contrast there is evidence that the administration of steroids, such as dexamethasone (16-α-methyl-9-α-fluoroprednisolone), leads to a continuing reduction of mean ICP and a marked diminution in the frequency and amplitude of pressure waves (Fig. 4).

These effects are usually accompanied by striking improvement in the patient's clinical condition (Galilich and French, 1961).

The precise mode of action of this agent is not clear; it seems probable however that it diminishes or prevents the cerebral oedema caused by damage to the blood brain barrier, resulting from recurrent hypoxic episodes. It may thus provide a more effecti-

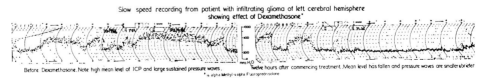

Fig. 4.

ve means of maintaining adequate cerebral circulation, pending more radical measures to deal with the primary pathological condition.

REFERENCES

BREBBIA, D. R. AND ALTSHULER, K. Z. (1965) Oxygen consumption rate and electroencephalographic stage of sleep. *Science*, **150**, 1621–1623.

CLARK, L. C., MISRAHY, G. A., AND FOX, R. P. (1958) Chronically implanted polarographic electrodes. *J. Appl. Physiol.*, **13**, 85–91.

COOPER, R. (1963) Local changes of intra-cerebral blood flow and oxygen in humans. *Med. Electron. Biol. Engin.*, **1**, 529–536.

COOPER, R. AND HULME, A. (1966) Intracranial pressure and related phenomena during sleep. *J. Neurol. Neurosurg. Psychiat.* **29**, 564–569.

GALILICH, J. H. AND FRENCH, L. A. (1961) *Amer. Prac. Dig. Treatm.*, **12**, 169–174.

HULME, A. AND COOPER, R. (1966) A technique for the investigation of intracranial pressure in man. *J. Neurol. Neurosurg. Psychiat.*, **29**, 154–156.

INGVAR, D. H. AND LUNDBERG, N. (1961) Paroxysmal symptoms in intracranial hypertension, studied with ventricular fluid pressure recording and electroencephalography. *Brain*, **84**, 446–459.

KANZOW, E. (1965) Changes in blood flow of the cerebral cortex and other vegetative changes during paradoxical sleep periods in the unrestrained cat. In: *Neurophysiologie des états de sommeil.* M. Jouvet (Ed.), pp. 231–240 (Colloques Internationaux du Centre National de la Recherche Scientifique, No. 127) Paris.

KAWAMURA, H., AND SAWYER, C. H. (1965) Elevation in brain temperature during paradoxical sleep. *Science*, **150**, 912–913.

KETY, S. S. (1965) *Relationship between energy metabolism of the brain and functional activity.* Paper read at Association for Research in Nervous and Mental Disease, December 1965.

LUNDBERG, N. (1960) Continuous recording and control of ventricular fluid pressure in neurosurgical practice. *Acta psychiat. scand.*, **36**, suppl. 149.

MOSKALENKO, YU. E., COOPER, R., CROW, H. J., AND WALTER, W. GREY, (1964) Variations in blood volume and oxygen availability in the human brain. *Nature*, **202**, 159–161.

PORTER, R., ADEY, W. R., AND KADO, R. T. (1964) Measurement of electrical impedance in the human brain. *Neurology*, **14**, 1002–1012.

RECHTSCHAFFEN, A., CORNWELL, P., AND ZIMMERMAN W. (1966) Brain Temperature variations with paradoxical sleep. *Proc. Lyon Symp. Sleep Consciousn.*, December 1965.

ROBINSON, B. W. AND TOMPKINS, H. E. (1964) Impedance method for localizing brain structures. *Arch. Neurol. (Chic.)*, **10**, 563–574.

The Effects of Halothane and Trichloroethylene on Cerebral Perfusion and Metabolism and on Intracranial Pressure

D. G. McDOWALL, W. B. JENNETT, AND J. BARKER

University Department of Anaesthesia, Western Infirmary, and Institute of Neurological Science, Glasgow

Halothane (Wollman *et al.*, 1964; McHenry *et al.*, 1965; McDowall, 1967) and trichloroethylene (McDowall, 1966) dilate the cerebral blood vessels and the degree of vascular dilatation is proportional to the concentration of the drug administered. Whether cerebral blood flow increases or not and, if so, by how much depends on the extent of the fall in blood pressure produced by the anaesthetic. For example, 0.5% halothane increases the blood flow through the cerebral cortex of the dog by 16% in the first 20 minutes but with more prolonged administration flow returns to near the control value. 2% halothane results in a 24% increase in cerebral cortical blood flow while 4% halothane reduces blood pressure so markedly that cerebral cortical flow is at or below control values (see Fig. 1).

These anaesthetic drugs also depress the aerobic metabolism of the brain and lead to a fall in cerebral oxygen consumption. This effect, at least in the case of halothane, is also proportional to the concentration of the drug administered; 0.5% halothane lowers the oxygen uptake of the cerebral cortex of the dog by 14% while 2% halothane causes a fall of 33% (see Fig. 1). These appreciable reductions in cerebral oxygen requirements may render partial protection to the brain during periods of surgical interruption of cerebral perfusion.

Since halothane increases flow while reducing oxygen uptake, the oxygen content of

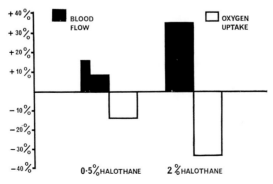

Fig. 1. The influence of 0.5% and 2% halothane on cerebral cortical blood flow and oxygen uptake (reproduced by kind permission of the Editor of the British Journal of Anaesthesia).

References p. 86

cerebral venous blood rises during anaesthesia with this agent. Some workers have attempted to assess the adequacy of cerebral perfusion from the level of jugular venous oxygen content (Wells *et al.*, 1963; Lyons *et al.*, 1964). This approach is certainly valid for the normal cerebral circulation but it is doubtful whether it can be extended to clinical situations in which localised regions of tissue ischaemia exist. Such ischaemic areas may not contribute enough blood to the jugular venous drainage for their plight to be reflected in jugular venous oxygen measurements. It must also be remembered that "luxury perfusion" of marginal areas around ischaemic foci will "falsely" elevate the level of jugular venous oxygen content. In a similar way, measurements of total cerebral blood flow may be totally misleading if used as indices of satisfactory regional perfusion within the brain. For example, the fact that halothane increases total cerebral blood flow should not be accepted as evidence that this drug is indicated for anaesthesia in patients with localised cerebral ischaemia; in fact, halothane-induced cerebral vasodilatation may merely divert blood away from the ischaemic area and towards more normal brain.

The administration of halothane or trichloroethylene at constant arterial carbon dioxide tension leads to increases in lumbar CSF pressure in patients with normal cerebrospinal fluid pathways (McDowall *et al.*, 1966). It is believed that this is a reflection of increased cerebral blood flow and intracranial blood volume and is not the result of any change in the rate of CSF production. The basis for this conclusion rests on the demonstration, in dogs, that cerebral venous pressure measured in the superior sagittal sinus rises pari passu with the changes in pCSF. The extent of the increases of pCSF produced by halothane and by trichloroethylene in patients with normal CSF pathways is relatively small and almost certainly clinical unimportant. The mean rise with 0.5% halothane was 68 (S.D. $\pm$ 31) mm H_2O and with 0.9%

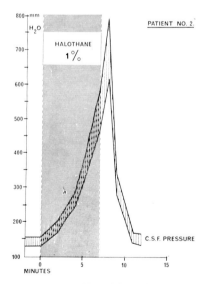

Fig. 2. Intracranial pressure changes produced by 1% halothane in a patient with a cerebral tumour (reproduced by kind permission of the Editor of the Journal of Neurosurgery).

trichloroethylene was 109 (S.D. $\pm$ 32) mm H$_2$O. The changes in pCSF with halothane were shown to be related to the existing arterial carbon dioxide tension. When this was low as a result of hyperventilation halothane had little influence on pCSF.

In some patients with intracranial tumours the situation is quite different in that both halothane and trichloroethylene lead to very large increases in intracranial pressure (Jennett *et al.*, 1967). The record of the intracranial pressure obtained in a patient with a frontal astrocytoma is shown in Fig. 2. It will be seen from this that the administration of 1 % halothane increased the intracranial pressure as measured by a cannula in the lateral ventricle from 155/130 mm H$_2$O to 800/620 mm H$_2$O; the pressure quickly returned to normal on withdrawing the halothane. The pressure changes produced by halothane in four patients with cerebral tumours recently studied are given in Table 1. It will be seen that in this group the pressure rise is 3 to 8 times greater than in the patients without intracranial lesions. It is believed that the sensitivity of patients with intracranial tumours to halothane-induced elevations of pCSF is due to the previous exhaustion by tumour growth of the mechanisms which normally compensate for fluctuations in intracranial blood volume. These mechanisms are believed to consist of volume redistribution between blood, brain and CSF.

It has not yet been established whether these intracranial pressure changes are great enough to be clinically disadvantageous. However, since on some occasions the intracranial pressure has risen to equal more than 80 % of the mean blood pressure, it would seem wise to assume meantime that patients with intracranial tumours should not be anaesthetised with halothane unless the arterial pCO$_2$ has first been lowered by hyperventilation. It may well be that in some patients with intracranial tumours halothane actually causes a secondary fall in cerebral blood flow consequent upon the induced intracranial hypertension. In this regard, the wellknown depression of systolic blood pressure by halothane is obviously also relevant.

In summary, halothane and trichloroethylene dilate the cerebral blood vessels and increase cerebral blood flow, provided that systemic blood pressure is not too greatly depressed. These drugs also cause considerable depression of cerebral oxygen uptake. As a result of this combination of flow increase and metabolic depression, cerebral venous oxygenation increases. As a result of the flow increase, cerebrospinal fluid pressure rises. This increase in pCSF may be so great in patients with intracranial

TABLE 1

THE EFFECT OF HALOTHANE ON INTRACRANIAL PRESSURE IN 4 PATIENTS WITH INTRACRANIAL TUMOURS

Patient	Control		Peak Halothane		Increase due to Halothane
	Syst./Diast.	*Mean*	*Syst./Diast.*	*Mean*	
1	180/160	167	520/460	480	313
2	155/130	138	800/620	680	542
3	168/108	128	537/281	366	238
4	382/232	282	690/455	533	251

References p. 86

tumours as to reduce cerebral perfusion. The value of hyperventilating patients with intracranial space occupying lesions prior to halothane or trichloroethylene administration is stressed.

REFERENCES

JENNETT, W. B., McDOWALL, D. G. AND BARKER, J. (1967) The effect of halothane on intracranial pressure in two patients with cerebral tumours. *J. Neurosurg.*, **26**, 270.

LYONS, C., CLARK, L. C., McDOWALL, H. AND McARTHUR, K. (1964) Cerebral venous oxygen content during carotid thrombintimectomy. *Ann. Surg.*, **160**, 561.

McDOWALL, D. G. (1966) Cerebral haemodynamics and metabolism during general anaesthesia. Contribution to Symposium on Tissue Perfusion at 2nd European Congress of Anaesthesiology. *Acta Anaesth. Scand.*, Supp. XXV, 307.

—, (1967) The effects of clinical concentrations of halothane on the blood flow and oxygen uptake of the cerebral cortex. *Brit. J. Anaesth.*, **39**, 186.

McDOWALL, D. G., BARKER, J. AND JENNETT, W. B., (1966) Cerebrospinal fluid pressure measurements during anaesthesia. *Anaesthesia*, **21**, 189.

McHENRY, L. C. JR., SLOCUM, H. C., BIVENS, H. E., MAYES, H. A. AND HAYES, G. J. (1965) Hyperventilation in awake and anesthetised man. *Arch. Neurol. (Chic.)*, **12**, 270.

WELLS, B. A., KEATS, A. S. AND COOLEY, D. A. (1963) Increased tolerance to cerebral ischemia produced by general anesthesia during temporary carotid occlusion. *Surgery*, **54**, 216.

WOLLMAN, H., ALEXANDER, S. C., COHEN, P. J., CHASE, P. E., MELMAN, E. AND BEHAR, M. G. (1964) Cerebral circulation of man during halothane anesthesia. *Anesthesiology*, **25**, 180.

Cerebral Blood Flow During Intracranial Hypertension Related to Tissue Hypoxia and to Acidosis in Cerebral Extracellular Fluids

N. ZWETNOW, Å. KJÄLLQUIST AND B. K. SIESJÖ

Neurosurgical Research Laboratory, University Hospital, Lund, and the Neurosurgical Clinic, University of Gothenburg, Sweden

When the cerebrospinal fluid pressure (*p*CSF) is progressively raised, causing a reduction of the cerebral perfusion pressure, the cerebral blood flow (CBF) is kept unchanged until the cerebral perfusion pressure (here considered to be the difference between the arterial pressure and the *p*CSF) is reduced to 40–50 mm Hg, i.e. the CBF shows autoregulation (Fig. 1) (Häggendal *et al.*, 1966). When the perfusion pressure is reduced below the figures given, and then subsequently released, a hyperemia ensues which is characterized by its long duration (1–3 h) (Fig. 2). The hyperemia has been studied with the diffusible isotope clearance method but it has also been fully verified by serial angiography (Aiba *et al.*, 1967). In addition, it has been shown that the hyperemia is accompanied by a damage to the blood-brain barrier (Petersén and Zwetnow, 1967).

Both the autoregulation of the flow during a progressive increase of the CSF pressure, and the prolonged hyperemia, may have important bearings on the basic problem concerning the regulation of CBF. Thus, we may ask if all these phenomena have a

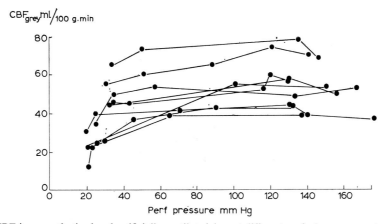

Fig. 1. CBF in anaesthetized and artificially ventilated dogs at different perfusion pressures induced by variations in CSF pressure. It can be seen that there was no significant variation of CBF in the individual dogs at perfusion pressures over 40–50 mm Hg, i.e. the CBF shows autoregulation.

common cause, or if different mechanisms are involved. In view of the present hypotheses regarding the regulation of CBF (Siesjö *et al.*, 1967) it seemed pertinent to investigate if the hyperemia could be connected with an extracellular acidosis, secondary to a tissue hypoxia. The present paper gives a preliminary account of experiments which show that the reactive hyperemia is accompanied by an extracellular acidosis, and by signs of a tissue hypoxia. However, the experiments also indicate that the autoregulation of the blood flow during moderate increases in the CSF pressure is concomitant with an extracellular lactacidosis.

METHODS

The experiments were performed on dogs, anesthetized with pentobarbital, immobilized with Celocurin and mechanically ventilated. The CBF was measured with a radioactive isotope clearance technique, using ^{133}Xe (Lassen *et al.*, 1963). The CSF pressure was increased by means of an infusion of an artificial CSF into the cisterna magna (Häggendal *et al.*, 1966). The CSF and the mean arterial pressures were continuously recorded. Arterial blood, blood from the superior sagittal sinus, and CSF were sampled and analysed for pO_2, pCO_2 and pH.

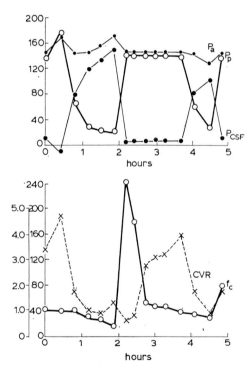

Fig. 2. CBF and cerebrovascular resistance (CVR) in anesthetized and artificially ventilated dogs during experimentally induced variations in cerebrospinal fluid pressure (P_{csf}). The upper part of the figure shows in addition to P_{csf} the mean arterial pressure (P_a) and the resulting perfusion pressure (P_p). In the lower part of the figure CBF in ml/100 g/min and CVR in mm Hg/ml/100 g/min are given. Note that after a reduction of the perfusion pressure to 10–20 mm Hg there was a marked and longlasting increase in CBF ("reactive hyperemia").

Lactate and pyruvate in blood and in CSF were measured enzymatically (see Granholm and Siesjö, 1967). Since the infused artificial CSF did not contain any lactate or pyruvate, but a bicarbonate concentration which sometimes differed from that of the CSF, a correction had to be applied to the samples withdrawn after an increase in the CSF pressure. This correction was obtained by adding a known concentration of inulin to the artificial CSF, and by determining the inulin concentration in the CSF samples withdrawn. The lactate/pyruvate ratio of the CSF samples were used as an index of the presence of a tissue hypoxia (Huckabee, 1958; Hohorst, 1960).

RESULTS

In all the experiments in which the CSF pressure was increased sufficiently to elicit a hyperemia, there was a decrease in the CSF pH, and an increased lactate/pyruvate ratio. Fig. 3 shows an experiment, in which the perfusion pressure was decreased from 140 mm Hg to 40 mm Hg during a period of about 15 min. Before the perfusion pressure was reduced control CSF samples showed a pH of 7.36 and two lactate/pyruvate ratios of 9.0 and 9.5 respectively. In CSF samples withdrawn directly after the pressure was released pH was lowered to 7.31 and the lactate/pyruvate ratio had increased to values around 18–19. Simultaneously with the decrease in the CBF after the hyperemia there was a progressive increase in the CSF pH, and a lowering of the lactate/pyruvate ratio. The experiment thus clearly shows that the reduced perfusion pressure, which

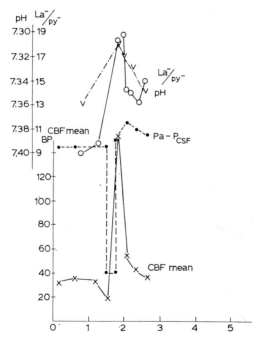

Fig. 3. Relationships between pH and lactate/pyruvate ratio (La$^-$/py$^-$) in the CSF, and the cerebral blood flow (CBF mean) in an anesthetized dog after a temporary increase in the CSF pressure which lowered the cerebral perfusion pressure (P_a–P_{csf}) from 140 to 40 mm Hg. Note the decrease in the CSF pH, and the increased lactate/pyruvate ratio, which accompanied the reactive hyperemia.

References p. 91–92

gave rise to the reactive hyperemia, also caused a marked acidosis and a marked increase in the lactate/pyruvate ratio in the CSF.

The next figure (Fig. 4) illustrates an experiment in which the cerebral perfusion pressure was lowered in steps from about 110 to about 40 mm Hg. When the perfusion pressure was decreased to 80 and 50 mm Hg, respectively, no hyperemia ensued. In spite of this, however, there were signs of an increased lactate concentration, and possibly an increased lactate/pyruvate ratio, in the samples withdrawn after the pressure was released. When, finally, the perfusion pressure was reduced to 40 mm Hg, giving a pronounced decrease in CBF, a large hyperemia followed, paralleled by a progressive CSF acidosis, and by very marked increases in the lactate/pyruvate ratio and in the lactate concentration. In this experiment the normalization of CBF was not paralleled by a corresponding normalization of the CSF pH, the CSF lactate concentration, or the CSF lactate/pyruvate ratio. This experiment thus shows that when the decrease in the perfusion pressure is of sufficient duration and magnitude, there is a progressive extracellular acidosis and a continuously elevated lactate/pyruvate ratio at a time when the flow has returned to normal. It is quite apparent that at this point, there is no longer any relation between the extracellular acidosis and the cerebral blood flow i.e.

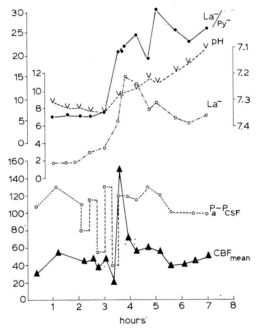

Fig. 4. Changes in CBF and in the pH, the lactate concentration, and the lactate/pyruvate ratio of CSF in an anesthetized dog, in which the cerebral perfusion pressure was reduced to 80, 55 and 40 mm Hg, respectively, by means of appropriate increases of the CSF pressure. During the first two reductions of the perfusion pressure (P_a–P_{csf}) there were no significant changes in CBF or in the pH or the lactate/pyruvate ratio (la$^-$/py$^-$) of the CSF but a significant increase in the lactate concentration. After the perfusion pressure had been reduced to 40 mm Hg for 15 min a marked reactive hyperemia ensued, lasting more than an hour. The hyperemia was accompanied by a fall in CSF pH, and a rise in the lactate/pyruvate ratio of the CSF. However, in this experiment the CSF changes persisted in spite of the normalization of CBF.

an uncoupling has taken place, which may be due to a cerebral edema.

An increased lactate concentration, an increased lactate/pyruvate ratio, and a decreased pH were sometimes observed in the CSF even after minor reductions in cerebral perfusion pressure, too small to cause any significant lowering of the CBF, or any reactive hyperemia. This strongly suggests that a glucolytic formation of lactic acid may be an important factor behind the cerebral blood flow autoregulation even within its "physiological" ranges.

CONCLUSIONS

The present experiments have unequivocally shown that a reduction of the cerebral perfusion pressure, which gives rise to a reactive hyperemia, is also accompanied by a reduced CSF pH and by an increased concentration of lactate, as well as by an increased lactate/pyruvate ratio in the CSF. In another paper (Siesjö, Kjällquist, Pontén and Zwetnow, this volume p. 93) we have shown that the CBF varies directly with the CSF H^+ at constant CO_2 tension. In view of the results obtained in the two papers the following conclusions can tentatively be put forward:

1. When the cerebral perfusion pressure is decreased due to an increased intracranial pressure the CBF is maintained within a considerable pressure range. This autoregulation might be due to a temporary extracellular lactacidosis, i.e. the CBF is regulated by means of metabolically released H^+.

2. When the cerebral perfusion is reduced to 50–60 mm Hg there are signs of a marked tissue hypoxia, and a pronounced extracellular acidosis. This acidosis probably causes the prolonged hyperemia, following the normalization of the perfusion pressure.

3. Sometimes, after a pronounced and longlasting decrease in cerebral perfusion pressue, the CBF returns to normal after a reactive hyperemia in spite of a progressive lactacidosis. The uncoupling between CBF and extracellular H^+ in such instances might be due to cerebral edema.

REFERENCES

AIBA, T., LANNER, L., STATTIN, S., WICKBOM, I. AND ZWETNOW, N. (1967) Effects of increased intracranial pressure on cerebral circulation, studied with serial angiography and isotope elimination technique. To be published.

GRANHOLM, L. AND SIESJÖ, B. K. (1967) Lactate and pyruvate concentrations in blood, cerebrospinal fluid and brain tissue of the cat. *Acta Physiol. Scand.*, **70**, 255–256.

HOHORST, H. J. (1960) *Der Reduktionszustand des Disphosphopyridin-Nukleotidsystems in lebendem Gewebe.* Inauguraldissertation, Marburg.

HUCKABEE, W. E. (1958) Relationship of pyruvate and lactate during anaerobic metabolism. I. Effects of infusion of pyruvate or glucose and of hyperventilation. *J. Clin. Invest.*, **37**, 244–254.

HÄGGENDAL, E., LÖFGREN, J., NILSSON, N. J. AND ZWETNOW, N. (1966) Die Gehirndurchblutung bei experimentellen Liquordruckänderungen, *Verhandl. Intern. Neurochirurgen-Kongress, Bad Dürkheim.*

LASSEN, N. A., HØEDT-RASMUSSEN, K., SØRENSEN, S. C., SKINHØJ, E., CRONQVIST, S., BODFORSS, B. AND INGVAR, D. H. (1963) Regional blood flow in man determined by krypton[85]. *Neurology*, **13**, 719–727.

PETERSÉN, I. AND ZWETNOW, N. (1967) Blood-brain barrier damage and prolonged cerebral hyperemia following changes in cerebral perfusion pressure; an experimental EEG study. *Experientia*, in press.

SIESJÖ, B. K., KJÄLLQUIST, Å., PONTÉN, U. AND ZWETNOW, N. (1967) Extracellular pH in the brain and cerebral blood flow. This volume, p. 93.

Extracellular pH in the Brain and Cerebral Blood Flow

B. K. SIESJÖ, Å. KJÄLLQUIST, U. PONTÉN AND N. ZWETNOW

Neurosurgical Research Laboratory, the Hospital of Lund, the Department of Neurosurgery, University of Lund and the Department of Neurosurgery, University of Gothenburg, Sweden

Situations which are associated with an increased cerebral blood flow (CBF) (for references, see Sokoloff, 1959) also lead to the accumulation or the formation of acids, or of potential acids like carbon dioxide. Thus, CO_2 is accumulated in *hypercapnia*, and lactic acid in *hypoxia*. During increased functional activity as in arousal CO_2 accumulates, while in *epileptic seizures* both CO_2 and lactic acid apparently contribute to the increased CBF. However, although all these observations may suggest that the extracellular pH governs tissue perfusion, direct proof thereof has been lacking. The present paper consists of two parts. In the first part, the regulation of extracellular pH in respiratory and nonrespiratory acid-base changes will be reviewed and related to known data on cerebral blood flow (regarding the regulation of cerebral blood flow in hypoxia, see Zwetnow *et al.*, this symposium, p. 87). In the second part, preliminary experiments will be reported which for the first time directly establishes the dependence of CBF upon extracellular pH.

CHANGES IN EXTRACELLULAR pH RELATED TO CEREBRAL BLOOD FLOW

During the first minutes of an *acute hypercapnia* the increased CO_2 tension will be associated with increased concentrations of CO_2, H_2CO_3 and H^+, but not of HCO_3^- since the CSF lacks efficient buffers against CO_2. Due to the low buffer capacity a given increase in pCO_2 will give a relatively large decrease in pH. In sustained hypercapnia (Fig. 1), however, pH is slowly regulated towards intermediate values due to a slow increase in the bicarbonate concentration (Swanson and Rosengren, 1962; Bleich *et al.*, 1964; Pontén and Siesjö, 1965). This increase is probably due to the increased plasma/CSF HCO_3^- gradient, to the increased CSF/plasma potential (see Held, *et al.*, 1964), and to a small extent to a decreased lactate production in the tissue, but it is questionable if active transport of H^+ is involved (Kjällquist and Siesjö, in press).

The fact that CBF increases in hypercapnia is no proof that extracellular H^+ regulates the flow since hypercapnia leads to an increase also in the dissolved CO_2, which could have an independent action, or an effect on the metabolism or the excitability of the cells (see Krnjević *et al.*, 1965) which triggers the perfusion changes. However, in view of the regulation of CSF pH it would be interesting to know the rela-

References p. 97–98

tion between the CO_2 tension and CBF in sustained hypercapnia when the CO_2 tension and the concentration of dissolved CO_2 are upheld but when the CSF pH is definitely higher than in the acute phase.

Hypocapnia during hyperventilation leads to CSF changes which are opposite to those in hypercapnia, and to a reduction of CBF, but it has been reported that both the CSF pH and the flow are quicky normalized (Severinghaus, 1965). The normalization of CBF when the CSF pH is regulated towards normal values strengthens the assumption that the tissue blood flow is related to extracellular H^+, and not to any other factor which accompanies the altered CO_2 tension.

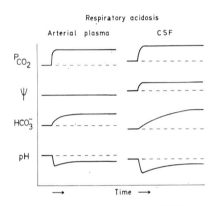

Fig. 1. Schematic diagram denoting acid-base changes in arterial blood and CSF in respiratory acidosis.

Arterial plasma: When the CO_2 tension is increased the plasma bicarbonate is immediately increased due to the buffer action of the blood proteins. However, due to renal retention of bicarbonate, and possibly to tissue buffering there is a further slow increase in the plasma bicarbonate. As a result of the increase in the plasma bicarbonate the initial acid shift in plasma pH will be gradually and partly compensated.

CSF: The CSF pCO_2 is normally 6–7 mm Hg higher than the arterial pCO_2. When the plasma pCO_2 increases there is a corresponding but slightly smaller increase in the CSF CO_2 tension (PONTÉN and SIESJÖ 1966). Due to the lower buffer capacity of the CSF the increase in the CO_2 tension will initially give a larger pH shift in CSF than in arterial plasma. The slow increase in the CSF bicarbonate will, however, slowly bring the CSF pH to an intermediate value. The increase in the CSF bicarbonate is probably entirely due to the passive influx of HCO_3^- along an electrochemical gradient. Accordingly the electrical potential difference between CSF and plasma (Ψ) is also seen to increase, and to remain increased during the hypercapnia (KJÄLLQUIST and SIESJÖ, in press). The straight potential line in the plasma diagram indicates that plasma is regarded as the zero reference point for the potential difference. The principal plasma and CSF changes during hypocapnia are the reverse ones to those seen during hypercapnia but there are indications that the pH is even better regulated (SEVERINGHAUS, 1965), possibly due to an increased glycolytic formation of lactic acid.

We may now ask why *nonrespiratory acidosis and alkalosis* do not cause any significant changes in CBF, as reported by Harper and Bell (1963). This is, however, easily explained if we keep the assumption of an inverse relation between CBF and extracellular pH (Fig. 2). Thus, even in chronic nonrespiratory acid-base changes there are very small changes in CSF pH (Mitchell *et al.*, 1965; Posner *et al.*, 1965; Fencl *et al.*, 1966; Pontén and Siesjö, in press). The stability of CSF pH is due to the fact that less than 50% of the plasma bicarbonate change is reflected in the CSF, and that the CO_2 tension changes in a direction that opposes the primary H^+ change (Fencl *et al.*, 1966). The restricted bicarbonate changes in the CSF have been assumed to be the result of an active transport of H^+ or HCO_3^- between CSF and plasma, but our results indicate that the potential changes are mainly responsible for keeping the CSF bicarbonate close to the normal values (Kjällquist and Siesjö, in press). At any rate, if we believe that extracellular pH and CBF are related we would not expect to find CBF significantly changed in nonrespiratory acid–base disturbances.

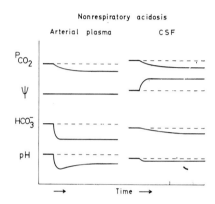

Fig. 2. Schematic diagram denoting acid-base changes in arterial blood and CSF in nonrespiratory acidosis.

Arterial plasma: When the plasma bicarbonate is decreased there is a corresponding fall in plasma pH. However, since lung ventilation will increase, the pCO_2 falls and partly compensates the pH fall due to the decrease in the bicarbonate.

CSF: The primary CSF event is probable an influx of H^+ into the extracellular fluids of the brain which triggers the increase in ventilation. Due to the slow penetration of H^+ to the large cavities the decrease in pCO_2 caused by the increased ventilation may temporarily give a paradoxical alkaline shift in the CSF pH (FENCL *et al.*, 1966) while the pH in true extracellular space changes slightly in acid direction as indicated in the Figure. In the chronic state there will be small but significant changes also in the CSF pH in the same direction as in blood (FENCL *et al.*, 1966, PONTÉN and SIESJÖ, in press). The restricted pH changes are due to the pCO_2 changes and to the fact that only apart of the plasma bicarbonate changes are reflected in the CSF. The relative stability of the CSF pH is probably not due to an active H^+ transport but to the creation of an electrical potential gradient which opposes influx of H^+ into the CSF (KJÄLLQUIST and SIESJÖ, in press). This gradient is due to an increase in the CSF/plasma potential which is upheld in chronic acid–base changes (GOODRICH, 1965; KJÄLLQUIST and SIESJÖ, in press).

The plasma and CSF acid–base changes in nonrespiratory alkalosis are the opposite to those in acidosis but the stability of the CSF pH is possibly even more marked than in acidosis (FENCL *et al.*, 1966; PONTÉN and SIESJÖ, in press).

CHANGES IN CBF AFTER EXPERIMENTALLY INDUCED VARIATIONS OF THE CSF HCO_3^- CONCENTRATION

The facts related above indicate that there is a parallelism between extracellular H^+ and CBF. This parallelism which has also been verified in measurements on the exposed cat cortex (Betz, this symposium, p. 99) has prompted Skinhöj (1966) to revive and extend the hypothesis of extracellular pH as the prime factor governing the cerebral circulation (see also Severinghaus, 1965; Pontén and Siesjö, 1965). Evidence of this hypothesis has, however, been lacking due to the experimental difficulties of varying the extracellular H^+ at constant CO_2 tension. Thus, due to the slow diffusion of ions between the CSF and the true intercellular phase (Rall *et al.*, 1962; Pappenheimer *et al.*, 1965), and to the dependence of the CBF on the experimental procedures, special techniques must be used which permit a long-lasting change in the CSF H^+ concentration, and minimal damage to the tissue.

In an attempt to prove unequivocally that CBF varies directly with the extracellular H^+ concentration we are presently using ventriculocisternal perfusion in anaesthetized and immobilized dogs, varying only the HCO_3^- and Cl^- concentrations of the artificial CSF. This technique, which has been used to describe quantitatively the relation between extracellular pH in the brain and lung ventilation, allows CSF pH to be varied independently of the CO_2 tension (Pappenheimer *et al.*, 1965; see also Davson, 1967). The CSF has been measured by means of the inert gas clearance method, using gamma-emitting ^{133}Xe (Lassen *et al.*, 1963; Häggendal *et al.*, 1966).

Figs. 3 and 4 show the results obtained in two of the dog experiments. In the first experiment (Fig. 3) which was conducted under pentobarbital anaesthesia the flow increased significantly when the normal artificial CSF (HCO_3^- = 25 mequiv./l was exchanged for an acid solution (HCO_3^- = 10 mequiv./l), but there was no decrease in flow when perfusing with an alkaline solution (HCO_3^- = 40 mequiv./l). In the next experiment (Fig. 4), in which the animal was under deep phenobarbital anaesthesia, the flow followed the H^+ concentration both in CSF acidosis and alkalosis. We are presently studying the extent to which different experimental conditions, including various forms of anaesthesia, influence the results. However, the experiments have so far unequivocally shown that CBF varies directly with the extracellular H^+ at constant CO_2 tension. These findings, which will be reported in full elsewhere, have corroborated the unique importance of CSF for the homoeostasis of the brain and ought to stimulate to an even more intense study of the CSF composition in neurology and neurosurgery.

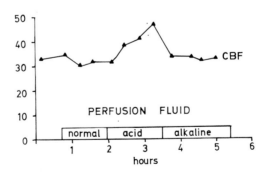

Fig. 3. The relation between CSF pH and CBF (ml/100 g/min) during ventriculocisternal perfusion in an artificially ventilated dog under pentobarbital anaesthesia. The artificial CSF perfused (see PAPPEN-HEIMER *et al.*, 1965) contained 25 ("normal"), 10 ("acid") or 40 ("alkaline") mequiv. HCO_3^-/l, and the chloride concentrations were varied reciprocally to give a constant osmolarity. Note increase in CBF when the acid fluid was perfused.

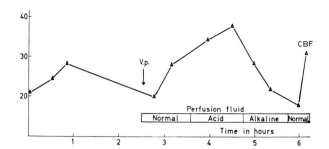

Fig. 4. The relation between CSF pH and CBF during ventriculocisternal perfusion in an artificially ventilated dog under deep phenobarbital anaesthesia (see Fig. 3). The lactate/pyruvate ratio and the lactate concentration in the CSF which were measured in order to check the redox state of the tissue did not show any noticeable changes during the perfusion except for a transient increase in the lactate/pyruvate ratio after the puncture of the side ventricle (v.p.). The experiment clearly indicated that the CBF varied directly with the CSF H^+ activity.

REFERENCES

BLEICH, H. L., BERKAMN, P. M. AND SCHWARTZ, W. B. (1964) The response of cerebrospinal fluid composition to sustained hypercapnia. *J. Clin. Invest.*, **43**, 11–16.

DAVSON, H. (1967) *Physiology of the cerebrospinal fluid.* Churchill, London.

FENCL, V., MILLER, T. B. AND PAPPENHEIMER, J. R. (1966) Studies on the respiratory response to disturbances of acid-base balance, with deductions concerning the ionic composition of cerebral interstitial fluid. *Amer. J. Physiol.*, **210**, 459–472.

GOODRICH, C. (1965) Effect of chronic acidosis and alkalosis on rat CSF-blood potential. Physiologist, **8**, 178.

HARPER, A. M. AND BELL, R. A. (1963) The effect of metabolic acidosis and alkalosis on the blood flow through the cerebral cortex. *J. Neurol., Neurosurg. Psychiat.*, **26**, 341–344.

HELD, D., FENCL, V. AND PAPPENHEIMER, J. R. (1964) Electrical potential of cerebrospinal fluid. *J. Neurophysiol.*, **27**, 942–959.

HÄGGENDAL, E., LÖFGREN, J., NILSSON, N. J. AND ZWETNOW, N. (1966) Prolonged cerebral hyperemia after periods of increased cerebrospinal fluid pressure in dogs. *Intern. Neurochir. Kongr. Bad Dürkheim.*

KRNJEVIČ, K., RANDIČ, M. AND SIESJÖ, B. K. (1965) Cortical CO_2 tension and neuronal excitability. *J. Physiol.*, **176**, 105–122.

LASSEN, N. A., HØEDT-RASMUSSEN, K., SØRENSEN, S. C., SKINHØJ, E., CRONQVIST, S., BODFORSS, B. AND INGVAR, D. H. (1963) Regional cerebral blood flow in man determined by krypton[85]. *Neurology*, **13**, 719–727.

MITCHELL, R. A., CARMAN, C. T., SEVERINGHAUS, J. W., RICHARDSON, B. W., SINGER, M. M. AND SHNIDER, S. (1965) Stability of cerebrospinal fluid pH in chronic acid-base disturbances in blood. *J. appl. Physiol.*, **20**, 443–452.

PAPPENHEIMER, J. R., FENCL, V., HEISEY, S. R. AND HELD, D. (1965) Role of cerebral fluids in control of respiration as studied in unanaesthetized goats. *Amer. J. Physiol.*, **208**, 436–450.

PONTÉN, U. AND SIESJÖ, B. K. (1965) Brain tissue carbon dioxide changes and cerebral blood flow measurements. In: *Regional Cerebral Blood Flow*, D. H. Ingvar and N. A. Lassen (Eds.). *Acta Neurol. Scand.*, suppl. **14**, 129–134.

—, (1966) Gradients of CO_2 tension in the brain. *Acta Physiol. Scand.*, **67**, 129–140.

—, (1967) Acid-base relation in arterial blood and cerebrospinal fluid of the unanaesthetized rat. *Acta Physiol. Scand.*, in press.

POSNER, J. B., SWANSON, A. G. AND PLUM, F. (1965) Acid-base balance in cerebrospinal fluid. *Arch. Neurol.*, **12**, 479–496.

RALL, D. P., OPPELT, W. W. AND PATLAK, C. S. (1962) Extracellular space of brain as determined by diffusion of inulin from the ventricular system. *Life Sci.*, **2**, 43–48.

SEVERINGHAUS, J. W. (1965) Role of cerebrospinal fluid pH in normalization of cerebral blood flow in chronic hypocapnia. In: "Regional Cerebral Blood Flow." Ed. by D. H. Ingvar and N. A. Lassen. *Acta Neurol. Scand.*, suppl. **14**, 116–120.

SIESJÖ, B. K. AND PONTÉN, U. (1966) Factors affecting the cerebrospinal fluid (CSF) bicarbonate concentration. *Experientia*, **22**, 611–614.

SKINHØJ, E. (1966) Regulation of cerebral blood flow as a single function of the interstitial pH in the brain. *Acta Neurol. Scand.*, **42**, 604–607.

SOKOLOFF, L. (1959) The action of drugs on cerebral circulation. *Pharmacol. Rev.*, **11**, 1–85.

SWANSON, A. G. AND ROSENGREN, H. (1962) Cerebrospinal fluid buffering during acute experimental respiratory acidosis. *J. appl. Physiol.*, **17**, 812–814.

The Significance of Cortical Extracellular pH for the Regulation of Blood Flow in the Cerebral Cortex

E. BETZ

Physiologisches Institut Marburg/Lahn (Germany)

Since changes in vascular resistance within circumscribed regions of the brain cannot always be equated with changes of vascular resistance in the whole brain, we measured the effects of variations in the acid-base balance in a small circumscribed region on the suprasylvian gyrus. Local changes of the acid-base equilibrium do not affect the surrounding vessels in the same way as they do the region in which the local acid-base

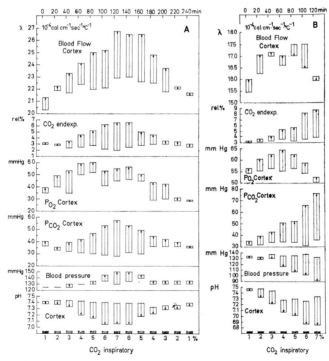

Fig. 1a. Cat, anesthetized with Nembutal (25 mg/kg). Local cerebral blood flow and P_{O_2} of the right suprasylvian gyrus. P_{CO_2} and pH of the left suprasylvian gyrus. Systemic blood pressure measured in the aorta and endexpiratory CO_2 concentration during respiration of air with CO_2, which was applied in periods of 10 min duration in various concentrations. Between the single CO_2 applications there were intervals of 10 min. — 1b. The same measurement values as in Fig. 1a. In higher CO_2 concentrations the blood pressure was decreased.

References p. 102

changes have taken place. Changes in total brain blood flow in most instances influence the local blood flow in a measurable way, whereas the reverse is not certain.

The increase of local cerebral blood flow during inhalation of CO_2 is caused by a dilatation of cerebral vessels and in many cases by an additional increase in systemic blood pressure. As a consequence of these effects, disturbances in the blood-pressure reactions have an influence on cerebral blood flow in atmospheres with high CO_2-concentrations.

In Fig. 1 the effect of CO_2-inhalation is shown. CO_2 was applied for periods of 10 min, and the CO_2-concentrations were gradually changed with intervals of 10 min between periods. Flow was recorded with heat clearance devices, endexpiratory CO_2-content with an infrared absorber, the cortical CO_2 pressure with a Teflon-covered pH-electrode[1], cortical oxygen pressure with a 10-wire platinum electrode[3], cortical pH with a flat glass-electrode. In Fig. 1a cortical blood flow increases with increasing CO_2-concentration, whereas in Fig. 1b blood flow is decreased during application of high CO_2-concentration, depending on the fall of systemic blood pressure recorded in the aorta. This example was chosen in order to demonstrate that it is better to use the local vascular resistance, instead of local blood flow, as a measure for the direct effects of changes in acid-base balance on local cerebral circulation.

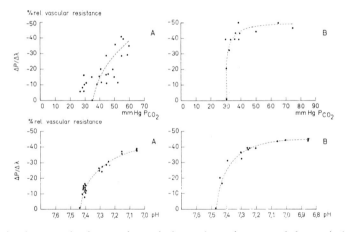

Fig. 2a. Relation between the decrease in cortical vascular resistance and the cortical P_{CO2} (upper graph), and between the decrease in cortical vascular resistance and the cortical extracellular pH (lower graph). The two graphs are based on the values obtained from Fig. 1a. — 2b. The same relations, but obtained from Fig. 1b. The percentage of change of the rel. resistance is calculated from the relation between flow change (measured in terms of heat clearance ($\Delta \lambda$)) and changes in arterial blood pressure (Δp). The value 0% rel. resistance is the initial value. The changes in resistance are compared with this initial value. Jugular venous pressure changed only very slightly in the experiments.

In Fig. 2 the changes in local vascular resistance are plotted against the cortical P_{CO_2} in the two experiments shown in Fig. 1a and 1b. Here it is seen that the vascular resistance is diminished during the increase of CO_2, but the measured values scatter considerably. In the same experiments the cerebral cortical vascular resistance was plotted against the extracellular cortical pH (Fig. 2b). The two graphs indicate that cerebral vascular resistance corresponds better to the extracellular pH changes than to the cortical P_{CO_2}.

The relations between pH and resistance demonstrate that a certain degree of acidosis is reached on the brain surface, the vessels have their maximal diameter and cannot dilate further. Blood flow, however, may increase during this phase. This depends then on the effective local blood pressure.

With the same combination of measuring devices we studied the effects of bicarbonate-infusions, HCl-infusions, hyperventilation and hypoxia. Table I summarizes the results.

As one can see, the cortical vascular resistance in these experiments always changes in the same direction as the extracellular cortical pH. Cortical blood flow reacts opposite to the cortical pH-changes, but only if the blood pressure remains constant. Cortical vascular resistance did not correspond in all experiments to the changes in cortical P_{CO2}, arterial pH, endexpiratory CO_2, or cortical P_{O2}. In edema of the whole cerebral cortex the cortical resistance is changed by the increased water content of the tissue. Increases of CO_2 concentrations in the air cause only very small changes of flow, but the normal relation between resistance and cortical pH is disturbed.

Fig. 3 shows the effects of CO_2 inhalation on the cortical blood flow with increasing cerebral edema, and Fig. 4 the correlation between cortical vascular resistance and cortical pH in this experiment. The acidosis caused a small and transient increase of

TABLE I

Reaction of cerebral cortical vascular resistance, extracellular cortical pH, arterial blood pH, cortical blood flow (blood pressure constant), cortical P_{CO2}, cortical P_{O2} and endexpiratory CO_2-content during various changes of the acid-base equilibrium. The arrows indicate the directions of deviation 6 min after the onset of the changes caused by inhalation of CO_2 or intravenous injection of 1/3 mol HCl or 3 min breathing 2% O_2 and 98% N_2 or hyperventilation or intravenous injection of 100 mg NaHCO₃ in anaesthetized cats (25 mg/kg Pentobarbital).

	Cerebral vascular resistance	Extra-cellular pH (cortex)	pH Arterial blood	Blood flow (cortex)	P_{CO_2} (cortex)	P_{O_2} (cortex)	CO_2-content (endexpiratory)
Acute respiratory acidosis (inhalation of CO_2)	↓	↓	↓	↑	↑	↑	↑
Acute metabolic acidosis of the blood (injection of HCl)	↑	↑	↓	↓	↓	↓ or =	↓
Cerebral acidosis after hypoxia	↓	↓	↑	↑	↓	↑	↓
Acute respiratory alcalosis (hyperventilation)	↑	↑	↑	↓	↓	↓	↓
Acute alcalosis of the blood (injection of NaHCO₃)	↓	↓	↑	↑	↑	↑ or =	↑

References p. 102

flow. Between the applications of CO_2 flow decreased beyond its initial value. Hyperventilation caused a further decrease in blood flow, in cortical P_{O2}, and in cortical CO_2. The cortical pH increased during the first stages of hyperventilations, but decreased after some time.

The effects of hyperventilation may be different if the edema affects only a small and circumscribed area of the cortex, because of the above-mentioned significance of the reactions of collateral vessels.

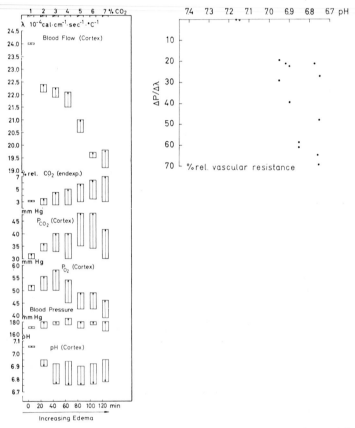

Fig. 3. Cat, anaesthetized with Nembutal (25 mg/kg). The cat has a visible edema of the cortex. The experiment was conducted in the same way as in Fig. 1.

Fig. 4. Correlation between the extracellular cortical pH and cortical vascular resistance in the animal (Fig. 3) with cerebral edema.

REFERENCES

ARNDT, H., BRINK, H., LÜBBERS, D. W. UND MAAS, A. H. J. (1966) Untersuchungen zur Stabilität, Empfindlichkeit und Linearität der P_{CO2}-Elektrode. *Pflügers Arch. ges. Physiol.*, **288**, 282–296.

LOESCHKE, H. H. UND BERNDT, E. (1967) *Die Säure-Baseregulation des Liquors.* in: Hämodynamik, Säure-Basen- und Elektrolyt-Haushalt im Liquor- und Nervensystem. Symposium. Frankfurt/M. (in press).

SCHMAHL, F. W., BETZ, E., DETTINGER, E. UND HOHORST, H. J. (1966) Energiestoffwechsel der Großhirnrinde und Elektroencephalogramm bei Sauerstoffmangel. *Pflügers Arch. ges. Physiol.*, **292**, 46–59.

The Mechanism of Action of Carbon Dioxide in the Regulation of Cerebral Blood Flow

M. N. SHALIT*, S. SHIMOJYO, O. M. REINMUTH,
W. S. LOCKHART, Jr.**, AND P. SCHEINBERG

Department of Neurology, University of Miami School of Medicine, Miami, Florida (U.S.A.)

The response of cerebral circulation to changes in arterial CO_2 tension is well known and has been confirmed in numerous experiments and clinical observations. Nonetheless, the mechanism of action of this gas is not completely understood although certain theories are presently generally accepted.

The dilatation of the cerebral vessels following an increase of arterial CO_2 tension has been said to be the result of the direct action of the gas on the smooth muscle of the cerebral arterial wall. Reviewing previous pertinent work it was somewhat surprising to discover that no direct demonstration of the effect of CO_2 on the cerebral arteries had been described. The only investigation quoted in various reviews dealing with this subject is the work of Cow (1911) who observed that isolated segments of carotid artery dilate when CO_2 is added to the Ringer's solution in which they are immersed. We believe that this experiment is inadequate evidence to support the conclusions so widely drawn. Our principle objection is the fact that Cow used the carotid artery which, in our opinion, is not a proper representative of the end arterial branches of the cerebral vessels. Moreover, Cow did not specify if he used the intra- or extra-cranial portion of the carotid artery. This distinction is important since Cow sharply distinguished between the "carotid artery" and "cerebral artery" in describing the opposite effect of epinephrine on these vessels. Apparently, Cow did not intend at all to demonstrate the effect of CO_2 on cerebral vessels themselves, although his observations have been so interpreted many times since as one of the main evidences for the direct effect of CO_2 on the cerebral vascular smooth muscle.

Regarding the importance of this point, we have designed an alternate method of testing *in vivo* the effect of changes of the intra-luminal CO_2 tension on the blood flow through distal branches of the cerebral vessels. In nine dogs we cannulated one of the main branches of the middle cerebral artery and perfused it with arterial blood of various CO_2 tensions, keeping the perfusion pressure at a constant level. It was found that an increase of the perfusion blood CO_2 tension from low levels of about 25 mm Hg to high levels of about 70 mm Hg *decreased* the perfusion rate 20–40%.

---

* Research fellow Department of Neurosurgery, Hadassah University Hospital, Jerusalem, Israel.
** Department of Neurosurgery, University of Miami School of Medicine, Miami, Florida (U.S.A.).

References p. 106

When the CO_2 tension of the perfused blood was reduced back to the low level the perfusion rate usually returned to its former level. An increase of the perfusion blood CO_2 tension *never* resulted in an increase of the perfusion rate. On the other hand, an increase of systemic arterial P_{CO_2} was followed by a significant increase of the perfusion rate, although the P_{CO_2} in the perfused vessels did not change. This phenomenon was observed also in cases where the perfusion pressure was reduced to levels below systemic arterial pressure, indicating that the increase of perfusion rate was a consequence of decreased resistance in the perfused vessels rather than escape of blood through the dilated collaterals into the surrounding vessels (Figs. 1 and 2).

The possibility of a neural regulatory mechanism for the cerebral circulation has been widely assumed to be negligible or non-existent because of failure of autonomic denervation or stimulation to affect cerebral blood flow significantly. Moreover, according to a review by Wolff (1936), the cerebral vasodilating effect of CO_2 persists after decerebration, spinal transection and section of various cranial nerves.

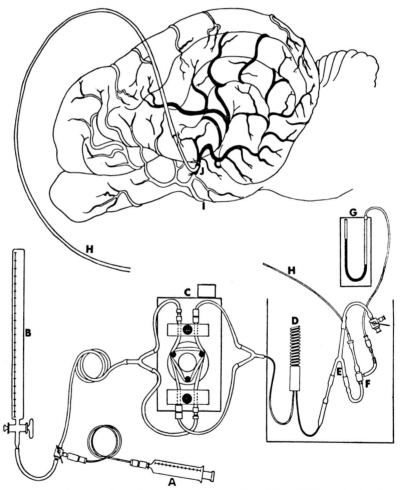

Fig.1 . Perfusion experiment by cannulating branches of the middle cerebral artery.

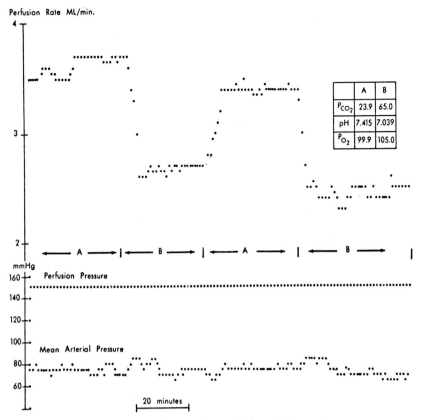

Fig. 2. Relation between P$_{CO_2}$ and the perfusion rate.

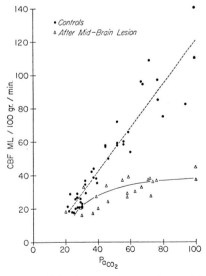

Fig. 3. Relation between the cerebral blood flow and systemic arterial P$_{CO_2}$ after midbrain lesions and control animals.

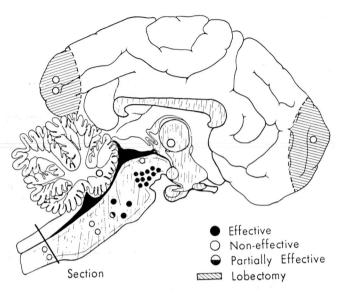

Fig. 4. Effectiveness of brain lesions on the response of CBF to systemic arterial P_{CO_2} alterations.

On the other hand, the existence of a rich supply of nerves which accompanies the major arteries of the brain, the pial vessels, and those vessels that dip back into the cortex should not be ignored. The absence of clear demonstration of their function is not an adequate reason to assume them functionless. Furthermore, in spite of the obvious importance of the observations of Wolff, it is disappointing to discover that Wolff refers to them all as "unpublished observations".

In order to obtain further information concerning this important problem we studied in 18 dogs the response of the cerebral blood flow (measured by the nitrous oxide method) to altered arterial P_{CO_2}, following lesions at various levels of the brain stem. It was found that following a lesion in the mid brain, the pons, and the upper part of the medulla the response of the cerebral circulation to CO_2 diminished significantly or disappeared. By the use of Cooper's cryosurgical system, reversible lesions in areas in the mid brain could be achieved there by producing concomitant variations in the response of the cerebral circulation to changes in the arterial CO_2 tensions (Figs. 3 and 4).

It is suggested, therefore, that the response of the cerebral circulation to changes in arterial CO_2 tension is not due to a direct effect of this gas on the smooth muscle in the cerebral arterial walls, but depends upon a neural reflex mechanism which can be interrupted or impaired by lesions in certain levels of the brain stem.

REFERENCES

Cow, D. (1911); Some reactions of surviving arteries. *J. Physiol.*, **42**, 125.
Wolff, H. G., (1936); The cerebral circulation. *Physiol. Rev.*, **16**, 545.

Influence of Systemic Blood Pressure on Blood Flow and Microcirculation of Ischemic Cerebral Cortex: a Failure of Autoregulation[*]

ARTHUR G. WALTZ[**] AND THORALF M. SUNDT, JR.[***]

Mayo Clinic and Mayo Foundation, Rochester, Minnesota (U.S.A.)

Previously[1] we described the changes of the superficial microvasculature and microcirculation of the frontal and anterior parietal regions of the cerebral cortex of cats and squirrel monkeys (*Saimiri sciurea*) which we observed and photographed after acute occlusion of the ipsilateral middle cerebral artery, exposed by an extradural approach with the aid of an operation microscope[2]. Early ischemic changes in cortical surface vessels included darkening of the blood in surface veins and venules, a decrease in the velocity of the flow of blood through arterial and venous channels, and aggregation of formed elements of the blood, producing "sludging" and stasis. Occasionally dilatation of arteries and arterioles was associated.

A few minutes to a few hours after occlusion, pallor of the cortex developed because of the disappearance of small surface vessels. Cortical pallor, either focal or generalized, was the earliest definite sign of cortical ischemia. Once pallor was established, spontaneous recolorization of the cortex rarely occurred.

Constriction or "spasm" of superficial cortical arteries and arterioles frequently accompanied ischemia. It was not determined whether the constriction was truly a response to ischemia or simply an artefact[1]. White thrombi, composed largely of platelets, often formed in veins. Rarely, venous blood became distinctly reddish, particularly in areas (focal or generalized) in which ischemic changes were progressing. Late ischemic changes included collapse of venous and arterial vessels and stasis or disappearance of the column of blood from larger vessels.

Ischemic changes occurring in the superficial cortical microvasculature and microcirculation after occlusion of the ipsilateral middle cerebral artery probably were representative of the process of cerebral infarction[1]. In our studies ischemic changes occurred regularly after arterial occlusion, even though systemic blood pressure remained at normotensive levels. There was considerable variation from animal to animal and between the two species. In general, ischemic changes in the surface vessels

[*] This investigation was supported in part by Research Grants FR-5530 and NB-6663 from the National Institutes of Health, Public Health Service.
[**] Cerebrovascular Clinical Research Center, Section of Neurology.
[***] Fellow in Basic Neurological Sciences, Mayo Graduate School of Medicine (University of Minnesota), Rochester.

References p. 111–112

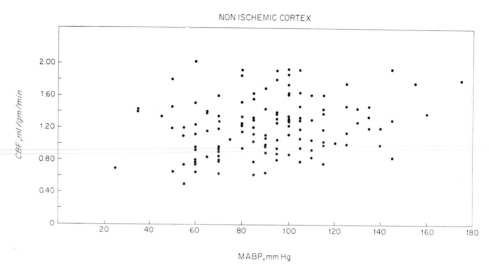

Fig. 1. Effect of changes of mean arterial pressure on blood flow of cerebral cortex of cats.

of the frontal and anterior parietal areas of the brain were more severe in squirrel monkeys than in cats. In cats occlusion of a middle cerebral artery more often produced an infarct deep in the brain or in the temporal lobe[2].

The variation of effects between species was confirmed by measurements of cortical blood flow by determination of the rate of clearance from the cortex of radioactive krypton-85 injected into the brachiocephalic artery or aortic arch. When measured over the frontal and anterior parietal areas after occlusion of the ipsilateral middle cerebral artery, cortical blood flow in squirrel monkeys was found to be too low to be calculated; in cats, blood flow after occlusion was reduced to about one half the pre-occlusion value[3].

All observations of the superficial cortical microvasculature and microcirculation and measurements of cortical blood flow which we describe subsequently in this paper were made in the areas of the brain mentioned above: the frontal and anterior parietal regions.

Influence of Hypotension

In our studies of the superficial cortical microvasculature and microcirculation after occlusion of the ipsilateral middle cerebral artery, hypotension occasionally occurred spontaneously during the surgical procedure, before or after arterial occlusion, or the systemic blood pressure purposely was lowered by the removal of blood from a femoral artery. Hypotension did not produce a qualitative change in the response of the superficial cortical microcirculation to ischemia. When hypotension occurred, ischemic changes developed in cortical vessels more quickly and were more severe than if blood pressure was maintained at normotensive levels. The character of the ischemic changes, however, was not altered.

In a separate series of experiments in cats we measured blood flow (by the krypton-

85 clearance method) in the cortex made ischemic by occlusion of the ipsilateral middle cerebral artery. As stated above, when systemic blood pressure remained at normotensive levels, cortical blood flow was reduced after occlusion to about half the pre-occlusion value. When systemic hypotension was produced by the intravenous injection of small amounts of sodium nitroprusside or trimethaphan camsylate (Arfonad), an additional reduction in cortical blood flow took place, often to values too low to be calculated by the method.

We did not find a "threshold" level of hypotension below which the flow of blood through the ischemic cortex decreased precipitously. Rather, in the ischemic cortex the reduction in systemic blood pressure appeared to result in a passive reduction in the flow of blood, as determined by observation of the severity of ischemic changes in surface vessels or by measurement of the clearance of krypton-85 from the cortex.

The response of the ischemic cortex to systemic hypotension was different from the response of the cortex of the cerebral hemisphere opposite the occluded middle cerebral artery. In the nonischemic cortex, blood flow remained relatively unaffected by hypotension until very low levels of blood pressure were reached (approximately 50 mm Hg mean arterial pressure, as measured by a manometer or strain gauge through a catheter placed in a femoral artery or the abdominal aorta). In the ischemic cortex, autoregulation of cortical blood flow for variations in blood pressure was impaired or abolished. The vascular mechanisms responsible for autoregulation of flow either were severely damaged by ischemia or had reacted maximally to ischemia and hence could not respond further to hypotension.

Influence of Hypertension

Elevations of systemic blood pressure, occurring spontaneously or produced by the intravenous injection of phenylephrine (Neo-Synephrine), usually did not influence changes in the microcirculation or blood flow in the cortex made ischemic by occlusion

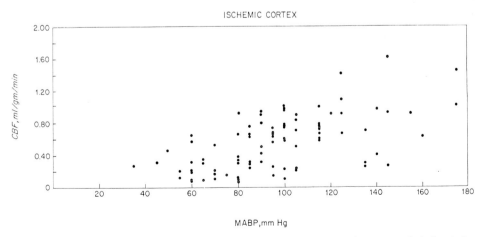

Fig. 2. Effect of changes of mean arterial blood pressure on blood flow of cortex made ischemic by occlusion of middle cerebral artery.

of the ipsilateral middle cerebral artery. Ischemic changes in surface vessels were not retarded or lessened, and values for blood flow calculated from the ischemic cortex were not increased by hypertension. However, when a slight rise in systemic blood pressure occurred in the presence of platelet thrombosis in veins, venous hemorrhage often developed.

The failure of cortical blood flow to increase in consonance with increasing systemic blood pressure probably was not caused by autoregulation of flow for variations in pressure. It seems more likely that cortical blood flow (through channels collateral to the occluded middle cerebral artery) already was maximal in response to ischemia and hence could not respond further to hypertension.

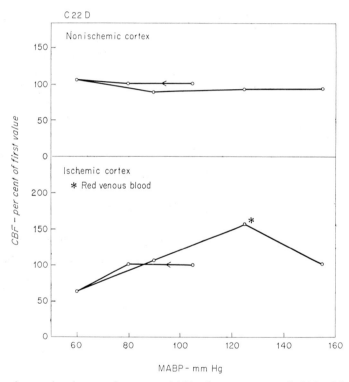

Fig. 3. Effect of successive changes of mean arterial blood pressure on cortical blood flow in one cat.

Occurrence of "Red Venous Blood" With Variations in Systemic Blood Pressure

As stated above, blood flow through the ischemic cortex (measured by the krypton-85 clearance method) was further reduced when systemic hypotension was produced by the intravenous injection of sodium nitroprusside. If the blood pressure was then allowed to return to normotensive levels by discontinuation of the use of sodium nitroprusside, cortical blood flow often would approach or exceed the values found for the ischemic cortex before hypotension. When systemic blood pressure increased from hypotensive levels and the cortical blood flow increased, the unusual phenomenon of reddening of blood in veins was seen.

Lassen[4], at this Congress, has stated that "luxury perfusion" of the brain, manifested by red venous blood, indicates a disturbance of autoregulation for oxygen availability and utilization. In the experiments we are reporting, when the cortical blood flow increased more oxygen apparently was supplied to the ischemic, partially damaged tissue than could be used, resulting in a higher venous oxygen saturation and red venous blood. We have reported previously[1] that red blood at times is seen in surface veins in ischemic cortex without known variations in systemic blood pressure. In both situations the lack of response of autoregulatory mechanisms to increased cortical venous oxygen saturation may have been the result of ischemic damage or deficiency of an essential substance other than oxygen (such as glucose) or an excess of a metabolite (such as carbon dioxide).

CONCLUSIONS AND SUMMARY

In cats and squirrel monkeys occlusion of a middle cerebral artery produces ischemic changes in the ipsilateral superficial cortical microvasculature and microcirculation. These ischemic changes, which probably are representative of the process of cerebral infarction, include darkening of venous blood, slowing of the velocity of the flow of blood, aggregation of formed elements of the blood, pallor of the cortex, dilatation or constriction, or both, of arterial vessels, formation of white (platelet) thrombi in veins and venules, reddening of the blood in veins and collapse of vessels. Blood flow through the ischemic cortex, measured by the krypton-85 clearance method, is markedly reduced.

Systemic hypotension, spontaneous or produced by drugs or the removal of blood, speeds the development and increases the severity of ischemic changes in the microcirculation, but does not alter the character of such changes. Hypotension after arterial occlusion results in a further reduction of cortical blood flow which appears to be passive, indicating a failure of autoregulation of flow. Autoregulation may fail because of tissue damage or because there is a maximal response to ischemia.

Systemic hypertension, spontaneous or produced by drugs, does not influence ischemic changes in the microcirculation, except for the fact that when platelet thrombi are present in veins, venous hemorrhage often occurs. An increase in systemic blood pressure does not produce an increase in blood flow through the ischemic cortex, except when hypotension previously has been present. In the latter instance, blood in veins may become redder, also indicating a failure of autoregulation of cortical blood flow.

REFERENCES

1 WALTZ, A. G. AND SUNDT, T. M., JR. (1967) The microvasculature and microcirculation of the cerebral cortex after arterial occlusion. *Brain* (In press).
2 SUNDT, T. M., JR. AND WALTZ, A. G. (1966) Experimental cerebral infarction: retro-orbital, extradural approach for occluding the middle cerebral artery. *Mayo Clin. Proc.*, **41**, 159–168.

3 WALTZ, A. G., SUNDT, T. M., JR. AND OWEN, C. A., JR. (1967) Effect of middle cerebral artery occlusion on cortical blood flow in animals. *Neurology*, **16**, 1185–1190.
4 LASSEN, N. A. (1967) On the regulation of cerebral blood flow in diseases of the brain with special regard to "the acute brain syndrome" characterized by luxury perfusion. This volume pp. 121–124.

Disturbances of Gas Metabolism in Patients with Occlusive Cerebrovascular Disease

E. RAUDAM, R. ZUPPING AND A. E. KAASIK

Department of Neurology and Neurosurgery of the Tartu State University, Tartu, Estonian S.S.R
(U.S.S.R.)

INTRODUCTION

One of the key questions in cerebral vascular pathology is the problem of brain gas metabolism. The physiological details of brain circulation and gas metabolism have been widely studied both in experimental animals and men; the results of those investigations have been exhaustively reviewed[1-4]. Considerably less work has been devoted to the investigation of gas metabolism of the brain tissue and of lung gas exchange in the conditions of cerebrovascular disease. Nevertheless, the general changes in lung ventilation, in cerebral blood flow and, accordingly, in cerebral oxygen metabolism, which take place in patients with occlusive cerebrovascular disease, have been determined rather well[5-12]. At the same time, almost no attention has been paid to the secondary changes which no doubt occur in brain gas metabolism already after the beginning of the stroke. Furthermore, the qualitative differences in the cerebral gas exchange pattern, which definitely exist between the patients with transitory ischemic attacks (TIA) on one hand and with cerebral infarctions (CI) on the other, have not yet been investigated in properly selected series.

The purpose of this paper is to summarize observations in this field, which have been obtained in our department during recent years. Here only a brief review of the main results is given. Elsewhere, most of the data have been reported in some more details[13-19]. The main aim of this study was to characterize the general derangements of gas metabolism both of the whole body in general and of the brain tissue specifically. An effort was made to find out the probable correlations between the location and extension of brain damage on one hand and disturbances of ventilation and brain gas metabolism on the other. Hence, the lung ventilation and both arterial and cerebral venous blood gases were investigated.

MATERIAL AND METHODS

Measurements of gas metabolism of the whole body, especially of the brain tissue, have been performed in a total of 159 patients. 15 elderly persons without cerebrovascular abnormalities constituted a control group (CG) for laboratory technique. The patients

References p. 118–119

were examined clinically and followed up in an effort to obtain as much clinical information as possible for correlative purposes. Carotid arteriography was performed to visualize the cerebral circulation. Clinically, 120 of all the 159 investigated patients, had brain infarctions; 39 transitory ischemic attacks. In 21 cases complete occlusion or severe narrowing of the extracranial part of the carotid arteries was diagnosed arteriographically. Patients with CI were of various degrees of severity; during the acute stage of the ailment 22 of them died. The others showed more-or-less remarkable recovery.

For investigating lung ventilation and pulmonary gas exchange, the exhaled air was gathered in the sack of Douglas. The pulmonary ventilation (PV l/min) was subsequently measured by means of a gas-meter. The PV was calculated according to STPD (0°C and 760 mm Hg) and the gas analysis was performed by the Haldane method. The oxygen consumption (O_2C ml/min) and the carbon dioxide release (CO_2R ml/min) were calculated according to the data obtained by the measurement of PV and the analysis of the exhaled air by the gas measurement.

Both internal jugular veins and the brachial artery were punctured and blood samples were drawn simultaneously. The blood gas analysis was carried out by the manometric method of van Slyke. Oxygen saturation percentage (O_2S %) of arterial (A) and cerebral venous (VJ) blood, arterial and cerebral venous carbon dioxide content (ACO_2 and $VJ CO_2$, respectively), the arteriovenous oxygen and carbon dioxide difference ((A-V) O_2 vol% and (V-A) CO_2 vol%, respectively), the brain RQ and oxygen utilization coefficient (O_2UC) were calculated. All patients with CI were investigated within the very first days of the ailment and subsequently at the end of every week for about five weeks. The sufferers from TIA were, as a rule, investigated on one occasion only. For statistical evaluation of the data obtained, the Student's *t*-criterion was used.*

RESULTS

Table I presents the mean values of the pulmonary ventilation and gas exchange for the entire period of investigation obtained in the various groups of the subjects studied.

The results presented in Table I indicate that the results obtained in TIA patients were within the normal limits. The respiratory rate was considerably increased in cases of CI with damage of only the brain hemispheres, where the ventilation was more superficial than in patients with TIA. In patients with brain stem compression a considerable hyperventilation was noticed. In the development of hyperventilation both the increase of respiratory rate and of the tidal volume played an important part. At the same time, the increase of PV was in close correlation with the decrease of ACO_2 ($r = -0.891$). A close correlation was also revealed between the increase of CO_2R and the decrease of ACO_2 ($r = -0.429$). In comparison with patients who had only damage

---

* The ranges of veracity to the arithmetical mean were calculated according to the formula $u = t_5\% m$, where u are the ranges of veracity; $t_5\%$ is the Student's criterion with the probability of 5 per cent and m is the mean error of the arithmetic mean.

TABLE I

MEAN FIGURES OF PULMONARY VENTILATION AND LUNG GAS EXCHANGE

Index of data	Clinical groups; $\bar{x} \pm u$		
	TIA	CI	
		I	II
PV l/min	6.8 ± 0.6	6.5 ± 0.2	10.7 ± 1.6
Respiratory rate	16.2 ± 1.2	19.3 ± 0.4	25.8 ± 2.5
Tidal volume	438 ± 5.6	353 ± 17	425 ± 67
O_2C ml/min	232 ± 22	194 ± 5	247 ± 31
CO_2R ml/min	204 ± 21	173 ± 5	226 ± 42

I Patients with damage of the brain hemispheres only; II Patients with brainstem compression.

of brain hemispheres, the cases with the brain stem compression showed more intensive O_2C from the inhaled air.

Table II presents the mean values of cerebral gas metabolism for the whole period of investigation.

In all patients the decrease of the O_2S was more intensive in the cerebral venous than in the arterial blood. This change was most marked in patients with CI. The oxygen A–V difference was, therefore, increased in both clinical groups.

TABLE II

MEAN DATA OF CEREBRAL GAS METABOLISM

Index of data	Clinical groups; $\bar{x} \pm u$		
	CG	TIA	CI
A O_2S %	95.4 ± 1.06	94.9 ± 1.18	91.07 ± 0.83
A CO_2 vol %	45.09 ± 1.10	44.79 ± 0.78	42.79 ± 0.65
VJ O_2S %	64.8 ± 2.23	56.2 ± 3.21	53.1 ± 1.04
(A–V) O_2 vol %	6.15 ± 0.44	7.78 ± 0.64	7.49 ± 0.20
(V–A) CO_2 vol %	6.13 ± 0.46	7.54 ± 0.70	6.61 ± 0.20
RQ	1.00 ± 0.004	0.97 ± 0.04	0.88 ± 0.02
O_2 UC	0.32 ± 0.017	0.41 ± 0.02	0.42 ± 0.02

Since O_2UC was considerably increased both in patients with TIA and CI, the increase in (A–V)O_2 was caused by an increased consumption of oxygen from the blood unit circulating through the brain vascular network. It appeared that in patients with TIA their brain gas metabolism was almost completely compensated by the aforementioned increase of (A–V)O_2 since there was an equivalent increase in (V–A)CO_2. The RQ of the brain remained normal. This equilibrium was disturbed when the brain infarction developed.

For patients with CI the presence of arterial hypoxemia and hypocapnia was also characteristic. Due to the arterial hypoxemia, $(A–V)O_2$ in patients with CI was somewhat lower than in TIA cases ($r = 0.41$). Comparatively more pronounced cerebral venous hypoxemia in CI patients might be due to the decrease of A O_2S in this group; but there was no correlation between these data ($r = 0.09$). At the same time, a close correlation between the severity of arterial hypocapnia and cerebral venous hypoxemia was revealed ($r = 0.72$). Similar correlations were disclosed between the severity of arterial hypocapnia on the one hand and the increase of $(A–V)O_2$ ($r = —0.89$) and O_2UC ($r = —0.64$) on the other.

In the cases of CI, the most marked changes in pulmonary ventilation and lung gas exchange were noticed during the very first days of the ailment. Both arterial hypoxemia and hypocapnia were most severe at the beginning of the disease; then there was a tendency to normalize, which was especially noticeable in cases with good recovery. Nevertheless, it was important that some degree of arterial hypoxemia was present even at the end of the acute stage of the illness. The cerebral venous hypoxemia was likewise most severe during the very first days of the disease; at the end of the first week of the disease VJ O_2S greatly increased but remained on the subnormal level till the end of the period of investigation. The A–V oxygen difference was also most increased on the first day of the ailment; then it gradually decreased but remained considerably high at the end of the investigation. Neither the RQ of the brain, nor the oxygen consumption coefficient normalized completely in patients with brain infarctions.

Relatively more frequent and superficial breathing was noticed in older patients and in cases with congestive heart failure. Both arterial and cerebral venous hypoxemia were also somewhat more expressed in the latter cases. Respectively, the cases with the congestive heart disease showed more marked decrease of VJ O_2S and VJ CO_2 than the other patients with CI.

The analysis showed that hyperventilation was most severe in the cases with a fatal outcome of the disease. Likewise, the severity of both arterial hypoxemia and hypocapnia were in remarkable correlation with mortality. In patients with a fatal outcome, the average A O_2S was $87.2 \pm 2.71\%$, A CO_2 38.53 ± 1.72 vol%, which was considerably less than in surviving cases. In the latter group, $(A–V) O_2$ was much more increased than in surviving cases (8.27 ± 0.69 vol% and 7.36 ± 0.20 vol%, respectively). Despite the increased utilization of the oxygen of the blood unit circulating through the brain, cerebral hypoxemia was continuous and the average RQ of the brain was only 0.78 ± 0.04 in the lethal group.

The A O_2S and A CO_2 were highest in patients with superficial infarctions of the cerebral hemispheres ($92.9 \pm 0.70\%$ and 43.98 ± 0.68 vol%, respectively) and lowest in cases with secondary brain stem damage ($88.2 \pm 2.42\%$ and 35.2 ± 2.3 vol%, respectively).

Table III presents the data obtained in 12 patients with CI before and after the administration of a gas mixture containing $7\% CO_2$ and $93\% O_2$. All investigations were performed during the first week of the disease.

The results presented in Table III indicate that the increase of both arterial and cerebral venous blood oxygen saturation was statistically significant after the inhala-

TABLE III

MEAN VALUES OF CEREBRAL GAS METABOLISM BEFORE AND AFTER THE ADMINISTRATION
OF 7% CO_2

Index of data	$\bar{x} \pm u$	
	Before CO_2	After CO_2
A O_2S %	87.9 ± 2.75	94.2 ± 2.62
A CO_2 vol. %	41.12 ± 1.79	44.01 ± 2.24
VJ O_2S %	50.5 ± 5.14	64.1 ± 2.18
(A–V) O_2 vol. %	7.77 ± 1.13	6.25 ± 1.19
(V–A) CO_2 vol. %	6.02 ± 0.09	6.29 ± 0.69
RQ	0.79 ± 0.09	1.01 ± 0.06
O_2UC	0.42 ± 0.06	0.31 ± 0.02

tion of the afore-mentioned gas mixture. At the same time the markedly increased (A–V)O_2 and the considerably decreased RQ of the brain normalized under the action of carbon dioxide.

A series of 21 patients was operated on the carotid arteries. The method of operation used was the thrombendarterectomy with subsequent patch graft arteriplastics. In 8 cases the blood flow via the occluded artery was restored. On successfully operated patients the investigation of the brain gas metabolism was repeated 3 weeks after the operation and this revealed quite normal data of cerebral gas metabolism.

COMMENTS

The analysis revealed that the hyperventilatory pattern of respiration in patients with CI was not caused by systemic changes in the body, i.e. arterial hypoxemia, congestive heart failure, pneumonia and metabolic acidosis. Hyperventilation was caused mainly by the damage of the upper brain stem. That conclusion coincides with the data of others, who have found that damage to the upper brain stem regions results in augmentation and acceleration of breathing[5,6].

The arterial hypocapnia was mainly connected with the increased CO_2 R in overventilating patients. However, it seems reasonable to believe that hypocapnia is partially enhanced by the metabolic disturbances in old patients, by disturbances of general circulation etc.

In the genesis of arterial hypoxemia, the most important part is played by the disturbances of the perfusion — ventilation ratio in the lungs. That mechanism has been suggested by various authors[20,21] and the data of this work seem to confirm it. Nevertheless, an important contribution to the development of arterial hypoxemia may be connected with the derangement of oxygen diffusion in the lungs.

The present study revealed that in patients with the occlusive cerebrovascular disease, the most characteristic change of the brain gas metabolism was the increased consumption of oxygen from the blood unit circulating through the brain. It was reflected in the decrease of cerebral venous oxygen saturation and in the increase of both A–V oxygen difference and O_2UC. These changes should be considered as compensational reactions in the conditions of decreased cerebral blood flow. It has been widely recognized that the occlusive process in brain vessels itself plays a major role in causing the increase of cerebrovascular resistance and, consequently, the decrease of cerebral blood flow[7–9]. The afore-mentioned view is supported by the fact that brain gas metabolism normalized after the restoration of adequate blood flow via the occluded carotid artery. At the same time, there seem to be very important secondary changes both in the cerebral blood flow as well as in the brain gas metabolism, which depend on the brain damage itself. The arterial hypocapnia caused by hyperventilation contributes to the further reduction of cerebral blood flow. This was shown in "physiological" conditions more than 20 years ago[22]. The present study suggests that even the rigid vessels of patients with occlusive cerebrovascular disease react to the vasoconstrictive stimulus of arterial hypocapnia. Furthermore, after the inhalation of 7 per cent CO_2, the increase of cerebral venous oxygen saturation was statistically significant and, since the cerebral metabolism remained unchanged following CO_2 inhalation[22], it indicated increased cerebral blood flow. This suggests that cerebral vessels of stroke patients react adequately to the vasodilatative stimulus of carbon dioxide.

SUMMARY AND CONCLUSIONS

This paper is a review of some of the studies performed at Tartu State University on the pulmonary ventilation, general and cerebral gas exchange in patients with occlusive cerbrovascular disease.

The restricted blood flow to the brain in patients with TIA appeared to be compensated by the increased oxygen consumption from the blood unit circulating through brain. That equilibrium is disturbed when brain infarction develops. In cases with secondary involvement of the upper brain stem a marked central neurogenic hyperventilation occurs. Severe respiratory hypocapnia follows which in its turn causes secondary restriction of the brain oxygen supply.

Both arterial hypoxemia and hypocapnia are in close correlation with mortality and most of the stroke patients with an unfavourable outcome of the disease "breathe themselves to death".

Timely surgical restoration of the blood flow via the occluded artery normalizes the brain gas metabolism. The inhalation of the gas mixture containing 7 % CO_2 permits temporary normalization of cerebral gas metabolism, but most likely only in the unaffected region of the brain.

REFERENCES

1 LASSEN, N. A. (1959) Cerebral blood flow and oxygen consumption in man. *Physiol. Rev.*, **39**, 183–238.
2 SOKOLOFF, L. (1959) The action of drugs on the cerebral circulation. *Pharmacol. Rev.*, **11**, 1–85.
3 INGVAR, D. H. (1963) *Studies of the regional metabolism and circulation of the cerebral cortex*. In:

Selective Vulnerability of the Brain in Hypoxaemia, J. P. Schadé and W. H. McMenemey (Eds.), Oxford, pp. 55–61.

4 HARPER, A. M. (1965) Physiology of cerebral bloodflow. *Brit. J. Anesth.*, **37**, 225–235.

5 PLUM, F. AND SWANSON, A. G. (1959) Central neurogenic hyperventilation in man. *Arch. Neurol. Psychiat.*, **81**, 535–549.

6 PLUM, F. (1960) Neural mechanisms of abnormal respiration in humans. *Arch. Neurol.*, **3**, 484–487.

7 SCHEINBERG, P. (1958) A critical review of circulatory physiology as it applies to cerebral vascular disease. *Ann. Int. Med.*, **48**, 1001–1016.

8 AIZAWA, T., TAZAKI, Y., GOTOH, F. (1961) Cerebral circulation in cerebrovascular disease. *Wld. Neurol.*, **2**, 635–648.

9 SOKOLOFF, L. (1961) Aspects of cerebral circulatory physiology of relevance to cerebrovascular disease. *Neurology*, **11**, 34–40.

10 EKBERG, R., CRONQVIST, S. AND INGVAR, D. H. (1965) Regional cerebral blood flow in cerebrovascular disease. *Acta Neurol. Scand.*, Suppl. **14** (Regional Cerebral Blood Flow) 164–168.

11 LASSEN, N. A. AND INGVAR, D. H. (1966) *Regional cerebral blood in apoplexy: studies of its patophysiology, using 8 to 16 external detectors with the Xenon-133 method.* Contribution to the 3. International Symposium on Cerebral Circulation. Salzburg, October 18–21.

12 MEYER, J. S., GOTOH, F. AND EBIHARA, S. (1966) Influence of cerebrovascular disease and state of consciousness on cerebral metabolism. *J. Amer. Geriat. Soc.*, **14**, 205–220.

13 ZUPPING, R. (1964) Arterial blood oxygen in patients with acute cerebrovascular disorders. *Transactions of Tartu State University, Tartu*, **163**, 161–167 [Russian with a German summary].

14 ZUPPING, R. (1965) Lung ventilation and CO_2 exchange in patients with cerebral hemorrhage. *Voprosi Klin. Nevrol. i Psihiatr. Tartu*, **5**, 74–78 [Russian].

15 ZUPPING, R. (1965) *Pulmonary ventilation, lung gas exchange and arterial blood gases in the acute stage of cerebrovascular disorders.* Dissertation, Tartu [Estonian and Russian].

16 KAASIK, A. E. (1966) Brain oxygen metabolism in the acute stage of strokes. *Proceedings of the 4-th All-Union Conference on Biochemistry of the Nervous System.* Tartu, pp. 48–49 [Russian].

17 KAASIK, A. E., LAAS, T. AND RIVIS, E. (1966) Disturbances of carbohydrate and gas metabolism of the brain tissue in patients with acute cerebrovascular diseases. *Voprosi Klin. Nevrol. i Psihiatr. Tartu*, **6**, 71–80 [Russian with English summary].

18 KAASIK, A. E. (1967) Investigation of the gas metabolism of the brain in patients with occlusion of the carotid arteries in the neck. *Transactions of Tartu State University, Tartu* [to be published in Russian with English summary].

19 RAUDAM, E. AND KAASIK, A. E. (1967) Treatment of brain oxygen insufficiency in the acute phase of cerebral infarction. *Zurnal Nevropatol. i Psihiatr. (Moscow)* [to be published in Russian with a French summary].

20 NAERAA, N. (1963) Blood gases analysis in unconscious neurosurgical patients on admission to hospital. *Acta anaesth. Scand.*, **7**, 191–199.

21 FISCHER-WILLIAMS, M., TELERMANN-TOPPET, N. AND MEYER, J. S. (1964) Clinico-EEG correlation with arterial and jugular venous biochemical studies in acute neurological disorder. *Brain*, **87**, 281–306.

22 KETY, S. S. AND SCHMIDT, C. F. (1946) The effects of active and passive hyperventilation on cerebral blood flow, cerebral oxygen consumption, cardiac output, and blood pressure of normal young men. *J. Clin. Invest.*, **25**, 107–119.

On the Regulation of Cerebral Blood Flow in Diseases of the Brain with Special Regard to the „Luxury Perfusion Syndrome" of Brain Tissue, i.e. a Syndrome Characterized by Relative Hyperemia or Absolute Hyperemia of the Brain Tissue

N. A. LASSEN

Department of Clinical Physiology, Bispebjerg Hospital, Copenhagen, Denmark

In chronic diseases of the brain associated with diffuse derangement of function–with organic dementia–the metabolism and the blood flow are both reduced. This parallel reduction of both metabolism and flow is seen e.g. in senile dementia, in dementia following apoplexy and in neuro-syphilis (see Lassen, 1959).

It is generally believed that the reduced blood flow is caused by the reduced metabolic demand although the precise mechanism by which metabolism influences the perfusion is not known (Roy and Sherrington, 1890). It may be specifically stated that neither the tensions of oxygen nor of carbon dioxide allow us to understand this metabolic regulation since it is so perfect as to leave no adequate stimulus as remarked recently by Siesjö (1965). Chronic adaptive phenomena related to those described by Betz (1965) perhaps play a role.

Be this as it may, the characteristic feature of the above mentioned chronic disease states of the brain is that of a very perfect adjustment: the arterial pCO_2 is usually normal as well as the arterial pH; the cerebral venous blood has a normal composition, most notably the cerebral venous oxygen content is normal being about 6–7 vol. % lower than that of the arterial blood at normocapnia. In other words the oxygen saturation of cerebral venous blood is at its normal level of about 60% at normocapnia. This is so precisely because of the parallel reduction of metabolism and flow.

Recently attention has been focused on an entirely different type of brain syndrome: "The Luxury Perfusion Syndrome of Brain Tissue" as we have called it (Lassen, 1966). Many of the speakers at this symposium have mentioned this syndrome, and it is one of the main purposes of the present symposium to call it to the attention of neurosurgeons.

A patient recently studied by Ewald, Skinhøj, and myself (1967) may serve to illustrate this condition; it was a case of contusion of the brain in a 54 years old man 24 h after the incident he was in a semicomatose state without focal neurological defects and with hemorrhagic spinal fluid. The oxygen uptake of the brain was found to be subnormal in this patient, a finding correlating well to the clinical state of depressed brain function. But, the cerebral blood flow was *not* reduced but remained normal and this despite a moderate degree of hyperventilation ($ApCO_2 = 36$ mm Hg). Thus the remarkable finding in this subject was an arterio–venous oxygen difference of about 4 vol.% in a situation where normal man would have had one of about 8 vol.%. We may also simply describe the situation by saying that the cerebral venous blood was *too* red–had too high an oxygen saturation. Thus, the cerebral venous blood was not utilized of oxygen in normal fashion. In this sense luxury perfusion of the brain existed. The cerebral blood flow was normal but the demand for oxygen was subnormal. So, *relative* to demand, a state of *relative* cerebral hyperemia was present.

This condition of acute maladaptation of the cerebral circulation has been recorded previously but its possible significance not fully appreciated. Let it just be mentioned that Fazekas and coworkers in 1951 studied 4 patients with irreversible post-hypoglycemic coma. The arteriovenous difference over the brain was only 1 to 3 vol.%, i.e. extremely low. Unfortunately these authors did not report the arterial pCO_2 values, but, we know now that moderate hyperventilation usually accompanies such acute brain disorders.

Where can one expect to find this acute brain damage syndrome: in all cases of acute apoplexy one might well expect such reactions in the periphery of the lesion (centrally a definite reduction of blood flow supposedly occurs; Høedt-Rasmussen *et al.*, 1967; Ingvar, 1967). Waltz and Sundt (1967) saw evidence hereof on the cortex of monkeys subjected to experimental infarction. They reported that veins draining the focal area contained in many cases not dark red (over-utilized) but light red blood (luxury perfusion). Cronquist has commented on the same phenomenon in man (Cronquist, 1967). Also, one may expect to find this acute brain syndrome in a number of acute neurological syndromes such as traumatic brain injuries. Especially one may expect that neurosurgeons encounter this as they hardly can avoid to produce areas of stagnant hypoxia as described by Zwetnow (1967). Indeed, Zwetnow's recent studies of post hypoxic hyperemia constitute an already classical description of the "luxury perfusion" syndrome.

Two aspects of the acute cerebral syndrome deserved special emphasis: its relation to cerebral acid-base regulation and its relation to brain edema.

With regard to cerebral acid-base regulation the possibility of selective acidosis of the brain tissue as a part of the syndrome must be mentioned. Betz (1967) and Siesjö (1967) commented on this point of the present symposium. One may also note that in the patient with cerebral contusion just described the pH of the spinal fluid was normal to slightly acid despite the respiratory alkalosis. Thus acute and selective acidosis of the spinal fluid was found as also reported by Froman and Smith (1966) in similar clinical cases. In our patient a lactate concentration of 3 milliequivalents per liter of spinal fluid was found and this would seem to explain the acidosis adequately. Such acidosis of the central nervous system may, as said, well be an integral part of the acute syndrome and could explain the moderate hyperventilation that usually accompanies it. Treatment by hyperventilation often used in neurosurgical praxis perhaps only assists nature in normalizing brain pH.

The mechanism of brain edema is not well understood. We shall not claim to be able to give more definite pathophysiological data to clarify its pathogenesis. May it be allowed, nevertheless, to point out, that brain edema complicated exactly those acute brain disorders here discussed. Could it be that intra-cellular acidosis was an important factor in its production? More generally speaking a deranged metabolism upsetting the electrolyte transport over the membrane would lead to cellular edema as all cells must swell if the ion pumps. And, acidosis in the cells, by impairing enzyme activities could well depress the ion pump. Normalization of intracellular pH as may be the essence of the hyperventilation treatment, could then by facilitating the return of normal electrolyte pumping be a very important anti-brain-edema agent. These thoughts are not just meant as speculation: as must be the case for a hypothesis to be of practical value, it is a testable hypothesis. One may substantiate, respectively negate, their value simply by measuring the bicarbonate concentration in the brain. The opinion is therefore expressed that such measurements on experimental animals or on brain biopsies in man could perhaps lead to an important advance in our understanding of brain edema: is it, or is it not, commonly (or always?) associated with metabolic acidosis (= bicarbonate deficiency) of the affected tissue area?

In ending my brief presentation with such speculations I have attempted to put "the luxury perfusion syndrome" in a wider perspective. We shall be very interested to hear our clinical neurosurgical colleagues comments hereon, as they daily are encountering such patients. Of special importance is the fact that only very mild local compression of brain tissue seems able to elicit the vicious circle of acidosis–hyperemia–blood-brain barrier damage-edema–local compression-acidoses → (Brock, 1967). Gentleness of manipulation of the brain during neurosurgery is not only a desirable feature, no– it may well be of vital importance in deciding the outcome (failure or success) of the intervention.

REFERENCES

BETZ, E. (1965) Adaptation of regional cerebral blood flow in animals exposed to chronic alterations of pO_2 and pCO_2. *Acta Neurol. Scand. Suppl.*, **14**, 121.

—, (1967) The significance of cortical extra cellular pH for the regulation of blood flow in the cerebral cortex. (this volume, p. 99).

BROCK, M. (1967) Experimental "luxury perfusion" in the cerebral cortex of the cat. (this volume, p. 125).

CRONQUIST, S. AND LAROCHE, F. (1967) Transitory hyperemia in focal cerebral vascular lesions studied by angiography and regional cerebral blood flow measurements. *Brit. J. Radiol.*, **40**, 270.

EWALD, J., SKINHØJ, E. AND LASSEN, N. A. (1967) Unpublished observations.

FAZEKAS, J. F., ALMAN, R. W. AND PARRISH, A. E. (1951) Irreversible post-hypoglycemic coma. *Am. J. Med. Sci.*, **222**, 640.

FROMAN, C. AND SMITH, A. C. (1966) Hyperventilation associated with low pH of cerebrospinal fluid after intracranial haemorrhage. *Lancet*, **I**, 780.

HØEDT-RASMUSSEN, K., SKINHØJ, E., PAULSON, O., EWALD, J., BJERRUM, J. K., FAHRENKRUG, A. AND LASSEN, N. A. (1967) Regional cerebral blood flow in acute apoplexy with a demonstration of local hyperemia (the "luxury perfusion syndrome" of brain tissue). *Arch. Neurol.* (in press).

INGVAR, D. H. (1967) Regional cerebral blood flow in cerebrovascular disorders. (this volume, p. 57).

LASSEN, N. A. (1966) The luxury perfusion syndrome and its possible relation to acute metabolic acidosis localised within the brain. *Lancet*, **I**. 1113.

—, (1967) Cerebral blood flow and oxygen consumption in man. A review. *Physiol. Rev.*, **39**, 183.

ROY, C. S. AND SHERRINGTON, C. S. (1890) On the regulation of the blood-supply of the brain. *J. Physiol.*, **11**, 85.

SIESJÖ, B. K. (1965) Discussion on clinical studies of regional cerebral blood flow. *Acta Neurol. Scand. Suppl.*, **14**, 190.

SIESJÖ, B. K., KÄLLQUIST, A. AND PONTÉN, U. (1967) pH, pCO_2 and HCO_3 in extra- and intra-cellular spaces in the brain. (this volume, p. 93).

WALTZ, A. G., AND SUNDT, TH. M. (1967) Influence of systemic blood pressure on blood flow and microcirculation of ischemic cerebral cortex: A failure of autoregulation. (this volume, p. 107).

ZWETNOW, N. (1967) Experimental studies of the effect of changes in intracranial pressure on cerebral circulation and metabolism. (this volume, p. 87).

Experimental „Luxury Perfusion" in the Cerebral Cortex of the Cat

A comment to the Paper by N. A. Lassen

M. BROCK

Department of Neurosurgery, University of Mainz, Western Germany

Preliminary studies have been performed, on the changes of cortical rCBF (Krypton-85 Beta clearance technique) in response to a localized pressure (corresponding to about 10 mm Hg/cm²) applied to the cerebral cortex (suprasylvian gyrus) of 8 cats under Nembutal anesthesia (30 to 40 mg/kg body-weight) and artificial respiration (arterial $pCO_2 = \pm 28$ mm Hg).

It has been possible to establish that during the compression, (which has been applied for periods up to one hour and a half, to a circular region with a diameter of 1.1 cm by means of a specially developed device) rCBF undergoes an increase in the compressed region as well as in the regions surrounding it. No change in rCBF is found at regions as distant as the contralateral hemisphere. The increase of rCBF *at* the compressed site, during the compression, seems to be more marked in animals with higher blood (i.e. perfusion) pressure, and may be absent in cats with blood pressure of about 80 mm Hg. The augmentation of rCBF *around* the compressed area during the compression is always very marked, and after some time flow values over twice as high as the control values may be attained.

After the compression is discontinued, rCBF *at* the formerly compressed site may remain increased for some time but eventually starts diminishing (edema?) and–even in animals with relative high blood pressure — it becomes lower than the pre-compression values 2 to 3 hours after the compression has been discontinued, and only later start to decrease very slowly. During the entire length of our experiments (3 to 4 hours) we have not observed the hyperemia around the formerly compressed area to decrease back to the normal pre-compression values.

The electrocorticogram shows a marked fastening of the activity and an increase of the manual frequency index *around* the compressed area (during and after compression), and a slowing of the activity as well as a pronoced decrease in the frequency index *at* the formerly compressed area when rCBF at this site has fallen to subnormal values.

The above studies were performed by suggestion of Dr. N. A. Lassen (Copenhagen) in the laboratory of Dr. D. H. Ingvar (Lund). The electrocorticograms have been analysed by Dr. A. Hadjidimos.

Rheoencephalography: Present Status

F. L. JENKNER*

Department of Surgery, University of Graz, Graz (Austria)

Circulation in any organ is a composite event. It has many aspects depending on action of heart, state of great vessels, anatomy and physiology of branching of vessels in the respective part of the body. Hemodynamic and metabolic factors all interact to achieve optimal nutrition and function of organs. In evaluating cerebral circulation we have learned a great deal by arteriography and the nitrous oxide method. But there are details which are not observable by any technique designed to measure blood flow; the events around the propagation of the pulse wave and concomitant changes in pressure and volume. Theoretically, an observation of these events should supply us with information otherwise unobtainable. Optimally suited for giving information on this aspect of circulation is a special application of impedance methods (Geddes and Hoff, 1963). Thus we turn to electrical monitoring of cerebral circulation to see if such a method may be useful to neurosurgeons (and others) as an adjunct in diagnosis.

As we see from Table I, various applications of impedance techniques are known. Rheoencephalography (REG; Jenkner, 1962) is an electrical method which is a special application of those electrophysiological techniques long disregarded, namely the observation of changes in conductivity (or impedance). I shall not give you a highly theoretical nor mathematical exposé of basic studies having been undertaken during the last 40 years, as essential as these studies had been and are to further progress and understanding of the possibilities of this method. Rather I am going to show you if there is a clinical significance to the method and if so, in which areas we may gain clinical information of importance from the method of registering impedance changes in its application to the head. For this purpose a brief regard for cerebral hemodynamics and intracranial fluid dynamics is imperative as is attention to electrical conductivity of various tissue components of the intracranial space. Much original work has been done (Kedrow and Naumenko, 1954; Lifshitz, 1964).

In general, the possibility to monitor circulation electrically is based on the specific electrical resistance which for blood is very much smaller than for most other tissues. While the impedance of blood depends on an even distribution of corpuscular as well as ionic particles (Fricke and Morse, 1925; Kedrow and Naumenko, 1954; Sigman *et al.*, 1937; Velick and Gorin, 1940), in extremities this may be the con-

---

* Present address: *Doz. Dr. F. L. Jenkner, Fichtnergasse 22, A-1130 Vienna, Austria.*

References p. 133–134

TABLE I

TABULATION OF VARIOUS APPLICATIONS OF IMPEDANCE TECHNIQUE IN EXPERIMENTAL
AND CLINICAL MEDICINE AND IN BIOLOGICAL INVESTIGATIONS

Organ or system	Application	Subject	
Respiration	Impedance spirogram	roach, daphnia, frog	
	(Exp.) Bronchospirogr.	rat and man	
Circulation: heart	Stroke volume separately		
	for right and left heart	animal	
	Stroke volume/min	animal	man
	Recording of heart sounds	animal	man
Organs: brain	Rheoencephalography	animal	man
	Depth studies (e. g. Thalam)	animal	
	Exp.: circul. in single neurons	animal	
eye	Rheo-ophthalmogram	animal	man
liver	Liver rheogram		man
kidney	Kidney rheogram	animal	
Periphery:	Rheogram of extremities		
	pedicle flaps (norm and path.:		
	occl. ascl drug effect)	animal	man
Other applications:			
Nervous system:	Effect of arousal, sleep and		
	anesthesia on nerv. function	animal	
	Conduction studies on fibers	animal	
	Conductivity of living brain		
	to assess tumor edema, etc.		man
Gastro-intest. tract:	Intestines rec'd perist.	animal	man
	Liver observ. on mechan. icterus		man
	Salivary glands secretion stud.	animal	
G. U. tract:	Kidney study on sodium excr. reabsorp.	animal	
	Bladder registration of emptying	animal	man
	Uterus reg. of contract. during labor	animal	man
Muscles:	Impedance myogram tremogram	animal	man
	Energy expenditure studies	animal	
Tongue	Motion studies for speech therapy		man
Eye	Impedance electro-oculogram for		
	nystagmus, ocular movements	animal	man
Various other applications:			
Changes of	Psycho-galvanic reflex	animal	man
basal impedance	Estrous activity; thyroid fct		man
of skin with:	Seasonal influence		man
Temperature	Record free of artefacts, easy accurate		
	calibration possible	animal	man
Fluid flow	In heart lung machine		
	Flow determination in various		experimental
	fluids and as drop meter		

necting link between circulation and impedance (Geddes and Hoff, 1963); this does not apply to intracranial circulation (contrary to a recent statement by others). Many reasons account for this: The 10% increase in conductivity seen in flowing blood is small compared to the electrical conductivity of cerebrospinal fluid being 250–500% better than blood which is of great importance since there are pressure and volume changes of pulse synchronous nature of CSF known to occur. Even distribution of particles within a vessel is achieved better by the propagation of pulse wave than by flow where the central core of fast motion disturbs the homogenicity of particles. Additionally intracarotid flow direction reverses from systole (to brain) to diastole (to heart!) very rapidly as may be observed on studying high speed angiographic motion pictures of the cervical internal carotid artery (Pirker, 1966): here one sees the gross counterpart to the intermittent motion of the blood column in arterioles and smaller vessels. Finally, correlations between REG and ballistocardiograms are relevant in this connection (Zouhar and Nevratal, 1966). Additionally, augmentation of changes in impedance (due to changes of intracranial pulse wave volume) by changes in volume of CSF (with its 250–500% better conductivity) makes those changes of impedance caused by extracranial pulse wave changes rather unimportant.

The importance of the pulse wave for REG is documented by two practical applications: measurement of pulse wave velocity and stroke volume in patients. It is understood because of two essential factors: (1) CSF impedance is less than half (or a third) that of blood. Changes in intracranial CSF-content are influencing intracranial impedance much more than changes in intracranial blood itself*. Due to (2) the fact that intracranial contents are encaged within an (almost) rigid container of (nearly) constant volume such changes of CSF-volume must take place to allow the volume of the pulse wave to enter the intracranial cavity. Pressure changes of CSF have been used to make relative estimations of blood volume shifts. Since the product of pressure and volume is a constant one, one may calculate from the pulsatile pressure changes the changes in volume which are responsible for these changes in pressure. We know the average volume of (a) intracranial space (b) intracranial blood and (c) intracranial "free space" (*i.e.* CSF, 3) and the changes of these volumes with age. We may therefore say that what we see as registration of changes in impedance (*i.e.* REG) represents those redistributions of volumes (of substances with differing specific electrical conductivity) which occur synchronously with the pulse wave propagation implying changing velocity of particles. Due to the changes of the named volumes with age, the changes of impedance (*i.e.* the REG-tracing) must also change with age, even without any pathology, vascular or other. There is ample evidence of such changes. Changes in CSF volume multiply the impedance changes of blood and present them in an integrated somewhat delayed fashion. Thus the redistribution of volume is apparently depending on the pulse wave volume and the term "relative pulse (wave) volume" in wide use for the extremities may also be applied to the intracranial (= cerebral) circulation by the use of REG: aside from depending on stroke volume and its changes it reflects elasticity (or rigidity) of vessel walls, patency (or obstruction) of lumen and changes in peripheral vascular resistance. These facts have been related to various parameters of curve phase by various authors. There is no space to elaborate on these unfortunately, but it should be mentioned that these correlations and measurements represent the basis for diagnostic applications of REG by many authors. From calculations of the impedance (or conductivity) of the overall

---

* Since all such changes are caused by the entering of the pulse wave into the cranial cavity they are desirable.

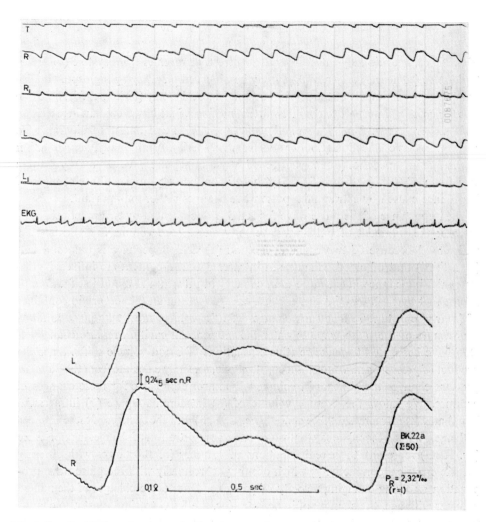

Fig. 1. Routine REG-tracing (upper half) and averaged curve arrived at by automatically averaging
100 curve phases using CAT 400 B and an x-y-recorder. By this enlarged registration, details of REG
are better visualized.

volume changes occurring intracranially we obtain information for (so-far) semi-
quantitative evaluation of an REG-tracing. We thereby gain information on and
insight into cerebral hemodynamic aspects otherwise inaccessible to us. After these
basic considerations we turn to practical applications of REG in medicine, with special
emphasis on our field, neurosurgery. First, let us look at a normal tracing (Fig. 1)
and the enlarged details of the sinusoidal phase of an REG which become better
evident by automatic averaging (Lifshitz, 1964). The start of a phase is clearly seen.
It occurs during the isometric phase of ventricular systole. The rising (anacrote)
part of the curve corresponds to the rapid (early) emptying of the cardiac ventricle
(Zouhar and Nevratal, 1966). The first peak is in constant temporary relationship
to the R-wave of the ECG (which conveniently is used to trigger the computer).

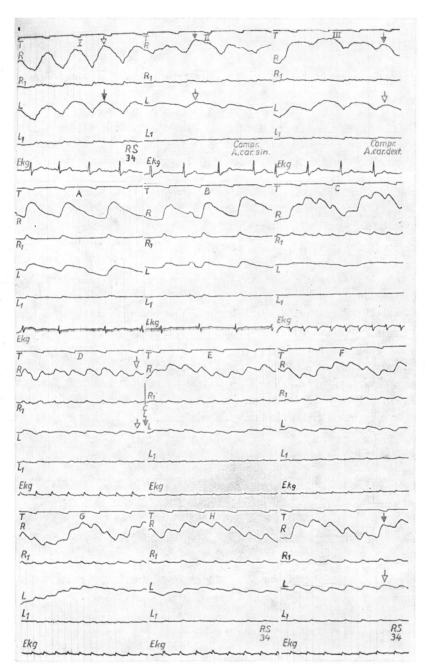

Fig. 2. REG-registration before, during and after carotid tie in case of infraclinoidal carotid aneurysm. Sections of continuous recording are shown: I–III = control and recordings during percutaneous rt. and lt. carotid compression. A = preoperative control, B = after approaching carotid bifurcation; C = immediately upon occluding common carotid artery (lt). Other lettered sample recordings follow (CL = definite tie placed). Pulse returns.

There follows a dip and a second peak (between these two there is the slow part of ventricular emptying (*l.c.*). From looking at one phase of the REG, it is evident that there are several details important for the evaluation of a tracing. However, not all apparatus commercially available do provide us with these details. Some models are not suited for our purposes.

There are 4 distinct groups of design of apparatus presently in use. Due to limitation in space, we can not go into these details here as we can merely mention that one or more of 9 different parameters of a curve phase are being used by various investigators to evaluate the REG. However, to all interested participants of this meeting, I shall gladly supply all desired information personally. It has to be mentioned that synchronous registration of EEG, ECG and other physiological parameters is possible with all principles of design using simple precautions. At present, there are at least 17 models of apparatus available commercially and many more experimental, pilot or institutional models are in use in various centers throughout the world.

Turning to practical aspects of REG, it must be stated first that irrespective of field studies (Lifshitz, 1964), which clearly demonstrate intracranial changes of impedance to be most important, the most essential testing of any method giving data on cerebral circulation is the registration during temporary clamping of various main vessels on occasions of carotid ties by neurosurgeons in the human. Fig. 2 provides this information (case of infraclinoidal aneurysm with common carotid tie, insufficient collateral circulation: when collateral blood supply is satisfactory, amplitude would remain constant while peak of phase would be delayed). This points out that an acute event is clearly defined by certain definite changes in the REG, while an occlusion of long standing may present difficulties when evaluating a curve. Examples of smaller vessel occlusions (m.c.a., a.c.a.) are given. Opposite changes in an REG tracing are observable in cases of a.-v. shunting, such as in carotid-cavernous

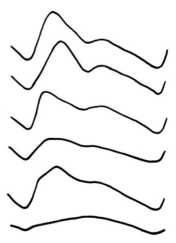

Fig. 3. Schematic drawings of various shapes of REG-curves (top to bottom): normal, vascular occlusion, a.-v. shunting, cerebral compression and arteriosclerosis, beginning as well as advanced arteriosclerosis.

Model Studies of the Circle of Willis:
Flow and Pressure Changes

WILLIAMINA A. HIMWICH AND M. E. CLARK

Thudichum Psychiatric Research Laboratory, Galesburg State Research Hospital, Galesburg, Illinois (U.S.A.), and Department of Theoretical and Applied Mechanics, College of Engineering, University of Illinois, Urbana, Illinois (U.S.A.)

The relative inaccessibility of the circle of Willis in the living animal as well as the technical difficulties of measuring simultaneous flow and pressure at a number of points has made it necessary to attempt studies of pressure and flow by means of a model. So far we have used a steady flow-rigid vessel model which has evolved through a fluid model, an electrical analog and a computer model. This model which is designed to conform with the circle of Willis in the dog has been evaluated by measurements made in the living animal[1–3]. Unfortunately, however, only pressure measurements have been obtained from experiments.

The model of the circle of Willis (Fig. 1) was designed using four basic criteria[1]: (a) a pressure drop of 115 mm Hg occurs across the system from the basilar-vertebral

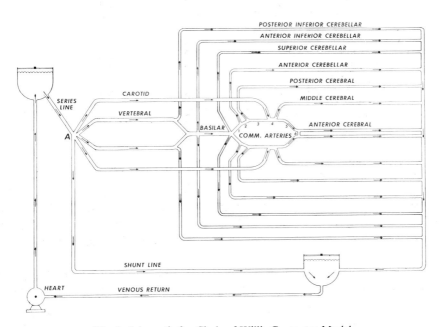

Fig. 1. Schematic for Circle of Willis Computer Model.

junction to venous return, (b) a total cerebral flow of 63 ml/100 gm of dog brain per minute occurs in the system, (c) an equal division of the afferent flow among the two carotids and the basilar artery, and (d) distribution of the efferent flow in accordance with the weight of brain irrigated by each vessel. In addition a physiologically feasible heart pressure of 135 mm Hg has been imposed as a work load.

In order to determine the difference in the hemodynamics in a model based on monkey instead of dog, we programmed a second computer model using data obtained from monkey brains (supplied through the courtesy of Dr. John S. Meyer of Detroit, Michigan, U.S.A.). For this model the criteria were the same as given above, except for the cerebral blood flow which was 51 ml/100 g of brain as taken from published data. As for the dog the actual diameters of the cerebral vessels of the monkey (Table I)

TABLE I

DIAMETERS OF CEREBRAL ARTERIES IN DOG AND MONKEY

Artery	Dog (mm) (10)	Monkey (mm) (7)
Right Vertebral	0.7	1.1
Left Vertebral	0.7	1.3
Basilar or Pons	1.1	1.5
Basilar at Circle	1.1	1.3
R. Anterior Cerebellar	0.6	0.5
L. Anterior Cerebellar	0.6	0.5
R. Posterior Cerebral	0.8	1.0
L. Posterior Cerebral	0.8	1.0
R. Posterior Communicating	0.7	0.6
L. Posterior Communicating	0.7	0.6
R. Internal Carotid	1.2	1.1
L. Internal Carotid	1.0	1.2
R. Mid. Cerebral	1.0	1.0
L. Mid. Cerebral	1.0	1.0
R. Anterior Communicating	0.8	0.8
L. Anterior Communicating	0.9	0.9
Anterior Cerebral	1.2	1.1

were used for construction of the model. Unfortunately, the use of blood flow figures from the literature result in total flow values which are not really comparable for the two species since for the dog figures are largely for cortical flow and in the monkey for whole brain flow. This situation arises because in the dog venous blood for cerebral blood flow determinations was taken from the sagittal sinus, in the monkey from the external jugular.

In order to have some measure of the efferent resistance which should be given to the various arteries arising from the circle the weight of brain tissue supplied by the various arteries (Table II) was used as reference. It is recognized that this is far from a perfect reference since there will be considerable difference in vascularity in white and

TABLE II

WEIGHT (GRAMS) OF BRAIN SUPPLIED BY CEREBRAL ARTERIES

Artery	Dog – (10)	Monkey – (7)
Anterior Cerebellar	3.7	11.6*
Posterior Cerebral	6.2	19.2
Middle Cerebral	16.9	44.8
Anterior Cerebral	7.6	10.5

* Derived value obtained from weight residue left after the weight of the other parts was subtracted from the total brain weight. This value was used in the computer program.

gray matter. However in the absence of actual flow data for each of the arteries, this basis for relating resistance appeared to us to be the best available. If the middle cerebral value is taken as 1 then the relative resistance figures for the posterior cerebral and the anterior cerebral in dog are 0.37 and 0.44 respectively. The figures relative to the middle cerebral for these arteries in monkey are 0.43 and 0.21, respectively. These differences emphasize the larger relative size of the hemispheres in monkey than in dog. We hope by comparing dog and monkey to evaluate how our model would function in predicting changes in cerebral circulation in man with proportionately even larger hemispheres.

The total flow and pressure of the models for the dog and for the monkey show very little difference between the two animals except for the flow in the anterior cerebral artery which is much lower in the monkey than in the dog (Table III, columns A and B). Pressure values are slightly higher at the carotid-circle and anterior cerebral-circle junctions for the monkey than for the dog. The second column under the heading *normal* translates the ml/min value into percent of total flow. Again there is considerable correspondence. However, the comparison of the percentage figures shows that in the monkey a greater percentage of flow leaves the circle through the anterior cerebellar, the posterior cerebral and the middle cerebral with correspondingly less passing out the anterior cerebral. In the monkey, therefore, we have a greater amount of flow going to the posterior and middle sections of the hemisphere and less to the frontal areas. The distribution proportions (Table II) of brain weight for the two animals would suggest this and of course the relative resistance figures used based on this table were responsible for the resulting flows. If the left carotid is occluded in either model the differences between the two are not very great, although the monkey model maintains somewhat higher flows throughout (Table III). These data demonstrate the ability of either model to maintain its usual pattern of flow regardless of the differences in original efferent distribution. It might be predicted that the prototype would show the same response unless factors such as metabolism override the response. The relative difference between models remains much the same although it becomes slightly less as the occlusions increase in number from one carotid to two carotids plus one vertebral.

Experiments conducted by Dr. Bruno Cucciniello of Naples, Italy while at the

TABLE III

COMPARISON OF CIRCLE OF WILLIS MODEL FOR DOG AND FOR MONKEY

Artery Flow	Normal* All Arteries Open (ml/min)		% of Total Flow (%)		Occlusions Left Carotid (%**)		Both Carotids (%)		Both Carotids and R. Vertebral (%)	
	A	B	A	B	A	B	A	B	A	B
Total System Flow	475.0	472.0			99.0	99.3	97.0	97.5	95.6	96.0
Total Cerebral Flow	46.54	44.14			89.2	91.7	68.6	72.4	53.9	56.0
Right Carotid	15.33	14.71	33,3	33.3	131.4	140.5	206.3	217.4	324.4	336.7
Right Vertebral	7.74	7.36	16.7	16.7	136.5	134.9	206.3	217.4	162.2	168.3
Basilar	15.84	14.72	33.3	33.3	136.5	134.9	75.9	79.8	59.7	61.8
Left Ant. Cerebellar	2.36	2.97	5.1	6.7	91.4	94.0	74.4	79.2	58.5	61.3
Left Post. Cerebral	4.02	4.90	8.6	11.1	90.3	93.6	66.2	68.7	52.0	53.2
Left Mid. Cerebral	11.39	11.50	24.5	26.0	84.8	88.3	66.2	68.7	52.0	53.2
Ant. Cerebral	11.01	5.40	23.7	12.2	88.4	90.7				
Junction Pressure (mm Hg)	A	B			A (%)	B	A (%)	B	A (%)	B
Carotid-Vertebral Origin***	132.9	132.9			100.0	100.0	100.1	100.0	100.1	100.1
Basilar-Vertebral	115.4	115.1			94.5	94.6	83.9	81.8	66.0	63.4
Left Carotid-Circle	106.3	113.7			84.7	88.2	66.2	68.7	52.0	53.2
Ant. Cerebral-Circle	102.5	112.5			88.4	90.7	66.2	68.7	52.0	53.2

* = A = Dog model, B = Monkey.
** = % = Ratio of Abnormal to Normal Flow or Pressure. 100% = actual values in normal column.
*** = Point A, Fig. 1.

TABLE IV

PREDICTED PROTOTYPE DATA FOR RIGHT MIDDLE CEREBRAL OCCLUSION IN DOG (A) AND MONKEY (B)

| Artery Flow | Normal | | | | Occlusions | | | | | |
| | All Arteries Open (ml/min) | | RMC* (%**) | | RMC and Lft. Car. (%) | | RMC and Rt. Car. (%) | | RMC and Lft. Vert. (%) | |
	A***	B	A	B	A	B	A	B	A	B
Total Cerebral Flow	46.54	44.14	79.2	76.4	71.2	71.1	73.5	72.6	77.0	74.4
Lft. Carotid	15.33	14.71	84.4	80.0			109.3	109.6	93.3	90.8
Rt. Carotid	15.53	14.71	70.5	66.5	99.3	101.3			79.7	77.6
Lft. Vertebral	7.74	7.36	82.3	83.1	114.7	112.3	111.2	108.6		
Rt. Vertebral	7.74	7.36	82.3	83.1	114.7	112.3	111.2	108.6	115.7	110.0
Lft. Ant. Cerebellar	2.36	2.97	103.9	102.9	96.3	97.9	97.6	98.6	100.1	99.1
Rt. Ant. Cerebellar	2.36	2.97	104.2	103.0	97.2	98.0	97.4	98.6	100.4	99.2
Lft. Post. Cerebral	4.02	4.90	103.9	103.0	95.4	97.6	97.7	98.6	100.4	99.3
Rt. Post. Cerebral	4.02	4.90	104.7	103.1	97.7	98.1	97.1	98.5	101.2	99.4
Lft. Mid. Cerebral	11.39	11.50	104.0	103.5	90.8	93.8	97.7	98.4	101.8	101.7
Rt. Mid. Cerebral	11.39	11.50								
Ant. Cerebral	11.01	5.40	105.9	104.7	95.5	96.9	96.6	97.9	103.6	102.8

| Junction Pressure | All Arteries Open (mm Hg) | | RMC* (%) | | RMC and Lft. Car. (%) | | RMC and Rt. Car. (%) | | RMC and Lft. Vert. (%) | |
	A	B	A	B	A	B	A	B	A	B
Basilar-Vertebral	115.4	115.1	102.7	102.7	97.8	98.1	98.4	98.7	97.7	98.5
Lft. Ant. Cerebellar-Circle	108.3	113.4	103.9	102.9	96.3	97.9	97.6	98.6	100.1	99.1
Rt. Ant. Cerebellar-Circle	108.3	113.4	104.2	103.0	97.2	98.0	97.4	98.6	100.4	99.2
Lft. Post. Cerebral-Circle	107.4	113.1	103.9	103.0	95.4	97.6	97.7	98.6	100.4	99.3
Rt. Post. Cerebral-Circle	107.4	113.1	104.7	103.1	97.7	98.1	97.1	98.5	101.2	99.4
Lft. Carotid-Circle	106.3	113.7	103.9	103.4	90.6	93.7	97.7	98.4	101.7	101.6
Rt. Carotid-Circle	106.3	113.7	107.4	105.7	100.2	99.8	95.3	97.1	105.1	103.8
Lft. Mid. Cerebral-Circle	105.8	113.4	104.0	103.5	90.8	93.8	97.7	98.4	101.8	101.7
Rt. Mid. Cerebral-Circle	105.8	113.4	107.7	105.9	100.3	99.9	95.6	97.3	105.4	104.0
Ant. Cerebral-Circle	102.5	112.5	105.9	104.7	95.6	96.9	96.6	97.9	103.6	102.8

* RMC = Right Middle Cerebral Artery.
** % = Ratio of Abnormal to Normal Flow or Pressure. 100% = values in normal column.
*** A = Dog model, B = Monkey.

References p. 143

Thudichum Laboratory show that in the living dog when the left carotid is occluded the pressure at the basilar-vertebral junction falls to 97% of its normal value. Occlusion of both carotids results in a rise in systemic pressure of 2.7% and practically no change at the basilar-vertebral junction. The models can do a fairly effective job of preserving basilar-vertebral pressure when only one carotid is occluded; beyond this point, however, they fail to approach the efficiency of the living animal.

The models can be used to analyze the response of the cerebral circulation to pathological conditions and thus lead to a better understanding of clinical cerebrovascular disorders. One condition of clinical interest is the complete occlusion by a thrombus of a middle cerebral artery. In the models, for monkey and for dog brain, one middle cerebral (the right) was occluded. All flow and pressure comparisons were made with those that occurred in the model with all efferent and afferent vessels open (*Normal*, Table IV). With the right middle cerebral occluded, blood flow fell most markedly in the right carotid (Table IV) especially in the monkey model, although flow was also decreased somewhat in the other inflow tubes. Normal flow was maintained in all the unoccluded efferent vessels and pressure throughout the circle remained normal.

Waltz *et al.*[4] have studied by means of radioactive krypton the changes in cortical blood flow in the cat and the squirrel monkey due to occlusion of one middle cerebral artery. As the authors do not specify the exact counting position over the hemispheres it is impossible to determine what effect posterior and anterior cerebral anastomoses with the middle cerebral may have had. It is nonetheless interesting that only the occluded side showed changes in blood flow following the occlusion as we have predicted from our model[3]. It would have been exceedingly interesting if the authors had also determined total blood flow. McHenry[5], however, has also shown that in infarctions of the middle cerebral artery or the internal carotid in man total CBF was reduced 13%. In our model we predicted a reduction of 11% in the dog and 13% in monkey following the occlusion of one middle cerebral artery[3]. The model can be used to help explain why a fall in total blood flow follows the removal of an efferent artery. The removal of an outflow increases the resistance of the system and therefore reduces blood flow.

With the right middle cerebral already occluded, the occlusion of the left carotid increased all remaining afferent flows, but total flow was further reduced. Even with this double occlusion, the left middle cerebral in the dog model was the only vessel whose outflow was decreased as much as 10%. At the same time the only junctions at which pressures fell this amount were in the region of the occluded afferent. The occurrence of a sink of pressure in this region can be attributed to the fact that the outflow under these circumstances in the left middle cerebral is derived principally from the right carotid. The drop in pressure must be such as to move flow around the anterior end of the circle and then posteriorly to the left middle cerebral. Causal analysis of the pressure percentages might indicate a pressure sink at the left carotid-circle junction (90.6%) when in terms of actual pressure it occurs at the left middle cerebral-circle junction. When the efferent and afferent occlusions both occur on the same side, it can be seen (Table IV) that there is a greater return to normality in both pressure and flow. The larger total flow which occurred indicates that less use was

TABLE V

PREDICTED PROTOTYPE DATA FOR RIGHT POSTERIOR COMMUNICATING OCCLUSION IN DOG (A) AND MONKEY (B)

Artery Flow	Normal				Occlusions					
	All Arteries Open (ml/min)		RPC* (%**)		RPC and Lft. Car. (%)		RPC and Rt. Car. (%)		RPC and Lft. Vert. (%)	
	A***	B	A	B	A	B	A	B	A	B
Total Cerebral Flow	46.54	44.14	99.9	100.0	89.2	91.6	86.0	90.6	96.8	96.6
Lft. Carotid	15.53	14.71	99.9	99.8			138.5	148.4	110.6	112.5
Rt. Carotid	15.53	14.71	103.4	98.7	134.3	141.4			108.8	106.4
Lft. Vertebral	7.74	7.36	96.5	101.5	133.3	134.0	119.7	124.0		
Rt. Vertebral	7.74	7.36	96.5	101.5	133.3	134.0	119.7	124.0	142.6	142.8
Lft. Ant. Cerebellar	2.36	2.97	100.7	99.8	92.0	94.1	95.2	95.9	95.0	93.7
Rt. Ant. Cerebellar	2.36	2.97	100.9	99.7	92.9	94.2	95.9	95.9	94.9	93.6
Lft. Post. Cerebral	4.02	4.90	100.6	99.8	90.8	93.8	94.5	95.6	95.4	94.0
Rt. Post. Cerebral	4.02	4.90	101.1	99.7	93.1	94.2	96.1	95.9	95.1	93.6
Lft. Mid. Cerebral	11.39	11.50	100.0	100.0	84.8	88.3	90.0	91.6	97.4	97.9
Rt. Mid. Cerebral	11.39	11.50	99.2	100.2	91.3	92.9	75.0	84.4	97.8	98.9
Ant. Cerebral	11.01	5.40	99.6	100.1	88.0	90.6	82.5	88.0	97.6	98.4
Junction Pressure (mm Hg)										
Basilar-Vertebral	115.4	115.1	100.5	99.8	95.0	94.7	97.0	96.3	93.5	93.4
Lft. Ant. Cerebellar-Circle	108.3	113.4	100.7	99.8	92.0	94.1	95.2	95.9	95.0	93.7
Rt. Ant. Cerebellar-Circle	108.3	113.4	100.9	99.7	92.9	94.2	95.9	95.9	94.9	93.6
Lft. Post. Cerebral-Circle	107.4	113.1	100.6	99.8	90.8	93.8	94.5	95.6	95.4	93.6
Rt. Post. Cerebral-Circle	107.4	113.1	101.1	99.7	93.1	94.2	96.1	95.9	95.1	94.0
Lft. Carotid-Circle	106.3	113.7	100.0	100.0	84.7	88.2	90.4	91.8	97.4	97.9
Rt. Carotid-Circle	106.3	113.7	99.2	100.2	91.4	93.0	74.7	82.2	97.8	98.9
Lft. Mid. Cerebral-Circle	105.8	113.4	100.0	100.0	84.8	88.3	90.0	91.6	97.4	97.9
Rt. Mid. Cerebral-Circle	105.8	113.4	99.2	100.2	91.3	92.9	75.0	84.4	97.8	98.9
Ant. Cerebral-Circle	102.5	112.5	99.6	100.1	88.0	90.6	82.5	88.0	97.6	98.4

* RPC = Right Posterior Communicating Artery.
** % = Ratio of Abnormal to Normal Flow or Pressure. 100% = values in normal column.
*** A = Dog model, B = Monkey.

References p. 143

made of the circle itself to redistribute the flow and since shorter resistance paths were involved the total flow was increased. When one vertebral was occluded, the total flow into the brain was slightly greater than with one carotid closed. Since the vertebral is a smaller vessel than the carotid its resistance to flow per unit length is larger. The criterion on afferent flow establishes that one carotid flow is equal to both vertebral flows. In this case efferent pressure and flows were maintained above the normal situation.

The above discussion of the occlusive patterns is in relation to the all open or normal pattern. The occlusion of a middle cerebral, however, immediately reduces the flow into the circle by approximately 10–15%. The effects of carotid or vertebral occlusion subsequent to the middle cerebral block are very similar to those which occur with the middle cerebral open. The previous closing of a middle cerebral, therefore, does not render the occlusion of a carotid or vertebral relatively more serious, although in terms of actual pressures and flows the decreases due to the loss of the middle cerebral are intensified. The combination of middle cerebral occlusion and the loss of a carotid inflow results in an additional reduction of flow of only 5–8%. In general it can be postulated that whatever the flow, it is distributed in the same relative manner as when all arteries are open; a demonstration of the anastomotic value of the circle.

As a second study of pathological conditions the right posterior communicating tube was occluded to simulate the absence or impatency of a posterior communicating. With all afferent arteries open and one posterior communicating closed, flows and pressures were essentially normal (Table V). If, with the right posterior communicating already occluded, the left carotid were closed, flows increased enough in the open inflow tubes to give an almost normal total flow. As might be expected the left middle cerebral had the largest reduction (15%); the anterior cerebral was reduced by 12% in the dog model. Corresponding values for the monkey model were 12% and 10% for the middle cerebral and the anterior cerebral respectively. If these flow data are compared with those obtained with the circle completely opened and the left carotid occluded (Table III), it can be seen that the changes are essentially the same in both conditions. These model data suggest that under these circumstances the closure of the posterior communicating makes essentially no difference in the ability of the circle to equalize pressure and flow.

Since the right and left carotids contribute equal amounts of resistance to the system it would seem to be immaterial, as regards the efferent flow, as to which carotid was occluded in the presence of an occluded right posterior communicating artery. The data (Table V) show a contradiction to this observation, however, since the flow in the ipsilateral middle cerebral drops 10% more in one case than in the other. The explanation for this decreased flow when both occlusions occur on the same side of the circle lies in the significant increase in pressure difference between open carotid and contralateral middle cerebral. In other words, the posterior portion of the circle aids in maintaining pressure at the middle cerebral if the occlusions occur on opposite sides of the circle. When both occlusions occur on the same side some of the communicating vessels on the anterior end of the circle pass considerable more flow (with concomitantly larger pressure drops) toward the defrauded distal middle cerebral (Fig. 2).

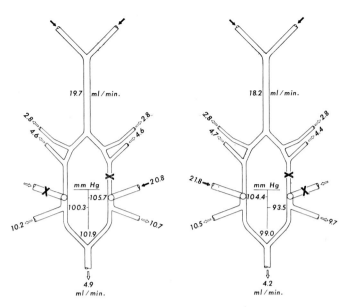

Fig. 2. Equalization in the Circle of Willis in the presence of a posterior communicating occlusion (monkey).

REFERENCES

1 HIMWICH, W. A., KNAPP, F. M., WENGLARZ, R. A., MARTIN, J. D. AND CLARK, M. E. (1965) The Circle of Willis as Simulated by an Engineering Model. *Arch. Neurol.*, **13**, 164–172.

2 CLARK, M. E., MARTIN, J. D., WENGLARZ, R. A., HIMWICH, W. A. AND KNAPP, F. M. (1965) Engineering Analysis of the Hemodynamics of the Circle of Willis. *Arch. Neurol.*, **13**, 173–182.

3 CLARK, M. E., HIMWICH, W. A., AND MARTIN J. D. (1967) Simulation studies of factors influencing the cerebral circulation. *Acta Neurol. Scand.*, **43**, 189–204.

4 WALTZ, A. G., SUNDT, T. M., JR. AND OWEN, C. A., JR. (1966) Effect of middle cerebral artery occlusion on cortical blood flow in animals. *Neurology*, **16**, 1190.

5 MCHENRY, L. C. (1966) Cerebral blood flow studies in middle cerebral and internal carotid artery occlusion. *Neurology*, **16**, 1145–1150.

Observations on Continuous Vascular Pulsative Phenomena in the Cerebral Cortex of Experimental Animals with Special Reference to the Effects of Closed *vs.* Opened Calvarium

ALBERT F. HECK

Department of Neurology, University of Maryland, School of Medicine, Baltimore, Maryland (U.S.A.)

Preliminary observations have been made on continuous recordings of change in optical density of the cerebral cortex and of the ipsilateral ear with vascular pulsation in anesthetized cats and in fully conscious monkeys with chronic implantation of transducers. The technique used employs fiber optic light guides implanted onto the surface of the cortex through openings in the skull and meninges[1]. The calvarium is reclosed with dental cement. Light guides are attached to the ipsilateral ear by means of teflon receptacles sewn to opposing surfaces. Change in light intensity with change in optical density of tissue is converted by a photocell to a voltage for polygraphic recording. The electrocardiogram is recorded simultaneously. In anesthetized animals, respiration is monitored by a nasal thermistor and pressures are recorded from the abdominal aorta (in millimeters of mercury) and from the inferior vena cava or right atrium (in centimeters of water) through catheters appropriately placed in femoral artery, femoral vein or right external jugular vein. Finally, in some experiments, pressure in the subarachnoid space at the site of implantation is recorded through polyvinyl tubing implanted with the fiber optic probe.

The times elapsed from ventricular excitation, that is from the QRS complex of the electrocardiogram, until arrival of the corresponding pulse wave in the brain, in the ear or in the aorta, and until occurrence of the next QRS complex are measured in milliseconds by means of a time-interval monitoring system previously described[2]. Time interval measurements are printed successively on paper tape in this manner by a digital printer. An electronic clock supplies the printer with diurnal or "clock" time in minutes and seconds at which the various time interval measurements are made. "Clock" time from the printer tape is correlated with the one second interval marker of the polygraphic recording. Measurements are referred to as the R-to-brain, R-to-ear, R-to-blood pressure and R-to-R times.

Pulse wave propagation time and its reciprocal, the pulse wave velocity, are dependent on the *relative* distensibility of the vascular wall[3-5]. Increase in propagation time corresponds to an increase in distensibility and, conversely, a shorter propagation time correlates with decreased distensibility of the vessel wall.

Time interval measurements are plotted against diurnal or "clock" time to provide continuous sampling of propagation times to brain, ear or aorta and of the intrinsic frequency of the heart beat — the R-to-R time. Instantaneous heart rate is calculated from R-to-R values by dividing into 60000 msec.

When plotted against diurnal time, propagation times and the R-to-R interval are found to fluctuate. In brain, fluctuation occurs irregularly from 6 to 18 times per minute. This activity is found to vary in two ways. It may vary in the mean level about which fluctuations take place. Or it may vary in the frequency at which fluctuations occur and in the duration over which an increase or decrease in propagation time persists. No consistent pattern is found at rest between fluctuation in propagation time and changes occurring with respiration in intracranial pressure or in systemic arterial or venous pressure.

Changes in optical density of cortex and ear occur at the same periodicity as does the heart beat. Aberrations in normal cardiac action as, for example, with ventricular extrasystole are clearly evident in both brain and ear simultaneously, but may differ in degree. Variation occurs in base line, wave amplitude and wave contour with changes in systemic arterial and venous pressures, in intracranial pressure and with respiration.

Animals in which the calvarium is closed exhibit a consistent phase difference in the initiation of pulsations in ear and in brain (Fig. 1). That of the ear precedes that of the brain. Behavior of propagation times in brain vs. ear are distinctly different. Propagation time to the brain is generally 40 to 100 msec longer than that to the ear, though

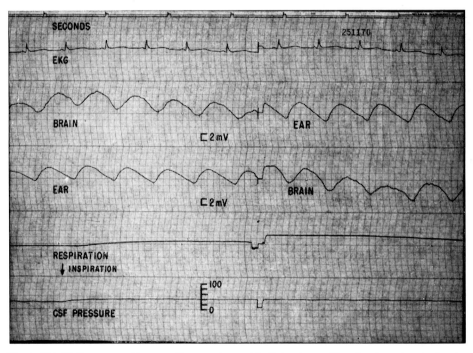

Fig. 1. Cat. Plethysmographic waves from cortex and ipsilateral ear with calvarium closed, showing phase difference in initiation of pulsations. CSF pressure in mm H_2O. Time base: 50 mm/sec. Recording was stopped and input cables to amplifiers reversed to demonstrate that phase difference is not pen artifact.

they may at times briefly approximate each other. The mean level of propagation time is found to vary at different periods in the same animal.

In animals where closure of the calvarium is never accomplished because of fluid leakage, and in animals in which a 2 cm defect in the skull and dura were made in the opposite parietal area, pulse waves from the brain tend to more closely resemble those from the ear in their contour and amplitude. Initiation and systolic peaks under these circumstances may be quite synchronous. Propagation time to either vascular bed is of the same magnitude, though differing in amplitude and frequency of fluctuation.

Integrity of the calvarium is *not*, however, the sole factor concerned in synchrony or asynchrony of brain and ear pulsation. In recording from cats in which cerebrospinal leakage occurred, initiation of brain and ear pulsations were synchronous. After placement of the 2 cm skull defect in the parietal area opposite, asynchrony was evident. Propagation time to brain and ear during the earlier recordings were found to be of the same magnitude. After placement of the 2 cm skull defect, the R-to-R time had decreased, heart rate was faster, and propagation time to the ear was also shorter. But propagation time to the brain were found to be remarkably stable despite introduction of the skull defect.

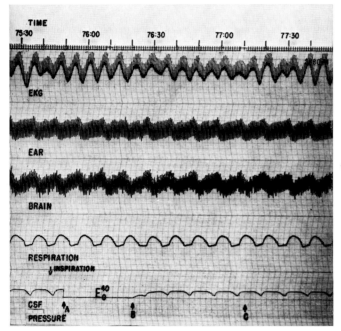

Fig. 2. Cat. Plethysmographic waves from cortex and ipsilateral ear. CSF pressure in mm H$_2$O. At "A" subarachnoid space opened to atmospheric pressure. System reclosed at "B" with return of CSF pressure to previous level at "C". Time base: 2 mm/sec.

Conversely, with the calvarium closed (Fig. 2), sudden opening of the subarachnoid space to atmospheric pressure at the site of the plethysmographic implantation by opening the pressure recording system at point "A" results in no change in brain pulse

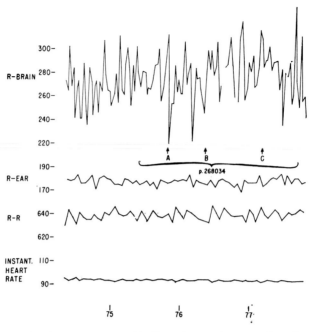

Fig. 3. Cat. Propagation times to cortex and ipsilateral ear and R-to-R times (msec) during events shown in Fig. 2. Transient decrease of R-to-brain time with opening subarachnoid space at A. Increase in mean level of R-to-brain time during reestablishment of CSF pressure from "B" to "C" with decrease in mean level following.

amplitude. Ear and brain pulses do *not* become synchronous during these brief periods. Reclosure of the system at point "B" results in gradual return of intracranial pressure to its previous level at point "C", but, again, no change is noted in the polygraphic recording. Propagation time to the brain (Fig. 3) may undergo transient decrease or increase at the time of opening at point "A". During the time subarachnoid pressure is returning to its previous level, there is usually, though not always a change in the mean level of propagation time, followed by a change in the opposite direction during the minute or so after subarachnoid pressure has been reestablished at point "C".

It should be emphasized that reduction of subarachnoid pressure from levels of 30 to 100 mm of water to zero pressure for these brief periods of time is within the range of change occurring under normal physiologic conditions, as for example, in changing posture from prone to erect.

Two classes of mechanisms are suggested as playing simultaneous roles in the demonstrated phenomena of cortical pulsation and of cortical vascular distensibility as monitored by the R-to-brain propagation time. One class of mechanism is concerned with the purely mechanical factors affecting this activity — intravascular pressure, tissue pressure, vascular transmural pressure and volume changes. The second class of mechanisms has not been touched upon at all in these data. These are the mechanisms concerned with local metabolic demand and feed back from brain tissues supplied by the vessels monitored.

These data suggest that where changes in intracranial pressure occur within the range of normal physiologic variation, mechanisms regulating cerebrovascular distensibility provide remarkable stability. In this, integrity of the calvarium may have an important though limited role, since by allowing for establishment of intracranial pressures which can vary widely above *and* below atmospheric pressure, integrity of the calvarium may allow for finer adjustment in vascular transmural pressure as this affects vascular distensibility. At atmospheric pressure, decrease in propagation time and in vascular distensibility appear to have a lower limit. At this lower limit, introduction of a skull defect of significant size causes no further decrease in propagation time. It is suggested that under these circumstances other mechanisms — metabolic, mechanical, or both — become engaged even more prominently in preserving the stability of the system.

ACKNOWLEDGMENT

This work supported by the U.S. Army Medical Research and Development Command under Research Contract. ±DA-549-193-MD-2229 and by The National Institutes of Health, NINDB Grant, NB-05077.

REFERENCES

1 HECK, A. F. AND HALL, V. R. (1964) A Technique for Differential Photoelectric Plethysmography of Brain and Ear. *J. Appl. Physiol.*, **19**, 1236.
2 HALL, V., CAGGIANO, V. AND HECK, A. F. (1965) An On-line System for Recording Physiologic Time Intervals. *Am. J. Med. Electr.*, **4**, 161.
3 HAMILTON, W. F., REMINGTON, J. W. AND DOW, P. (1945) The Determination of the Propagation Velocity of the Arterial Pulse Wave. *Am. J. Physiol.*, **144**, 521.
4 HAMILTON, W. F. (1962) *Measurement of the Cardiac Output*, in Handbook of Physiology: Circulation, Vol. I, Am. Physiol. Soc., Washington, D.C., pp. 555–557.
5 HARDUNG, V. (1962) *Propagation of Pulse Waves in Visco-Elastic Tubings*, in Handbook of Physiology: Circulation, Vol. I, Am. Physiol. Soc., Washington, D.C., pp. 107–135.

Neuropathology of Intracranial Haemorrhage

ZÜLCH K. J.

Cologne (Germany)

INTRODUCTION

Neurosurgical procedures influence the course of intracranial haemorrhages: (1) by surgical closure of the source of haemorrhage in many cases; (2) by removing the blood clot which is space occupying and the cause of perifocal oedema at the same time[1,2]. Indication to surgery is then closely related to pathogenesis[1]. Therefore it seems justified to discuss some of its details.

The following classification may serve as a basis for discussion.

A. Haemorrhages mainly due to localized causes

1. Trauma:

(a) Epidural haemorrhage. In the majority of cases it follows a traumatic lesion of the middle meningeal artery, rarely venous oozing in decreased intracranial pressure may be responsible. Site and extension of epidural bleeding may be explained by the anatomical fixation of the dura to the skull; therefore, the localization may be different from that of a typical subdural haematoma, whose predilection site in the free subdural fronto-temporo-parietal space is well known[3,4]. The epidural haemorrhage may on the other hand be more frontal, temporal or occipital-parietal (Fig. 1) according to the site of the fracture affecting a branch of the middle meningeal artery. The second, postoperative form arising from venous oozing into the epidural space is naturally related to the site of the surgical flap since we all know, how well the dura is fixed to the bone.

(b) Subdural (acute and chronic) haemorrhage including chronic subdural *encapsulated* haemorrhages can spread more easily than the epidural ones because of the open subdural space. Its predilection site is in the centre of the three great lobes that is over the fronto-temporo-parietal region (Fig. 2). This latter may be explained by the site and direction of the mass movements giving way to the blood clot. These lateral shifts are determined by the mobility of the brain[5,6] underneath the falx and its fixation at the base and by its internal structure (great fasciculi of the white matter). Its mobility is dependent then upon the local resistance of the brain tissue to compression or deformation by the haematoma. This, in turn, may be influenced by the pressure of the CSF, by the intraarterial pressure, and by fixation of the brain itself (pituitary stalk, vessels, nerves) to the skull[5,6].

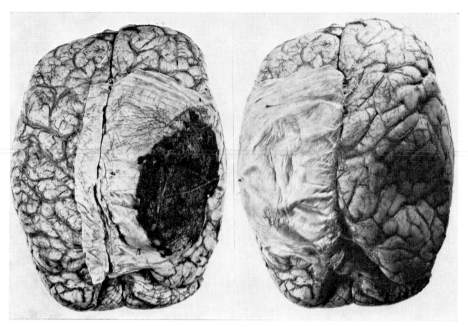

Fig. 1. Fresh epidural parietal haematoma.

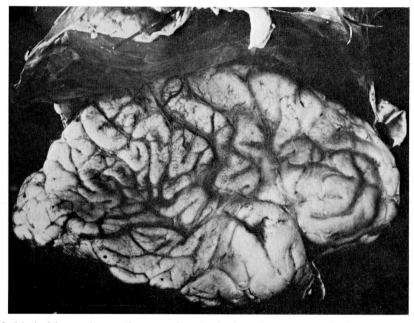

Fig. 2. Marked impression on the convexity of a brain with consequent displacement by an old
subdural capsulated haematoma (upper margin).

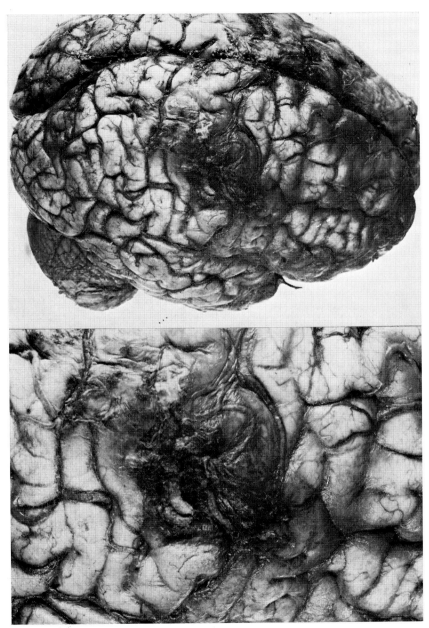

Fig. 3. Traumatic laceration of cortical arteries giving rise to acute subdural space occupying haematoma.

One point I ought to add in order to explain some figures from Dandy's "Surgery of the Brain". In rare cases the subdural encapsulated haematoma may be accompanied by a congenital arachnoidal cyst, a phenomenon which Dandy calls in his textbook on brain surgery, a "subdural hygroma" (Figs. 171, 172). We have also had such a patient, aged 48, who died in spite of the emptying of the subdural haematoma because

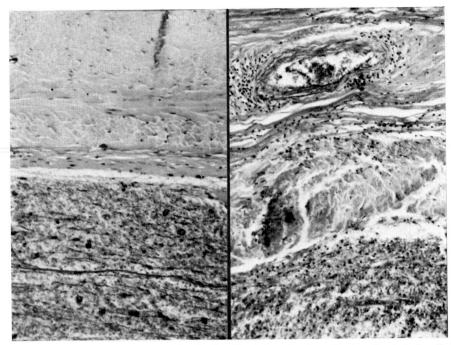

Fig. 4. Organization of the fresh blood film by fibroblastic invasion from the dura "endothelium". (a) From a healthy dura. HE, 125 ×. (b) in a dura with lymphoid infiltration and degenerative changes of the layers of the dura. HE, 125 ×.

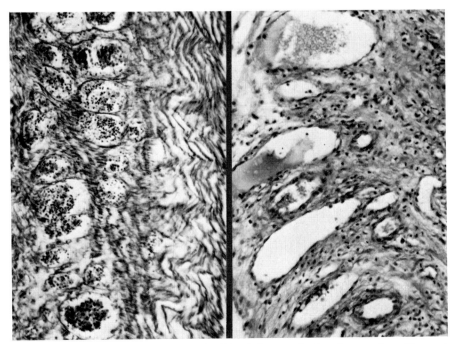

Fig. 5. Formation of new vessels in the organized blood clot near the dura in an angioma-like condensation. (a) HE, 125 ×. (b) Wilders impregnation, 125 ×.

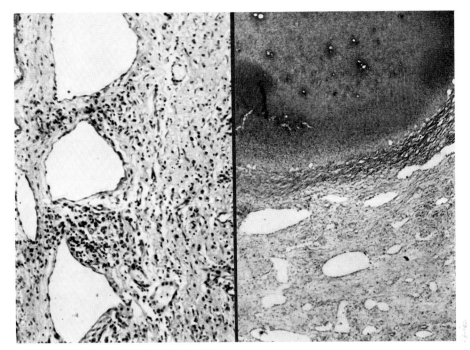

Fig. 6. (a) Great angioma-like vessels in the organized blood clot near the dura. HE, 125 ×. (b) Rupture of these vessels and formation of fresh haemorrhage. HE, 50 ×.

of a space occupying arachnoidal cyst in the Sylvian fissure underneath the haematoma, which was not recognized through the burr holes at surgery and was only revealed at autopsy. Usually a protrusion of the bone may indicate such a congenital cyst[7].

The acute traumatic subdural haematoma stems from a laceration of a major arterial vessel (Fig. 3) usually on the surface of the brain, as in our own case of a man aged 56. Here, if early and correctly diagnosed, surgery ought to be easy. The predilection site of this acute subdural haematoma corresponds to the subacute and chronical type.

These facts of a predilection site and a combination with other space occupying lesions seem to be of importance for roentgenology and echoencephalography in the diagnostic process of epidural and acute and chronic subdural encapsulated haematoma.

The fact of a predilection site of the subdural encapsulated haematoma is now better understood since we have a better insight into pathogenesis, where we distinguish between two forms: (1) a primary degenerative process of the dura, in the old-age group, called the true "pachymeningitis" or "pachymeningosis" of Virchow and (2) the posttraumatic subdural haematoma which is later encapsulated and is more common in younger people[3,4]. Macroscopically they both seem to be very similar processes. But there are histological differences in the dura. In pachymeningosis we find primary degenerative changes and/or lymphoid infiltration, whereas in the traumatic form the dura is unchanged or only secondarily affected. The various steps in the development of the encapsulated haematoma commence with a small blood film underneath (Fig. 4) the dura which becomes organized and forms capillaries and a cavernoma-like accumulation of vessels (Fig. 5) which may break and form small blood clots (Fig. 6). These blood clots attract cerebro-spinal fluid by osmosis according to the postulates of Gardner, who defined the inner membrane of the haematoma as an osmotic membrane. Thus, the small haematomas grow in size by taking up cerebro-spinal fluid. Then they tear other vessels in the granulation tissue. Thus new blood is added, the internal osmotic tension is reinforced and again cerebro-spinal fluid absorbed by increase of osmotic pressure: then these small haematomas unite, form a greater blood clot, and again new blood is added, thus the haematoma is steadily growing. At a certain moment it may be too big as to find reserve spaces in the internal and external spaces of the cerebro-spinal fluid, even though these spaces may be enlarged through atrophy of the aged brain. Finally the point of decompensation is reached, cranial pressure is beginning to rise, and neurological symptomatology will begin (Fig. 7).

This working hypothesis could be adopted not only for the posttraumatic form of subdural haematomas but for pachymeningosis as well if we only here presume that the first blood in the subdural space is not of traumatic origin from rupture of the bridge-

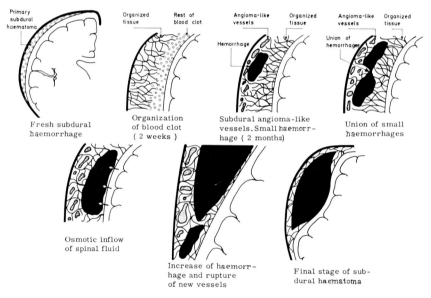

Fig. 7. Various stages of the pathogenesis of the capsulated subdural haematoma.

ing veins but comes from degenerative oozing on the internal surface — endothelium — of the degenerated dura. Thus, the thin primary blood film in the subdural space which is later transformed into a small granulation layer on the inside of the dura of one or both hemispheres can be of a twofold source: rupture of the bridgeing veins or oozing from the inside of the dura. As for the legal cases in the younger age group trauma may be regarded as the *main* cause whereas in older patients pachymeningosis, i.e., a primary degenerative process in the dura may be the lesion and forms therefore the main lesion, the formation of the haematoma in the pachymeningosis by a trauma being only secondary.

(c) Subarachnoid haemorrhage. Traumatic subarachnoid haemorrhage is usually associated with simultaneous subdural haemorrhage, whereas subarachnoid haemorrhage from aneurysms and angiomas tends to destroy and invade the surrounding brain tissue. Haemorrhage from ruptured saccular aneurysms penetrates into the neighbouring brain in a region typical for the site of the aneurysm; it is interesting to know that they, therefore, have a predilection site and thus form a very typical picture for each of the three great groups of the aneurysms of the basal arterial system. Thus we see a double-sided penetration of blood into the base of the medial frontal (Fig. 8)

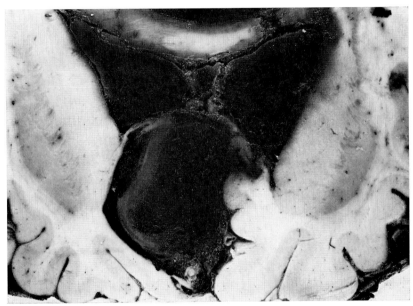

Fig. 8. Typical site of haemorrhage in a case of ruptured saccular aneurysm of the anterior communicating artery.

lobes from the ruptured aneurysms of the anterior communicating artery. In the posterior communicating artery we see a rupture (Fig. 9) into the temporal horn and finally we may find a haemorrhage in the Sylvian fissure breaking into the adjacent frontal and temporal lobe tissue in aneurysms of the middle cerebral artery (Fig. 10).

(d) Intracerebral haemorrhage (contusion, laceration of deep vessels of white matter). Posttraumatic intracerebral haemorrhage is usually subcortical and may be space occupying and therefore give rise to surgical emptying in the acute traumatic phase. Moreover it may be found as a special form in the old-age group as the so-called "Schwarzacher Markblutungen"; details of its pathogenesis are not yet quite clear (Fig. 11). The little traumatic pericapillary haemorrhage in contusion may enforce the significance of the local lesion by perifocal oedema. Haemorrhages into the mesencephalon and the pons are usually (Fig. 12) a consequence of an "axial shift" of the

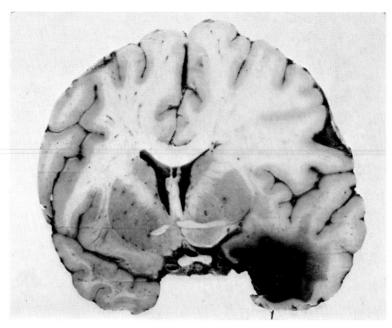

Fig. 9. Haemorrhage near the ruptured saccular aneurysm of posterior communicating artery. Typical localization.

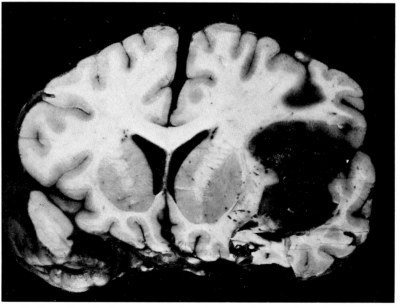

Fig. 10. Typical localization of haemorrhage in a case of ruptured saccular aneurysm of middle cerebral artery.

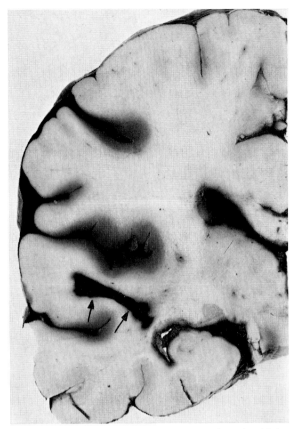

Fig. 11. Traumatic haemorrhage into the white matter. Acute subarachnoidal arterial haemorrhage by laceration, haematocephalus internus.

brain stem. This may be the following very acute hurling as in traumatism more commonly a consequence of an "axial shift" of the brain stem which may follow subacute shift in space occupying lesions in the supratentorial space[5]. In both cases tearing of the tips of the arteries and veins may be the consequence and this will result in periarterial or perivenous haemorrhages in the terminal parts of the vessels as shown by postmortem injection specimens.

2. Malformations and diseases of the intracranial vessels: Haemorrhages due to angiomas, malformations and saccular aneurysms.

Haemorrhage from angiomas may penetrate into the brain substance, into the subarachnoid space and into the ventricles through rupture of their walls.

A good many of cerebral mass haemorrhages particularly in younger people are seen in an *atypical* site which is easily distinguished from the typical hypertensive haemorrhages into the basal ganglia. The former have a predilection for the frontal parietal, or occipital region[1] and may be seen in the region between thalamus and quadrigeminal plate and even in the pons. They are usually encountered in younger

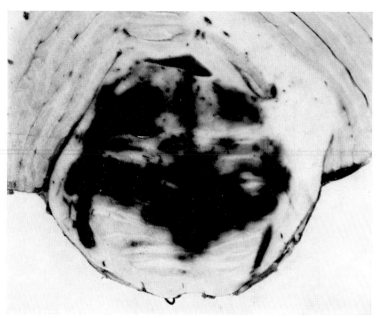

Fig. 12. Typical haemorrhages around bulbar veins and arteries in a case of marked "axial shift" in supratentorial tumour with gross brain oedema.

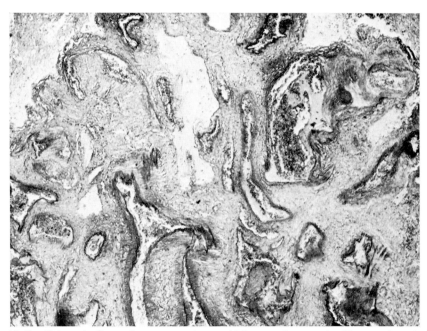

Fig. 13. Small (pea-sized) arteriovenous angioma which gave rise to a fatal haemorrhage (micro-angioma).

persons and caused very often by the rupture of a "microangioma" (Fig. 13), a term allowed in the clinical jargon. Morphologically it may correspond to the "telangiectatic" or "capillary angioma" or rarely to the cavernoma or even a small arteriovenous angioma. These we have seen particularly in the mesencephalothalamic region[8] (Figs. 401, 402).

3. Tumours:

Haemorrhage into tumours are met with mostly in oligodendrogliomas and glioblastomas, but also in cerebral metastases (hypernephroma, melanoma). They often form an alarming feature of the neurological symptomatology and may simulate a "stroke" particularly in older people. The pathogenesis of a rupture of these vessels is understandable in the huge disorderly fistulous vessels of glioblastomas (Zülch[8], Figs. 188 ff.). It is less well understood in the oligodendroglioma where, however, we may have calcification (Zülch[8], Fig. 112) and one should also try to understand the rupture of the friable larger vessels in metastases. Smaller haemorrhages into the necrotized parts of glioblastoma multiforme are part of its variegated picture and cause of the brownish and reddish colour of these tumours.

4. Cerebral infarctions:

Pericapillary haemorrhage in arterial infarction, mostly in the grey matter, is a typical feature of these softenings. They are explained by the endothelial damage of capillaries in the grey matter, where the oxygen-demand is five times higher than in the white substance and therefore cause an early lesion[9]. Haemorrhages in infarctions from venous obstruction, however, have their predilections in the white matter around the subcortical great veins and to a lesser extent also in the grey matter. Perivenous oozing around the great veins of the whole subcortical white matter including the corpus callosum in the case of fat embolism gives an almost specific pattern macroscopically[10]. The same perivenous haemorrhages, as seen for instance in penicillin and arsphenamine hypersensitivity, have a predilection site around the white matter of the ventricles.

5. Intracranial mass displacements:

Chronic or subacute space occupying lesions produce haemorrhage within the caudal brain stem similar to those in acute traumatic hurling. The mechanism is described above[5,6].

B. Cerebral haemorrhage mainly due to extracranial factors

(1a) Hypertensive–striate–haemorrhages:

Since the work of Guillaume attempts have also been made to evacuate typical mass haemorrhages surgically, i.e. the hypertensive haemorrhage of the older-age group, although in these cases irreversible rupture of the internal capsule is met with at the very beginning of the bleeding and usually leads to irreversible neurological symptoms like hemiplegia. Yet, in order to save life and to prevent perifocal oedema, which leads to an accentuation of the neurological syndrome, evacuation of the blood clot is con-

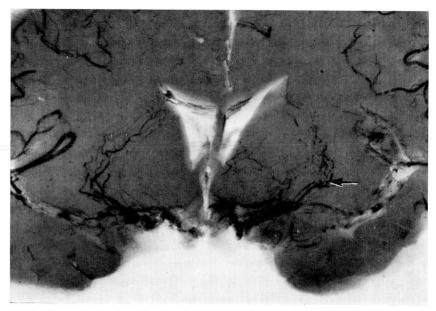

Fig. 14. Injection specimen of arteries of the basal ganglia. Arrow points to the probable site of rupture in case of hypertensive mass haemorrhage.

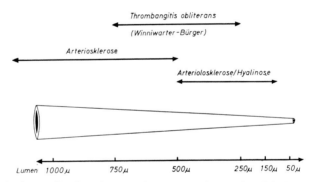

Fig. 15. Predilection of arterial disease according to size of the lumina.

sidered by some neurosurgeons, and it should be possible with a minor operation, i.e. a stereotactic suction, since we can exactly define the site of the bleeding vessel in more than 4/5 of all cases[1]. It lies a little above the knee (Fig. 14) of the lenticulostriate artery[9]. The pathogenesis of this hypertensive mass haemorrhage is still obscure although we know that hyalinosis (arteriolosclerosis) of the strio-lenticulate and lenticulo-optic artery is the predisposing factor. Hyalinosis follows long-standing hypertension, but the actual haemorrhage is usually provoked by an acute rise of blood pressure ("hypertensive crisis"). It is interesting to see how differently vascular diseases affect the arteries with regard to the size of their lumina. The sites of predilection of arteriosclerosis, for instance, range from the great brain arteries in the neck to the intracranial arteries of 1/2 mm inside diameter. Hyalinosis on the other hand, or

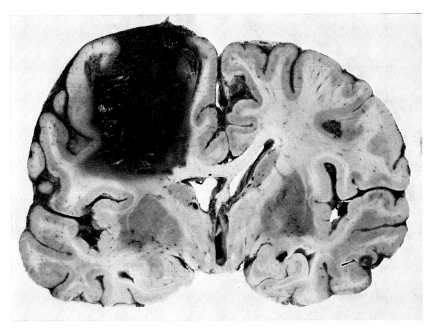

Fig. 16. "Atypical" haemorrhage without any relation to the lenticulostriate artery ("artery of apo-plexy").

arteriolosclerosis, is a disease of the *terminal* arteries particularly of those in the white substance, i.e. arteries around 250 μ size and beyond, whereas thrombangitis obliterans stands between both and affects vessels between 1 mm lumen and 250 μ [11].

With a little exaggeration one could say that these three major groups of arterial disease exclude each other by the size of the lumen of the affected arteries (Fig. 15). This change of arterial diseases in the course of an artery is particularly well seen in frontal sections through the lenticulo-striate artery, where in the horizontal plane of the anterior commissure arteriosclerosis stops and turns into the hyalinosis of the terminal branches met with in a more dorsal plane.

Yet, as in haemorrhages from very small branches of the middle meningeal artery, it seems still difficult to understand why from rupture of vessel of *1-mm* lumen, there may result enormous distortions and ruptures of the internal white matter with cavities the size of a fist;

(b) Atypical haemorrhages localized in paracapsular region (frontal, temporal, parietal) (Fig. 16) without local predilection occur mostly in younger people (see above). In occasional cases a small angioma in the subcortical white matter may be found as the cause of the haemorrhage (see above[9]) (Fig. 13).

2. *Pachymeningosis haemorrhagica:*

Chronic subdural encapsulated haematomas may not have a traumatic origin but result only from a previous degenerative lesion of the dura (see above).

References p. 165

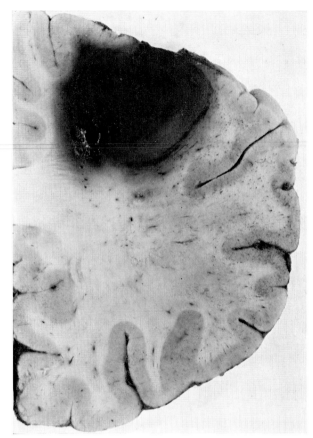

Fig. 17. Mass haemorrhage at the lower "frontier zone" of an infarct of the middle cerebral artery. It occurred after fibrinolytic (streptokinase) therapy.

3. Haemorrhages due to natural or iatrogenic disturbances of the coagulation system:
Cerebral haemorrhage resulting from changes in the blood coagulability without site of predilection may occur due to failures or unforeseen accidents in anticoagulation- or fibrinolytic therapy of thromboses of brain- or other arteries. Such haemorrhages are demonstrated by an own observation where during a typical regime of streptokinase, haemorrhages in the border line zones of an infarct occurred after thrombosis of the middle cerebral artery as a final and fatal complication. This haemorrhage was located in the frontier zone of the infarct, which very often itself is haemorrhagic by nature as was shown already by Virchow for the edge of the infarct (Fig. 17).

Thus, only the study of pathogenesis can lead to a rational therapy particularly if this is neurosurgical, i.e. consists of removal of the blood clot, because it can show the predilection site, the source of the bleeding vessel and the cause for its rupture.

REFERENCES

1 ZÜLCH, K. J. (1961) Zur Operation der intracerebralen Massenblutungen. Chirurgen-Kongress Leipzig. *Zbl. Chir.*, **86**, 350–359.
2 ZÜLCH, K. J. (1943) Hirnödem und Hirnschwellung. *Virch. Arch.*, **310**, 1–58.
3 ZÜLCH, K. J. (1950) Diskussion über das subdurale Hämatom. 2. Jahrestag d. Dtsch. Ges. Neurochir., Göttingen 1949. *Zbl. Neurochir.*, **10**, 305.
4 ZÜLCH, K. J. Histologische Untersuchungen bei chronischem subduralem Hämatom. *Hefte Unfallhk.*, **55**, 212–213.
5 ZÜLCH, K. J. (1959) *Störungen des intrakraniellen Druckes·* In Handb. der Neurochir., I/1. Springer-Verlag, pp. 208–303.
6 ZÜLCH, K. J. (1963) Les déplacements en masse dans les processus cérébraux expansifs et leurs rapports avec le siège et le genre de la tumeur — La classification des tumeurs cérébrales — Les altérations dues à l'hypertension intracranienne — Le "gonflement" et l'oedème cérébrale. *Acta Neurochir.*, **XI**, 161–193.
7 ZÜLCH, K. J. (1954) Betrachtungen über die Entstehung der frühkindlichen Hirnschäden auf Grund der klinischen und morphologischen Befunde. *Arch. Kinderhk.*, **149**, 3–27.
8 ZÜLCH, K. J. (1956) *Biologie und Pathologie der Hirngeschwülste*. In: Handbuch der Neurochirurgie, volume III, Springer-Verlag, Berlin.
9 ZÜLCH, K. J. (1961) Die Pathogenese von Massenblutung und Erweichung unter besonderer Berücksichtigung klinischer Gesichtspunkte. Kongr. Gesamtverb. Dtsch. Nervenärzte Köln 1959. *Acta Neurochir.*, *Suppl.* **VII**, 51–117.
10 ZÜLCH, K. J. (1965) Transsudation Phenomena at the Deep Veins After Blockage of Arterioles and Capillaries by Micro-Emboli. 3. Europ. Conf. Microcirculation, Jerusalem 1964. *Bibl. anat.*, **7**, 279–284.
11 ZÜLCH, K. J. (1967) *The Cerebral Form of v. Winiwarter-Buerger's Disease, Does It Exist?*. 8th Ann. Meeting Int. Coll. Angiology, Madrid, August 31st — September 5th 1966 (in press).

Occlusive Cerebrovascular Disease

PETER O. YATES

Professor of Neuropathology, Department of Pathology, University of Manchester (England)

Occlusive cerebrovascular disease is best considered under three headings corresponding to the clinical states of major fixed stroke, small stroke with fairly slow recovery, transient attack with apparently complete recovery.

The first state is usually associated with a major infarct. Five percent of these occur in the territory of the anterior cerebral, 55% in the middle cerebral, and 10% in the posterior cerebral artery; 25% occur in the cerebellum, and 5% in the brain stem. Why do we find such a discrepancy? The significance of atherosclerotic disease of the vessels of the circle of Willis has always been exaggerated, because we look at the arteries either from outside their walls or, if in cross section, then in the collapsed state. When we use a distending medium before fixation we see something quite different. Although there may be quite large atheromatous plaques, unless they are very rigid and calcified the lumen is often quite well preserved.

There are certainly differences in the amount of local atheromatous disease, but this is not the principal cause of major infarcts which lies, in fact, outside the skull. For the middle cerebral artery only about 10% of occlusions have a purely local cause, 10% are due to emboli from the heart, 30% to emboli from mural thrombus in the carotid arteries, and in 50% the occlusion is by extension of thrombus up an occluded internal carotid. Even in major infarcts it is not always possible to find an occlusion after a few days' survival (Moossy, 1959). Especially in cases of embolism the obstruction has been observed radiologically to break up and disintegrate peripherally (Sussman and Fitch, 1961).

Occlusion of an internal carotid artery itself is only significant in producing major infarcts if it is the second or even third extracranial artery to be severely stenosed or occluded. A moderately severe stenosis may offer almost total resistance to blood flow, if the pattern of flow changes from a laminar to a turbulent one because of irregularities and tortuosity of the remaining channel. Experimental evidence suggesting the contrary has been carried out in the dog (Hamilton, Holling and Roberts, 1963) and in man (Brice, Dowsett and Lowe, 1964). In both cases the hydrodynamically smooth internal contour of the constricted channel produced by clamps cannot be said to resemble a calcified, ulcerated, atheromatous surface.

It is very difficult to evaluate the role of stenosis or occlusion of extracranial cerebral arteries. Schwartz and Mitchell (1961) found an incidence of 40% in a carefully randomised series of general hospital autopsies, irrespective of the cause of death.

We have found (Yates and Hutchinson, 1961) that 90% of cases with cerebral infarction, which are not obviously due to embolism from the heart, have severe stenosis of the carotid or vertebral arteries. By contrast we found a lower than normal incidence of stenosis in cases with cerebral haemorrhage. Only one of these had a completely occluded carotid and that was on the opposite side to the haemorrhage. I have since come to the belief that carotid artery stenosis may protect one half of the brain from the effects of hypertension just as renal artery stenosis protects the kidney. One must conclude that excision of a carotid stenosis should be thought of as prophylactically removing a focus for thrombosis and embolism, and only of significance in improving cerebral blood flow if more than one extracranial artery is affected.

Small strokes are mirrored pathologically as small infarcts or cysts. One should differentiate between cysts which are the result of an old infarct and the dilated perivascular spaces which surround sometimes the whole length of striate arteries in the condition of état lacunaire. This latter condition is not directly due to occlusive vascular disease, but is a result of the pulsatile unfolding of arteries in hypertension (Hughes, 1965). We have found it in the brains of 40% of hypertensive patients, but only in 10% of those who were normotensive during their last illness.

Small infarcts or cysts are sometimes quite numerous, as many as 12 lesions less than 2 cm across being found in a single brain. Such lesions rarely lead directly to death, but can be found quite commonly in a routine survey of hospital necropsies. In our series of normotensive cases, predominantly aged over 35 years, dying from a wide variety of diseases, about 18% showed small infarcts or cysts. The cause of these small ischaemic lesions is not always clear, some being due to obstruction of local arteries by emboli; others are associated with severe disease of the vessels on the surface of the brain and perhaps obstruction of the mouths of penetrating arteries.

We have found only a slight increase in ischaemic lesions of the brain in hypertension. Thirty percent of a series of 100 hypertensives showed large or small infarcts or ischaemic cysts, compared with 23% of our age- and sex-matched series of normotensive controls. The hypertensive group did however contain a further large number 18% where the brain showed evidence of small haemorrhages and old pigmented cysts, lesions many of which probably represented minor strokes. Such small haemorrhages and corresponding cysts were not found in cases where the diastolic pressure had been below 110 mm Hg.

One may conclude that small strokes in normotensives, being always ischaemic in origin, might be benefited by anticoagulants; it would be unwise to include hypertensives in such a therapeutic trial, because only half of their small strokes will be due to vascular occlusion. Failure to recognise this fact might account for the confusing results that such trials have produced.

Transient ischaemic attacks may result from the passage through the small cerebral arteries of emboli of platelet thrombi or of atheroma crystals, some of which may obstruct an artery permanently. It is difficult to believe that occlusion of such very small vessels can produce many neurologically appreciable lesions. Anticoagulants may prevent some of these events.

Transient attacks may be produced in at least two ways when the neck is turned:

by obstructing an internal carotid which has a redundant loop; by nipping and distorting an atheromatous vertebral artery in cervical spondylosis. Resection of redundant loops of internal carotid artery, thought by Weibel and Fields (1965) to be primarily congenital, is reported as curing the ischaemic attacks.

Normally elastic vertebral arteries will have no difficulty in adjusting to distortions of the cervical vertebrae but stiffening by calcification may make this impossible. Unusual movements of the neck are now well known to precipitate attacks of vertigo and ataxia, and surgical removal of osteophytes is a well-recognised therapy. We have found osteoarthritic changes in the cervical spine sufficiently severe to distort the vertebral arteries in about half of all people over the age of 40 dying in hospital (Holt and Yates, 1966). It seems probable that a high proportion of the falls of old age may be due to this cause.

It is becoming clear that much of the blood intended for the brain may in disease be transferred to other areas. Blood flow may be fairly suddenly diverted to supply exercising arm muscles in the subclavian steal syndrome, or to a flushed face if the common carotid is occluded and blood refluxes from the internal to the external carotid system. Attacks caused in these ways are clearly amenable to surgical therapy.

All these possible mechanisms indicate the wide range of provocative tests which might be required clinically in order to clarify the basis of any individual case of occlusive cerebro-vascular disease.

REFERENCES

BRICE, J. G., DOWSETT, O. J. AND LOWE, R. D., (1964); *Br. med. J.*, **2**, 1363.
HAMILTON, R. W., HOLLING, H. E. AND ROBERTS, B., (1963); *Surg. Forum*, **14**, 418.
HOLT, SHIRLEY AND YATES P. O., (1966); *J. Bone Jt. Surg.*, **48B**, 3, 407.
HUGHES, W., (1965); *Lancet*, **2**, 19.
MOOSSY, J., (1959); *Neurology, Minn.* **9**, 569.
SCHWARTZ, C. J. AND MITCHELL, J. R. A., (1961); *Br. med. J.*, **2**, 1057.
SUSSMAN, B. J. AND FITCH, T. S. P., (1961); *Angiology*, **12**, 169.
WEIBEL, J. AND FIELDS, W. S., (1965); *Neurology, Minn.*, **15**, 7.
YATES, P. O. AND HUTCHINSON, E. C., (1961); *Cerebral infarction*. M.R.C. Special Report 300. London; H.M.S.O.

Quantitative and qualitative* methods in the study of cerebral blood flow

H. FISCHGOLD**, D. DILENGE et J. METZGER

(Paris)

We will expound the case of radiologists intent on defining the role of cerebral angiography in the wide field of basic and clinical research concerned with "Cerebral Blood Flow" (C.B.F.).

With regard to this very field, S. Kety wrote: "Much of the new information relating to the human cerebral circulation has been at the basic physiological level — in fact, it has been said that more basic knowledge in this area has been acquired through studies in man in the past twenty years than was ever gained in lower animals".

Kety's reference to those twenty years shows, however, he had in mind the study of blood flow by inert gas rather than cerebral angiography.

Indeed, Moniz introduced the latter forty years ago, whereas Seymour Kety undertook to measure cerebral blood flow by means of nitrous oxide twenty years later.

Does it follow that cerebral angiography has been of such slight avail in terms of basic research?

What is more, the perusal of current literature reveals a surprising standpoint: it is generally claimed that the measurement of CBF by the method of Kety and Schmidt is "quantitative" whereas the method of Moniz is only "qualitative". The distinction is thereby stressed between that which is quantitative, because leading to a numerical result, and that which is qualitative, expressed by an image. In fact however the latter method combines anatomical contours and their serial representation. If certain quantitative data, such as the timing of CBF, do not figure in an isolated image, they appear through the temporal succession of serial images.

---

* According to Littré, the foremost french linguist "quality" is the essence of a thing whereas quantity refers to "anything which can be measured or expressed in figures". If one reads in Littré the two pages concerning the definition of "quality" it seems obvious that the meaning of "quality" is manifold. On the other hand, in defining "quantity" Littré's only field of reference is chemistry.

It follows that if the method of diffusible gases is undoubtedly quantitative it seems far from established that angiography is qualitative. Whatever dictionary we open, "qualitative" makes no sense when referring to angiography. Cerebral angiography is a morphological and dynamic method.
** Adresse: 1e Rue Las Cazes, Paris VIe, France.

References p. 180

MORPHOLOGY AND DYNAMICS IMPLY QUANTIFIABLE PARAMETERS

Overstressing the contrast between the two techniques, it is even held that the method of Kety and Schmidt is dynamic whereas that of Moniz and Lima is .... static.

Obviously Seymour Kety whose works ally exactness and subtlety cannot be held responsible ... As for us, we feel this conflicting image of two necessary methods needs reconsideration.

By no means do we contest that *transit time and volume of CBF, cerebral vascular resistance* and *oxygen consumption* — as measured by the various techniques involving inert gases whether radioactive or not, breathed by the subject or injected intravenously or into the carotid artery, and monitored by external detectors placed over the head or the neck vessels — have been quantified to a degree allowing for satisfactory understanding between different workers.

But cerebral angiography — anatomical method if there is one — also provides quantitative data: *transit time, size of lumen, optical density*. And, as it is our purpose to show, the quantifiable information contained in an angiographic image largely remains to be evaluated.

Let us now proceed to the crux of the matter.

Doubtless, the evaluation of CBF by the method of inert gas must take into account diffusion within the cerebral tissue, through the blood-brain barrier, and even into the nerve cells. It follows that this method and those derived from it yield an index of cerebral metabolic activity and essentially of oxygen consumption.

On the other hand, contrast media used for cerebral angiography remain in the blood stream without permeating the brain tissue. Such is also the case for fluoroscein used in evaluating fore-arm to retina transit time, RISA [133]I or ^{51}Cr labelled erythrocytes.

Rather than to radioisotopic investigation by means of inert gases ([85]Kr or [135]Xe), cerebral angiography is more appropriately compared to those methods using non diffusible tracers.

If one takes heed of this distinction, it appears that the transit time of cerebral blood flow as measured by Greitz, injecting RISA [133]I into the carotid artery or by Nylin, using radioactive labelled erythrocytes, is numerically coherent with that measured by cerebral angiography.

In the normal brain, the transit time of non diffusible tracers and contrast media, expressed in seconds, depends on the sites of reference under consideration: carotid siphon — parietal veins — carotid artery — 'ugular vein and so forth.

Quantitative aspects of cerebral angiography

The timing and volume of CBF evaluated by inert gas, and the transit time measured by cerebral angiography are but two facets of the same coin. The elementary processes of cerebral metabolism can be called to witness the foremost aim and end result of cerebral blood flow is the conveyance of oxygen to the neurones.

Whenever this blood flow meets with increased intracranial pressure, whatever its cause may be, the CBF (measured by inert gas) falls and the transit time through the cerebral vascular bed is augmented (as is seen by delay in angiography).

When intracranial pressure is increased each oxygen - bearing erythrocyte has an increased transit time through the cerebral vessels. It follows that fewer RBC will yield their oxygen per unit time; CBF, of which O_2 consumption is an essential expression falls. The basic works of Greitz and of Tönnis and Schiefer exemplify this reasoning: CBF (measured by diffusible gas) and transit time (measured by angiography) can be referred to a common denominator O_2 consumption.

Greitz's figure 10 indicates that normal transit time between the carotid siphon and parietal veins varies from 3 to $5\frac{1}{2}$ sec. It increases to 7 sec and more in patients with cerebral tumor but not having choked discs. When cerebral tumor is accompanied by choked discs, transit time rises to over 8 sec.

Tönnis and Schiefer have shown that when cerebrospinal fluid pressure rises from 100 to 700 mm, blood flow measured with nitrous oxide, decreased from its normal value (over 50 ml/100 g/min) to less than 40 ml/100 g/min.

The prolonged transit time and the diminished CBF lead to a significant decrease of O_2 consumption passing from 3.3 ml/100 g of brain tissue in the normal individual to 3 and even less than 2 while intracranial pressure rises.

The correlation between CBF, angiographic transit and oxygen consumption is particularly outstanding in circulatory arrest as Riishede and Ethelberg, amongst others, have pointed out and as Gros *et al.* (Montpellier) have recently shown.

When intracranial pressure becomes critical, it entails:

– a sharp decrease of CBF
– the absence of filling of cerebral vessels during technically correct angiography
– the suppression of oxygen consumption
– the disappearance of all electrical activity on EEG

In Tönnis department, Frowein has drawn a parallel between prognosis in head traumas and blood oxygen tension: survival is significantly more frequent when oxygen tension is above normal in the jugular vein and less frequent when oxygen tension is inferior to normal. In the first case 22 out of 54 patients survived whereas only 8 out of 42 survived in the latter case.

These data should suffice to indicate the correlation between angiographic parameters and oxygen metabolism as it is estimated by CBF. This correlation is particularly striking in neurosurgical patients with increased intracranial pressure whether due to space-occupying lesions or to head trauma; it is not as constant in circulatory insufficiency or vascular diseases.

In the latter case, CBF and O_2 consumption vary according to the severity of the disease and depending on whether or not it is compensated. Transit time is also augmented, the delay being essentially arterial (Decker, Schiefer, Dilenge and col.). As far as we know this phenomenon has not, as yet, been studied in any large series of patients. But for reasons of safety and in the absence of surgical treatment, the method of diffusible gases seems better adapted to these patients.

Before closing our parallel between CBF measure and a method which yields a morphological representation of cerebral circulation by serial images, such as angiography, it must be stressed to what extent these methods differ with regard to regional measurement.

The use of inert and freely diffusible gas, since ^{85}Kr and ^{135}Xe have been introduced, can at best give information concerning an entire cerebral lobe. If such gross localization can be of use in vascular diseases and limited obstructions, it can by no means suffice to localize a neoplasm in view of surgery.

On the other hand, cerebral angiography is constantly gaining in discriminative power, both temporally and spatially:

temporally, excellent definition can now be obtained with 4 to 6 images per second seriography;

spatially: substraction allows identification of vessels of 400 μ diameter, thus broadening the field of angiographic interpretation to such vessels as branches of the ophtalmic artery, perforating arteries of the basal nuclei, and ever finer arteries of the brain stem and the cerebellum.

What is more, we are at present visualizing "irrigation units" which appear as contrasted cerebral tissue during the capillary phase of angiography, units which are considerably smaller than a cerebral lobe. In our department, such "units" have been observed in the thalamus and the cerebellum, whereas Greitz has observed them in the cerebral cortex.

Contribution of angiography to the study of cerebral blood flow

The contribution of cerebral angiography to the study of blood flow is not confined to morphology, however important this aspect has proven with regard to diagnosis of cerebral lesions. Its contribution in the field of cerebral hemodynamics has come to the fore as seriography has developped.

The gain in speed and automation acquired by this method now permits us to determine not only cerebral transit time as a whole, but even transit time of each successive circulatory phase.

These measurements are based on a better knowledge of the delay required by contrast media to progress through the various cerebral vessels, a knowledge which is fostered by ever finer methods of analysing the angiograms (substraction, densimetry, etc...) and by progress in the contrast media used and automation of its injection (Cisal II syringe). It is our experience that:

An increase in transit time is characteristic of certain degrees of increased intracranial pressure, especially when the latter is of sudden onset. Such is the case in some head injuries when associated with severe cerebral contusion. In these cases, slowing of blood flow, seemed to involve mainly the cortical and subcortical vascular bed since contrast in superficial veins was delayed in comparison with contrast in the deep median veins.

Nothwithstanding the commonly held opinion that in cerebral angiomas, transit time is shortened, we have observed in a certain number of such malformations a prolonged opacification of the afferent arteries, of the arteriovenous shunt itself or even of the efferent veins. There is as yet no satisfactory explanation for such observations.

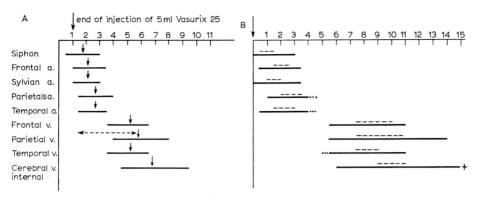

Fig. 1.(A) Time during which contrast medium is present can be measured for each artery and vein, for instance it fills the internal cerebral vein up till the 10th second.
(B) Under moderate hypothermia transit time is increased.

In several subarachnoid hemorrhages with hemiplegia, we have found evidence of increased transit time localized in the cerebral region presumably responsible for the paralysis. We have seen a concomitant constriction of feeding arteries, due to vasospasm. It has thus been possible to attribute hemiplegia to a degree of ischemia caused by diminished blood flow.

If we consider vascular diseases, transit time seems to increase whenever there is a sudden obstruction of a cerebral artery, an acute infarct with hemorrhage, or severe systemic hypotension.

Distal to a stenosis of the carotid artery, transit time seems to vary in accordance to blood flow. Thus in six of our cases increased transit time was accompanied by an altered EEG witness to the existence of hypoxia.

Last cerebral blood flow serving first and foremost as an oxygen carrier to the

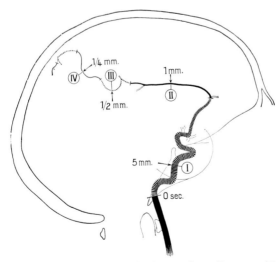

Fig. 2. Cerebral transit time and caliber of arterial lumen: for a diameter of 5 mm (internal carotid and anterior cerebral artery) the speed of flow is 465 mm/sec; decrease of speed parallel to decrease of caliber: for a diameter of 0.5 mm, speed decreases to 165 mm/sec.

neurones, we have compared some measurable parameters of angiography to oxygen consumption as it is influenced by moderate hypothermia. In this case (Fig. 1) angiography reveals a considerable increase of cerebral transit time. It should be noted that, for a given degree of hypothermia this angiographic parameter seemed to follow variations in oxygen tension as determined by artificial ventilation. What is more, these modifications of hemodynamics are accompanied by clearly visible modifications in the size of the lumen of cerebral vessels, a fact which once again brings to light the relationship between angiographic and blood flow parameters.

Advances in cerebral angiography automation and polygraph

Angiography however has gone a step further in matters of quantifiable information. Certain aspects of carotid angiography now imply further numerical operations, measurements and graphic representations.

We will just mention radiocinematography which provides us with several hundred frames per second. Sharpness of detail on each image is no doubt poor although constant advance is being made. The progression of the contrast medium along the vascular bed is striking as one looks at the film but we cannot interrupt its progression to select significant information. If we blow up any single frame, we will no longer have the fine details which can be observed on a seriogram. And the neurosurgeon requests one or more images to which he can refer in the operating ward.

While we await new progress in photographic technique, the analysis of dynamic phenomena and their graphic representation as space time functions require machines

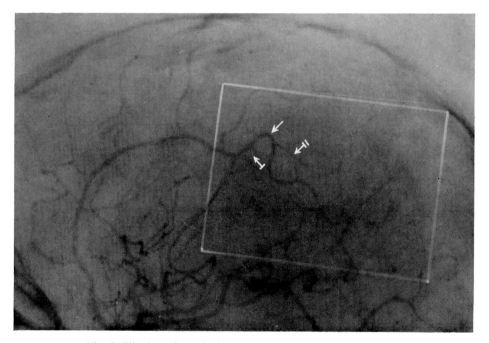

Fig. 3. Distal portion of a branch of the anterior cerebral artery.

allowing for integration such as those used by Ohlsson while charting progress of a minute contrast bolus in the aorta of a dog.

Using seriography at a rate of 4 images per second and substraction we have been able to measure the rate of progress of contrast media in the anterior cerebral artery and its finer branches.

Fig. 2 shows that transit time increases as the lumen of the vessel becomes finer. The rate of progress is 465 mm/sec for a vessel of 5 mm diameter decreasing to 165 mm/sec for a diameter of 0.5 mm. Poiseuille's formula is not, here, strictly applicable insofar as the diameter of the vessel is not the only variable. In any event it seems certain that speed varies in proportion with caliber.

It is, of course quite difficult to measure the diameter of a vessel of less than 0.5 to 0.6 mm.

We are not so ambitious as to search for those vessels of 0.05 mm diameter which form what we might call the vascular architectony of the brain, although they are perfectly distinguishable on G. Salamon's anatomical slides our purpose is to identify vessels in the range of 0.2 mm.

In this angiogram (Fig. 3) we have drawn a rectangle. In the following (Fig. 4) the

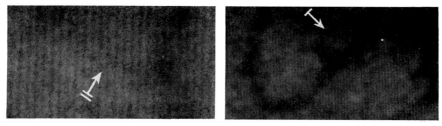

Fig. 4. × 4.5: the fine vessels ↓ have lost sharpness of détail since the grain of the film acquires opacity equal to that of the contrast medium.
Fig. 5. × 10.5: the branch is practically masked by the lines of the grid.

same rectangle is magnified four times as are the vessels opacified by contrast medium. But the grain of the film, now apparent, annuls for a large part the advantage of magnification. If we magnify ten times (Fig. 5), the grid now becomes visible and the fine vessels are no longer as distinct as on the original angiogram.

It was necessary we should become aware of such obstacles. Optical electronics and the laser will probably allow us to discard these factors which limit sharpness of detail and should provide us with an ever finer perception of angiographic detail.

Hilal, at the Neurological Institute of New York, has opened a most original outlook.

He separates the images to be analyzed into 150 to 200 minute squares, each of which is scanned by the light source of a microdensimeter. The radiological image is thereby transformed into a table of densimetrical values which are arranged according to position by the ordinator (Figs. 6 and 7).

The maximum density of each vessel can thus be determined on each angiogram of the seriography as well as the discrete differences in parenchymal density.

This astute method derives from the photography of Mars by a satellite using differ-

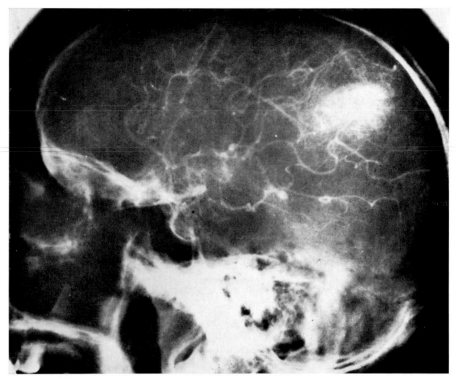

Fig. 6. Angioma injected by angiography (Courtesy of Dr. Hilal, New-York).

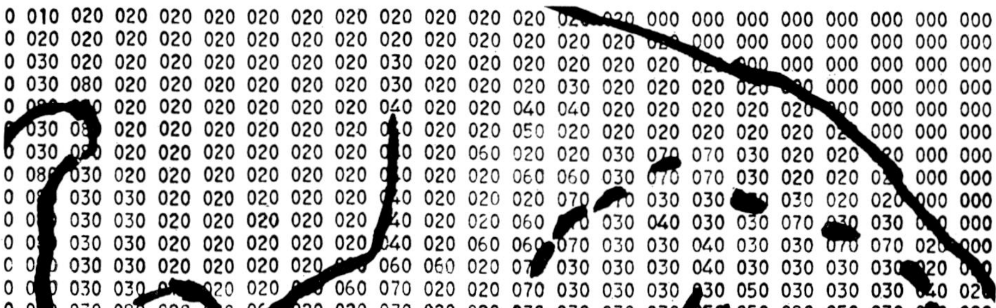

Fig. 7. The area occupied by the angioma is divided into 660 squares; a microdensimeter translates the density of each square into a figure; the apparatus organizes these figures in their spatial relationship according to corresponding density (Courtesy of Dr. Hilal, New-York).

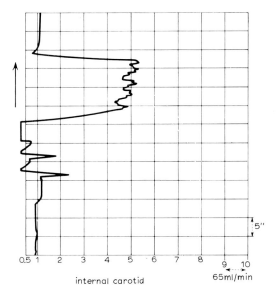

internal carotid   65ml/min

Fig. 8. Curve of carotid blood flow measured by the flowmeter (Massiot Philips). On the abscissa, each division corresponds to a flow of 65 ml/min; on the ordinate, each division corresponds to 5″.

ences in tone between pictures which were sent earthbound as coded numbers by digital television.

We will also draw attention to the value of polygraphic techniques whenever it is wished to bind cerebral angiography to a physiological or physiopathological situation represented by a subject. We can now record ECG as well as onset and end of injection of the contrast medium during angiography. For Greitz such simple graphic correlation has become routine during all angiographies. We are in the process of adding to these EEG and, only recently, the curve of intra-carotid pressure immediately after injection (yielding a profile lasting — for the overall duration of angiography — at least 5 or 6 seconds). Thus the progress of the contrast medium through the cerebral vessels during rapid seriography is monitored alongside with other parameters and transit time becomes but one of several functional transients which can be examined in correlation.

Lastly, we have adjoined to seriography and automatic injection another apparatus. It is a *flowmeter* which records the flow of a cold liquid injected at a determined temperature into the carotid, while a computer transforms the data into real value of carotid blood flow. The same needle, after percutaneous puncture, serves for injection of the contrast medium, for measurement of intra-carotid pressure during part of the angiography and for measurement of carotid blood flow immediately before or after the seriography. The information yielded by cerebral angiography is thereby associated with other quantifiable factors and this information can be correlated more readily with that concerning CBF. Furthermore this apparatus allows for measurement of jugular blood flow.

References p. 180

CONCLUSION

Any fact can be described in terms of quantity or quality. This is true of cerebral circulation, a hemodynamic process situated in the intracranial vascular bed.

Diffusible gases, whether radioactive or not, serve to measure blood flow, vascular resistance and oxygen consumption.

Cerebral angiography can be translated into measurement of cerebral transit time and diameter of vessels.

Furthermore cerebral angiography yields morphological information which is essential to diagnosis and to neurosurgery; cerebral angiography thus stands out as an *anatomical technique but not a qualitative one.*

The essential difference between radioactive diffusible gas methods and cerebral angiography (or non diffusible gas methods) is that the former permeate nerve cells whereas the latter do not leave the vascular bed.

For this reason, diffusible labelled gases which serve to measure oxygen consumption are more appropriately used in examining patients suffering from atherosclerosis for whom it may be preferable to avoid cerebral angiography. All the more so since this method can be of some inconvenience in vascular disease.

For the same reasons, cerebral angiography remains unsurpassed for the examination of patients with neurosurgical complaints. The quantifiable information yielded by this method has increased in the past years in adjunct to the anatomical data.

REFERENCES

DILENGE, D., PERILHOU, J., AUPHAN, M., FISCHGOLD, H., METZGER, J., DAVID, M. ET BOURRÉE, R. (1967) Mesure du débit carotidien au moyen d'un debitmètre à dilution thermique. *C.R. Acad. Sci. (Paris)*, **264**, 1514–1516.

GREITZ, T. (1956) A radiological study of the Brain Circulation by rapid serial Angiography of the carotid Artery. *Acta Radiologica*, Suppl. 140.

TÖNNIS, W. AND SCHIEFER, W. (1959) *Zirkulationsstörungen des Gehirns im Serienangiogramm.* Springer.

SYMPOSIUM (1965) Regional Cerebral Blood Flow. An International Symposium. *Acta Neurol. Scand.*, Suppl. 14.

SYMPOSIUM (1966) *Symposium International sur la Circulation Cérébrale.* Sandoz (Ed.).

STROKE (1967) Ed. by A. Engel and T. Larsson. Nordiska Bokhandelns Forlag. Stockholm.

The Application of the Subtraction Method to Cerebral Angiography

B. G. ZIEDSES DES PLANTES

Röntgen Laboratory, Wilhelmina Gasthuis, University of Amsterdam, The Netherlands

In this communication the application of the subtraction method to the examination in cerebral vascular lesions will be demonstrated.

The various technical subtraction procedures can be divided into two groups, namely the photographic and the electronic methods.

With the photographic method, the difference between two radiographs is visualized by covering one radiograph with a transparent positive print of the other. Fig. 1 shows how a separate picture of the opacified vessels can be obtained by covering a cerebral arteriogram with a transparent positive print of a plain radiograph which is made in exactly the same position. This positive print may be called the mask. The image which is seen after superimposition of the angiogram and the mask is rather dark. Therefore it is advisable to print the superimposed films on high contrast material. Fig. 1D is such a print.

The plain radiograph is the first film of the angiographic series. It is made before the injection of the contrast material is started.

Attention should be paid to the successive films being made in exactly the same position of the patients head. The slightest movement of the head will spoil the result of subtraction. Therefore the head is immobilised by means of a radiolucent box which is shown in Fig. 2.

The photographic method is the most reliable procedure. Besides the photographic method three electronic procedures are more or less successfully used. They are schematically shown in Fig. 3.

The method which is shown at the top has firstly been used by Holman and Bullard. The plain radiograph and the angiogram are placed before two television cameras, in this case two vidicons. The videosignal of the first vidicon is reversed, in other words, the negative television image is turned into a positive one. Then the video-signals of the two vidicons are fused and conveyed to a television monitor which shows the subtraction image. From technical reasons a good superimposition of the two television images is very hard.

An exact superimposition can be obtained with two other methods. The method of Borgman is drawn in the midst of the figure. The light of the flying spot of a cathode tube is optically divided by means of a semitransparent mirror. The beam of light is projected on the films. Thus the two films are quite synchronously scanned. The

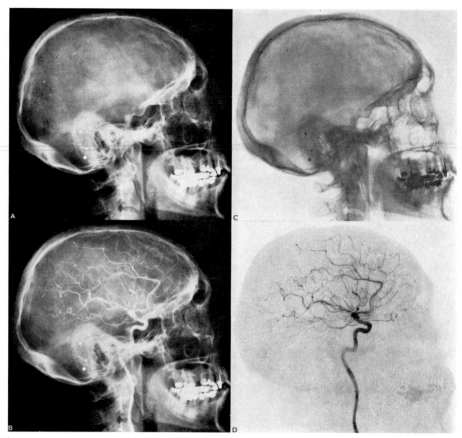

Fig. 1. The principle of the photographic subtraction method. A: Plain radiograph, B: Angiogram,
C: Transparent positive print of A, the "mask". D: Print which is made after superimposition of the
angiogram and the mask.

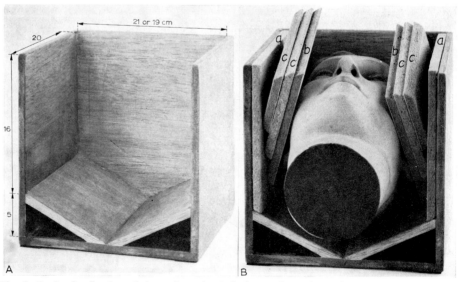

Fig. 2. Device for fixation of the patients head during angiography. It is made of balsawood or
cellotex. A: Indication of measures in cm, B: The patients head is wedged by means of cellotex plates,
aa: Plates to prevent sliding, bb: Plates touching three points of the patients head, cc: Plates for
wedging.

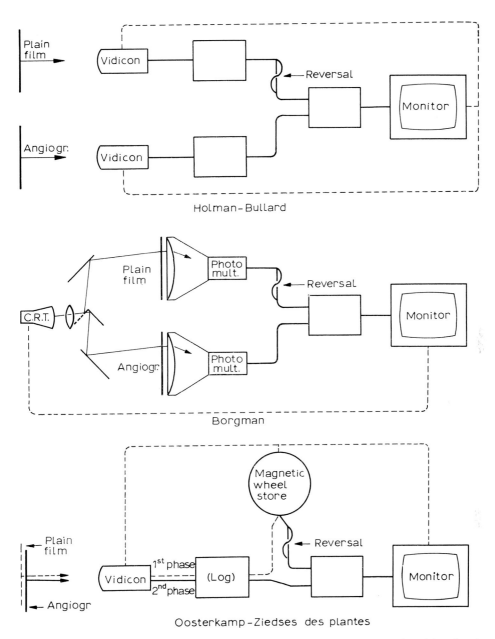

Fig. 3. Three different electronic procedures. The dotted lines indicate the synchronizing electric connections.

transmitted light is converted into electric signals by means of two photomultipliers. Reversal and fusion of the signals are carried out in the same way as shown before.

Theoretically this method supplies optimal conditions. Our experiments with this method however showed, that the light intensity was only good for bright radiographs.

Oosterkamp proposed the use of a magnetic memory. His method is shown near the bottom of the figure and will be explained by Oosterkamp himself. In this method the same television chain is used for both radiographs. Thus an exact superimposition is assured.

Up till now only the method with two vidicons is routinely used.

Fig. 4 shows a device for electronic subtraction. Fig. 5 is made to show the results which are obtained with the photographic and with the electronic method in the same case. Fig. 5A shows an angiogram in a man, 18 years, suffering from a traumatic carotid–cavernous fistula. Fig. 5B shows the result of the photographic procedure. Fig. 5C shows a photograph of the monitor image in electronic subtraction with the device which is shown by Fig. 4.

Up till now the resolution which can be obtained with electronic subtraction is inferior to that which can be obtained with photographic subtraction. Compensation by means of "close up" technics is possible.

Generally the subtraction procedure is not indispensable in the examination of intracranial haemangiomas or arterio–venous aneurysms. Still it provides clearer

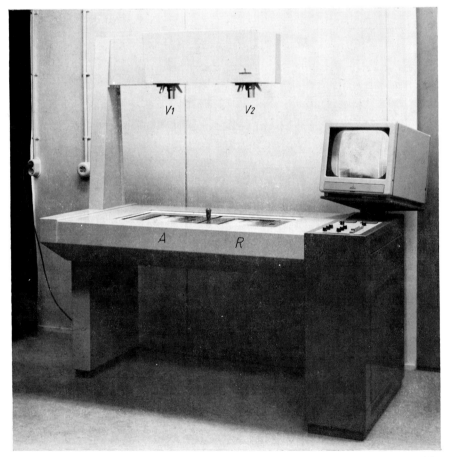

Fig. 4. Device for electronic subtraction. A: Angiogram, R: Plain radiograph, V_1 and V_2: Vidicons.

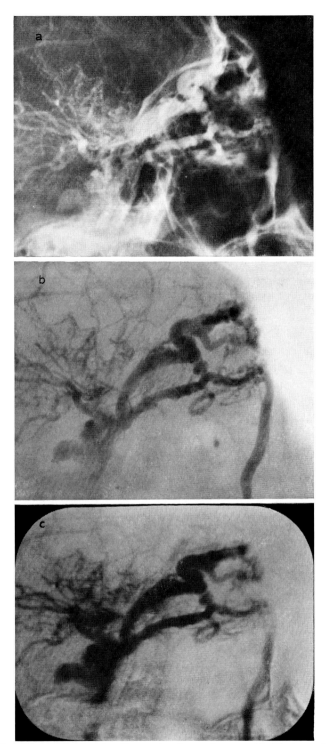

Fig. 5. Carotid-cavernous fistula. A: Conventional arteriogram, B: Photographic subtraction picture, C: Electronic subtraction picture.

pictures of the vascular pattern especially in the antero-posterior view.

The same applies to subdural and epidural haematomata.

The subtraction image provides optimal information in circular disorders in the posterior fossa.

The method has shown to be very useful in the study of the collateral circulation in obstructive lesions.

Fig. 6A shows a common carotid angiogram in a 60 years old man, suffering from a leftsided hemiplegia which started suddenly and improved gradually. The angio-

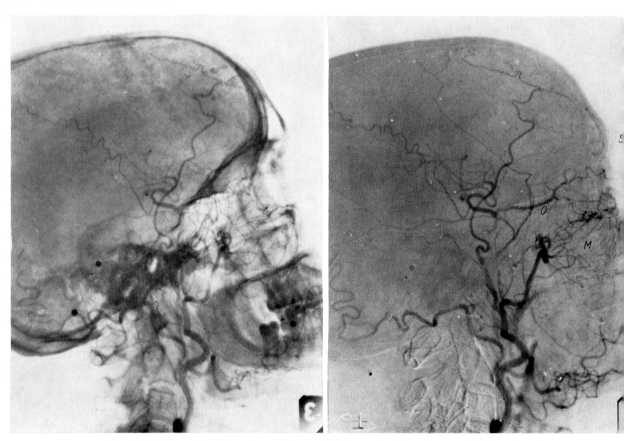

Fig. 6. Occlusion of the internal carotid artery. A: Conventional arteriogram, B: Subtraction picture showing collateral supply via the ophthalmic artery (O) by the facial artery (F), the maxillary artery (M) and the superficial temporal artery (S).

gram shows a complete occlusion of the internal carotid artery. The internal carotid syphon is filled via the ophthalmic artery. Fig. 6B is the subtraction picture. It shows clearly the collateral circulation via the facial artery, the maxillary artery and the superficial temporal artery.

Sometimes it has been possible to show direct collateral circulation from the maxillary artery to the carotid syphon.

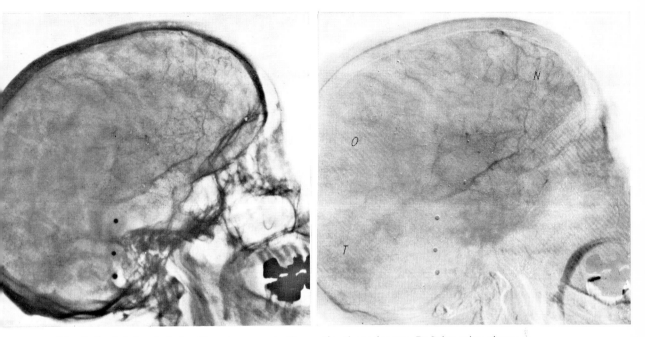

Fig. 7. Occipital metastasis of breast cancer. A: Conventional arteriogram, B: Subtraction picture, T: Tumour, O: Oedema and disturbed circulation, N: Normal vascular pattern.

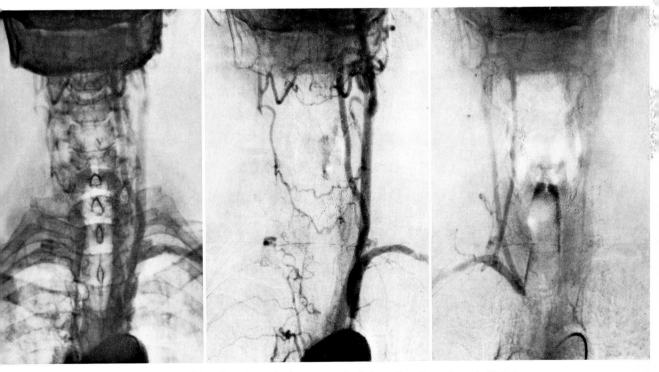

Fig. 8. Subclavian and carotid steal syndrom. A: Aortogram, B: Subtraction picture from A, C: Subtraction picture 5 seconds after injection, showing various collateral circulations.

It must be emphasized, that in such cases stereoscopical examination is necessary. All cases which are shown are analysed by means of stereoscopic examination.

The subtraction images may provide clear information about the circulation disorders, which are caused by braintumours.

Fig. 7A shows the conventional arteriogram in a metastasis of breast cancer, which is located in the occipital lobe. Fig. 7B represents the subtraction image. The tumour is supplied by the posterior cerebral artery. The parietal region shows impairment of the bloodcirculation and extensive oedema. The vascular pattern in the frontal and temporal regions is normal.

The subtraction method provides very good information on the vascular supply of brain tumours. Some examples are shown elsewhere.

The subtraction method may be successfully used in the study of steal syndroms. An example is shown in Fig. 8. The patient, a man aged 58 years, is suffering from progressive circulatory insufficiency of the right subclavian and the right internal carotid artery. The aortogram, Fig. 8A shows a complete occlusion of the brachio-cephalic trunc. The subtraction picture, Fig. 8B shows clearly various collateral circulations to the left external carotid artery. They are supplied by the right thyreo - cervical trunc, the costo - cervical trunc and the left external carotid artery. Fig. 8C is the subtraction picture of an angiogram which is made 5 seconds after the injection. It shows the collateral circulation from the left vertebral artery, via the right vertebral artery and the brachiocephalic trunc to the right common carotid artery.

REFERENCES

BORGMAN, J. (1960) Electronic Scanning for Variable Stars. *Publ. Kapteyn. Astr. Lab.* No. 58.
HOLMAN, C. B. AND BULLARS, F. E. (1963) The application of Closed-Circuit Television in Diagnostic Roentgenology. *Proc. Mayo Clinic*, **38**, 67
ZIEDSES DES PLANTES, B. G. (1935) Subtraktion. *Fortsch. Röntgenstr.*, **52**, 509.
— (1961) *Subtraktion*. G. Thieme Verlag, Stuttgart.
— (1963) Application of the Subtraction Method in Neuroradiological Examination. *Psychiat. Neurol. Neurochir.*, **66**, 480.

Official Discussion

P. FRUGONI

Via Aquileia 4, Padova (Italy)

When confronted with a patient suspected of having a cerebral vascular disorder, we face several and serious problems, particularly from a diagnostic point of view. Many of these problems invest neuroradiology, and among them the first to be solved is how to conduct the radiological study, so as to reach a prompt and exact diagnosis with the least possible number of examinations.

The clinical findings are often sufficient to indicate which is the radiological problem to be solved and to consent, from the beginning, an aimed radiological investigation. This may happen, for instance, if we suspect a vascular malformation or a vascular occlusion in a given district. In such a case, it is possible to carry out, from the very beginning, a radiological study selective enough to allow an exact diagnosis and, at the same time, to supply us with all information which may be necessary for a surgical attack upon the lesion.

A typical example of these aimed radiological techniques is given by the selective angiography of the external carotid artery, which is so useful for studying many vascular conditions. If we perform the angiography through the temporal artery by means of a small catheter (Dagradi and Pistolesi, 1966), it is possible for instance to visualize either a limited district of the external carotid circulation (Fig. 1) — or to visualize the whole district of distribution of the artery, as in this case of arteriovenous fistula between the cavernous sinus and a branch of the internal maxillary artery (Fig. 2). These cases do not refer strictly to a cerebral pathology, but they show particularly well what I mean.

Going back to what I was saying, the clinical findings, on the other hand, are not always sufficient to allow a presumptive diagnosis; in such a case it becomes necessary to resort to a preliminary general radiological study, which may focus the diagnostic problem. Radiological study "d'ensemble" which comes also useful inasmuch as the vascular disease is often a widespread one, as very rightly Prof. Almeida Lima has pointed out.

As preliminary orientative study, we have often used a right percutaneous brachial cerebral angiography, associated to simultaneous compression of the left cervical carotid artery. However, among the various techniques for cerebral panangiography, I actually believe 4-vessel angiography to be the best. I hope, therefore, that aortography may become a routine examination in neuroradiology and that its technique may be made simpler and safer.

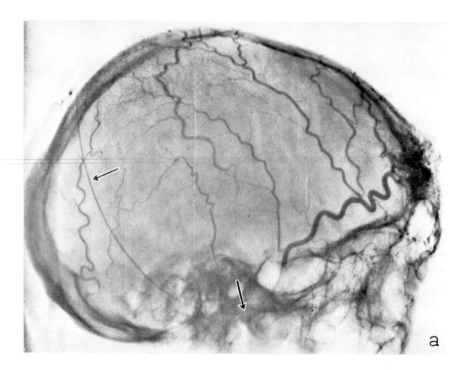

a

Fig. 1

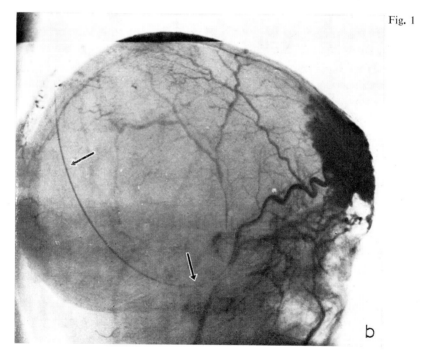

b

Image subtraction has often proven itself of great usefulness in all these radiological investigations, as Professor Ziedses des Plantes has so well demonstrated.

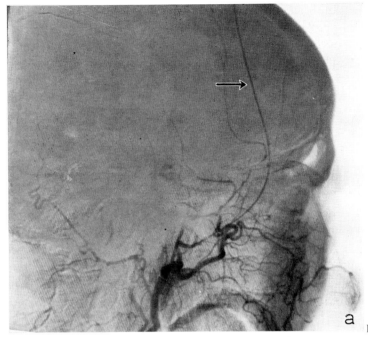

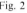

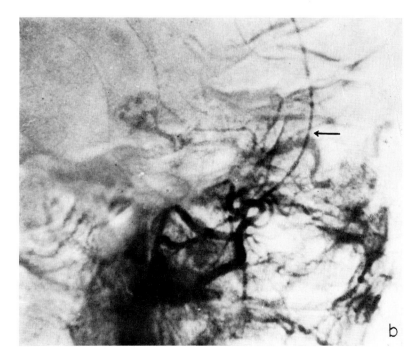

Fig. 2

Speaking about radiological investigations "d'ensemble" or anyway about methods that, in parallel to standard angiographic techniques, may increase our diagnostic possibilities, I believe that a great help may be derived from the studies that Professor Fischgold and his associates have reported in their extremely interesting presentation. It is not up to me, by the way, to comment on the great interest that radioisotopes do have in the study of cerebral vascular disorders, but I feel that in the future they will play a great role in this connection.

The reports we have heard have faced and greatly enlightened several very important problems. Other problems however remain, perhaps equally important, which may be worth mentioning. I am sure that our knowledge about cerebral vascular malformations and vascular occlusions will be much improved at the end of this Congress; but many questions will be left unanswered, concerning that numerous group of vascular conditions which stem out of a functional, rather than an anatomical disorder; conditions which are more difficult to document radiologically and which, above all, are more difficult to be interpreted; conditions which are ill-defined and are often — and wrongly — disregarded.

I am thinking, for instance, about those clinical syndromes which do have a definite vascular pattern, but in which the angiographic studies reveal only a generalized or a localized arterial spasm "sine materia" or anyway unexplainable. I am thinking about the marked slowing of cerebral circulation that we often see under different circumstances, the cause and significance of which escape our understanding; and so forth.

In Italy, in the past one or two years, some neurosurgeons (including myself) have noticed a definite increase in the number of cases of "pseudotumor cerebri", another clinical entity which is still ill-defined and that, in many instances, is probably caused by a disturbance of the venous circulation, particularly an occlusion of the dural venous sinuses. Many similar examples could be made.

As a neurosurgeon, I feel that the radiological study of cerebral vascular disorders still presents unsolved problems. Even the study of intracranial vascular malformations presents limitations that we all know and that my associates discussed two years ago, here in Madrid at the 5th Annual Neurosurgical Symposium (Ruberti *et al.*, 1965). I don't want to repeat now what was said at that time, but I wish to call attention upon the fact that the limitations of neuroradiology are even greater if we refer to that group of ill-defined vascular disorders, at times purely functional, that I pointed out before. Disorders which often, rather than the arterial, concern the venous cerebral circulation, which is not always studied with the attention it deserves. In this connection, some old techniques such as dural sinus venography, to-day rather neglected, may still be of help.

The study of disorders of the cerebral circulation demands in a special way a close cooperation between radiologists and surgeons, as the clinical findings are determinant in pointing out which is the particular diagnostic problem to be solved, while it is up to the radiologist to find the best way for solving it.

REFERENCES

DAGRADI, A., ET PISTOLESI, G. F., (1966); L'angiographie rétrograde de l'artère carotide externe par voie transtemporale, *Ann. Radiol.*, **9**, 603–615.
RUBERTI, R., GALLIGIONI, F., ET FRUGONI, P., (1965); Problèmes de neuroradiologie dans les lésions vasculaires cérébrales. *Acta Neurochir.* **13**, 145–185.

The EEG in Vascular Lesions

ORLANDO CARVALHO

Neurologist, Lisbon Civil Hospitals, Lisbon (Portugal)

If we go through everything that has been published on the subject of EEG in vascular lesions since the Berger case, to the numerous works of these last years, we feel shocked by the many efforts and most accurate and useful conclusions but, notwithstanding, we are astonished to find a lot of imagination there as well. Because we are speaking in Spain, we can gloss and say that the EEG owes a great deal to some "Don Quijote", with their genial strokes, sometimes fanciful, even delirious; but that the right and fruitful way has been built, step by step, by the positive mind, often sceptic, of many "Sanchos Panza".

Before coming into the general semeiology of EEG in vascular lesions, it is necessary to repeat what has been often stressed by many authors, but just as often forgotten, viz., that the EEG must be made part of the clinical data as a whole. Just as in any other complementary diagnostic method, it is the clinician only who can draw its importance from the whole clinical context.

In fact, it is possible to find out almost all the morphologic types of electric troubles in the EEG of the patients suffering from vascular affections of the CNS.

However, if a pathological record can be found, the changes are almost always slow. But, unfortunately, those are the same slow anomalies which are found in several other etiological lesions, mainly in brain tumours, which does not make our diagnostic problems easier. Such as Delisle stressed in his Thesis, regarding ischaemic lesions in the occlusions of internal and Sylvian carotid arteries, but also true about all other brain vascular affections, all the types of slow rhythms can be found, as they were described by Arfel and Fischgold in the cerebral tumours:

(1) Polymorphic delta activity, almost continuous and of large and average voltage, sometimes superimposed by alpha residues.

(2) Flat polymorphic delta activity, which slow voltage can reach the aspect of "electric silence", with disappearance of any faster frequency.

(3) Mixed delta activity, from 1,5 to 3 cycles per second, mixed to alpha frequencies or to "irritative" components, showing a rhythmic or, at least, a periodic aspect.

(4) Monomorphic delta activity, often with typical large voltage sinusoidal outbursts.

Without reverting to the discussion on the focal value of some, and marginal or

SOME TYPICAL CASES

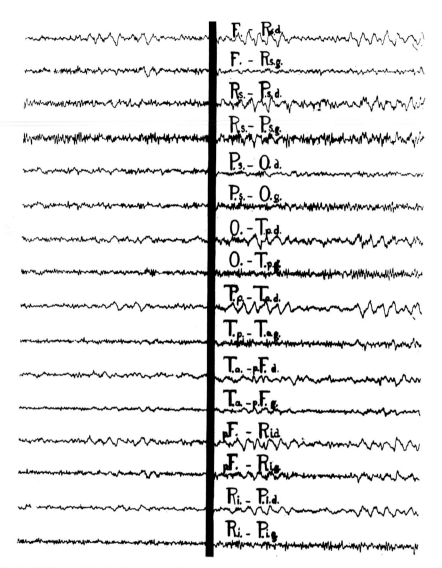

Fig. 1. CASE 1 — F. M., 68 years, male patient. Sudden appearance of a parieto-central syndrome of the left arm. Fundus of the eye with vascular sclerosis. Clinical diagnosis: cerebral thrombosis. EEG with an important focus of polymorphic delta (Fig. 1, left). Slight improvement of the clinical status. EEG one month afterwards: marked aggravation and extension of the alterations (Fig. 1, right) requiring an angiography which revealed a right parietal tumour. Operative and biopsy findings: multiform glioblastoma.

"at distance" of others, what is important is to find also in the vascular affections all the other EEG troubles described in cerebral tumours:

Alpha deficient changes: instability, slowing, asymmetry of amplitude, total absence. But, if these anomalies often appear on the side of the lesion, we must pay attention, because we may also find them on the opposite side and, if we do not have any tracing taken previous to the present affection, as it is usually the case, such alpha asymmetry could exist before, without any pathological significance.

The blocking response can be abolished from the sick side, as well as the answer to the rhythmical photic stimulation.

We often see irritative signs, chiefly of the more or less fast and ample spikes, sometimes of the spike-and-wave variant. There is often a unilateral increase of the fast rolandic rhythms and of the "rythmes en arceaux", but mostly on the opposite side.

The study of the sleeping records is very important on the point of view of localization. Besides the asymmetry of the slow rhythms of the different sleeping stages, we can see the activation of a slow, light or dubious focus. Already in 1948, Cress and Gibbs described a unilateral depression or abolition of the sleep spindles, and, later on, others found a reduction of the awakening reaction or of the K-complexes, on the affected side. Recently, Niedermeyer and Pribram also found the unilateral suppression of the vertex sharp waves, in a case of occlusion of the posterior branches of the right middle cerebral artery.

Quite certainly, the hyperpnoea activates, almost always, the slow or fast changes, and we can even have the chance of recording it during this test on a previous normal tracing.

Nevertheless, we must not forget the fluctuations of the electric troubles in some carotid thrombosis, the progressive aggravations in other ischaemic lesions, and the regressions, even temporary, in a tumour, after an intratumoural haemorrhage.

(2) Intracranial aneurysm: The practical problem is, almost always, the spontaneous subarachnoid haemorrhage. In the absence of other clinical findings, the occurrence of a focus of slow waves or of epileptic type potentials, an asymmetry of the rhythms or of the physiological reactivities, can reveal to the clinician the possibility of an aneurysm which should require angiography.

Some works have been made to try to find EEG signs capable of showing the precise site of the aneurysm (Roseman, Binnie, Dehing, etc.), but this is a question which may be considered an academical one by the neurosurgeons, much more interested as they are in the angiography, based on strong reasons. The major advantage of EEG in meningeal haemorrhage is the possibility of indicating to the neurosurgeon the site which should be submitted to angiography, if other clinical or complementary signs do not exist.

Perhaps the echoencephalography might be a simpler and more practical way of resolving the problem, but only in the cases where there is a formation of an haematoma with shift of the middle echo, which are far from the majority.

(3) In the traumatic vascular lesions the subdural haematoma is, almost always, our main difficulty. In spite of the fact that there are no more illusions about the value, frequency and constancy of voltage depressions and of localized "electric

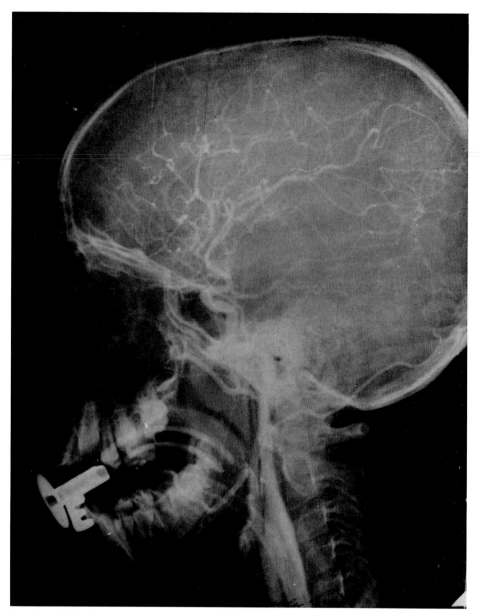

Figs. 2, 3. CASE 2 — L. D., 14 year old girl. Came to consultation because of her old paroxysmal headaches, with a serious recurrence the week before, of which she had almost recovered. Quite normal neurological examination, including fundus of the eye. Seemingly hysteric behaviour having led to the same diagnosis at a previous consultation. Nevertheless, an EEG was made because she lived far, in the province. This is the recording, requiring no words (Fig. 2). Angiography: Arteriove-nous aneurysm and haematoma of the left temporal lobe (Fig. 3).

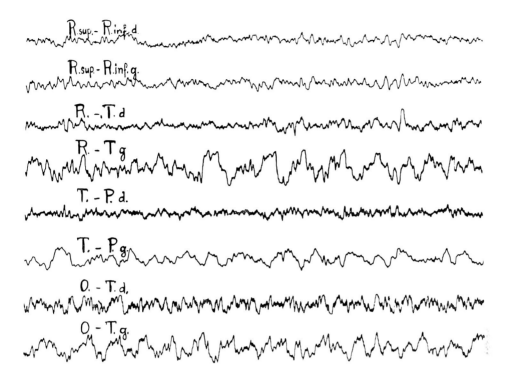

Fig. 3. Legend see Fig. 2, p. 196.

silence", for the diagnosis of the traumatic subdural haematoma, the EEG is still an indispensable complementary method in the treatment of cranial trauma, giving sometimes, in agitated and comatose patients, valuable help towards diagnosis, towards the choice of other complementary procedures, and even towards neuro-surgical intervention.

There again, the echoencephalography may show, in a simpler, faster and more accurate way, the site of haematoma, but by-pass a form which is not exceptional, *i.e.*, the bilateral haematoma.

CONCLUSIONS

The neurosurgeons have often been disillusioned by the so-called EEG negative results, even when the clinical symptoms and the pathologic lesions were spectacular. They have been known for long, the cases of "normal record" or "record not showing pathologic changes" in spite of a thrombosis of one large brain artery, in spite of a serious classical softening of the internal capsule, in spite of an advanced diffuse arteriosclerosis, in spite of the rupture of an aneurysm in the subarachnoidian space, etc. But everybody has now recognized that: it is possible to have lesions reaching

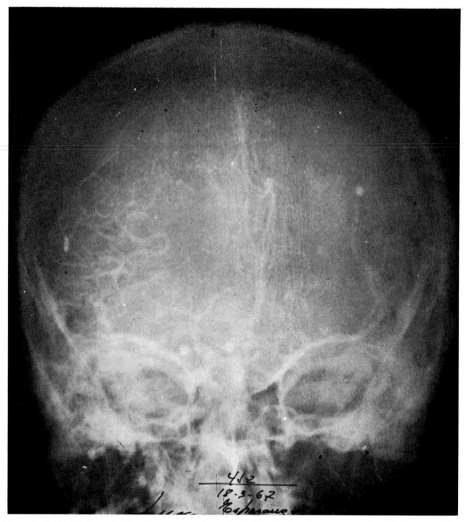

Figs. 4, 5. CASE 3 — L. S., 47 years, male patient. Headaches for some weeks. Under oto-rhino-laryngology treatment of a maxillary sinusitis. Progressive aggravation a week before. No focal clinical signs nor other intracranial hypertension signs. No cranial trauma. EEG focal polymorphic delta activity in the right fronto-temporal area (Fig. 5). Right carotid angiography: subdural haema-toma (Fig. 4).

structures which might be sensible to a clinical expression, without touching the systems which are responsible for the cerebral electrogenesis, or not changing the parameters we know about at present. This means that the "normal" tracings have reasons to stay normal, or else that we do not yet know to see farther. Perhaps we are still in a "pascalian" period of the neurophysiology, to confess that the EEG "has reasons which reason does not know".

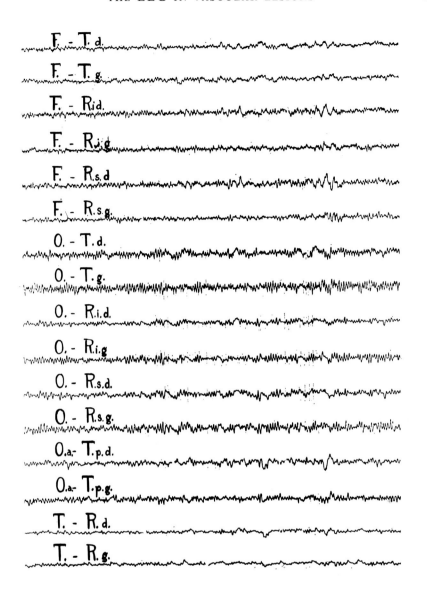

Fig. 5. Legend see Fig. 4, p. 198.

Of course it may often happen that the EEG does not bring any help to the problem put by the clinic of cerebral vascular lesions but it constitutes no additional inconvenience or danger to the patient. Almost always will it contribute to a more complete knowledge of the disease, better understanding of certain clinical symptoms, to confirmation of a localization, to a more accurate prognosis, etc. Only rarely will it be the only means to draw the attention to a diagnosis or to show a localization.

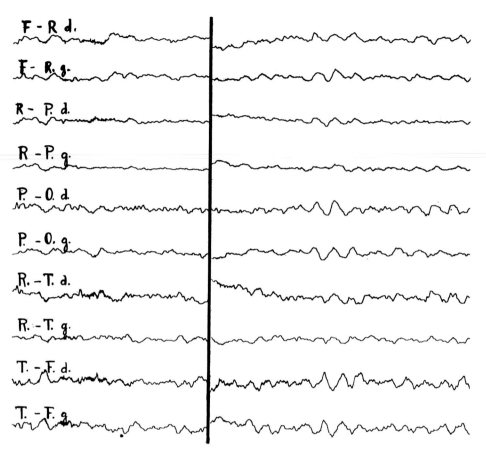

Fig. 6. CASE 4 — J. S., 54 years, male patient. A month before cranial trauma without loss of con sciousness. Two days before the recording, progressive numbness. The neurologic examination only showed slight aphasic signs. The EEG (Fig. 6 — two bits of the same recording) required an angio-graphy which did not show any "classic" signs of haematoma, nor deviation of the anterior cerebral artery. On the basis of the EEG, the surgical exploration revealed bilateral subdural haematoma.

Even if the subsidiary aspects are not considered important or useful, the fact that an EEG may be the decisive factor to save one of our patients, is sufficient reason to practise it always.

Gammaencephalography in Cerebral Vascular Accidents

D. OECONOMOS

Athens (Greece)

The visualization of cerebral infarcts and intracerebral hemorrhages by means of the radioisotopes has already proved to be a most valuable method for the diagnosis and in some way the prognosis of these conditions. On the other hand definite physio-pathological conclusions may be drawn when the results of gammaencephalography are closely compared to those of arteriography and electroencephalography.

There have been published already many contributions on the subject reporting the results obtained with a variety of isotopes such as ^{131}I, ^{74}As, ^{64}Cu, ^{203}Hg or ^{197}Hg (see references).

METHOD

^{197}Hg or ^{203}Hg labeled chlormerodrin, ^{99m}Tc and in a small number of cases RISA-^{131}I were used. Using a rectilinear photoscanner the patients were serially scanned in different time intervals following the administration of the drug. At the end of each scan the differential uptake of the lesion versus the normal brain was counted and its variations within time were compared to those of the photoscans. Many patients had had repeat scan series at different time intervals after the onset of their lesion.

MATERIAL

One hundred cases with circulatory insufficiency of the hemispheres were analyzed. The diagnosis was ascertained on clinical and EEG data and follow-up, once other etiologies had been excluded. Eighty two per cent of the patients have been submitted to serioangiography.

ONSET AND EVOLUTION OF ABNORMAL UPTAKE

Even in the first hours after the stroke the scans and/or the counting of uptake may show an increased concentration in a rather diffuse or localized manner over the affected hemisphere or area, but the isotopic focus is becoming better visualized the following days, the optimal time for visualization occurring between the 10th and 20th day. Later on the abnormal uptake decreases progressively and it disappears generally within 2 to 4 months, eventually in some cases much later. This regressive evolution is in favor of the ischemic nature of the lesion.

References p. 209

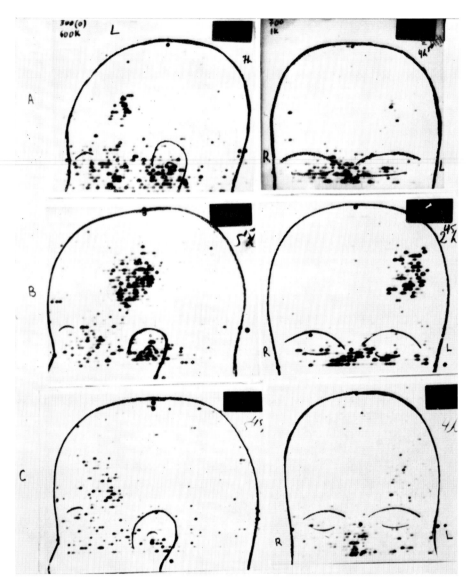

Fig. 1. (A) Posterior low frontal infarct; (B) Ascending frontal convolution infarct; (C) Low frontal (frontoorbital) infarct.

Intensity of uptake

Our results were graded as follows:

Grade 0 Negative

Grade   I Slight hyperactivity not exceeding 40% of the activity of normal brain

Grade II Moderate hyperactivity with differential uptake between 40–70%

Grade III With higher activity and differential uptake from 70–100%

Grade IV Very active focus with differential uptake higher than 100%.

Distribution of our material:

Grade   0 21% of cases
Grade   I 22% of cases
Grade II 27% of cases
Grade III 23% of cases
Grade IV 6% of cases

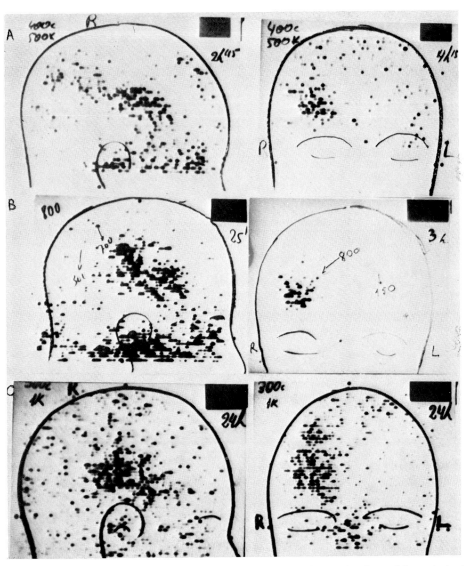

Fig. 2. (A) Infarct of parietal operculum and low parietal area infarct; (B) Infarct of frontoparietal operculum; (C) Extensive suprasylvian infarct.

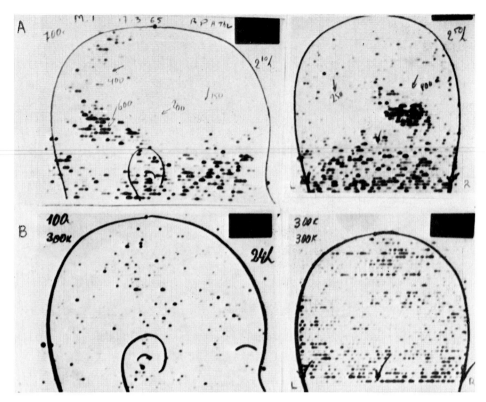

Fig. 3. (A) Infarct of the posterior cerebral artery territory; (B) Infarct at the anterior cerebral
artery territory.

This table shows that 50% of the lesions show a low or moderately increased concentration of isotope and that only 30% have an intense or high uptake. Our overall
positive results are about 79% while those obtained with [74]As amount to 90%
(Ojeman *et al.*, 1964).

1. *Configuration of the abnormal area*

Generally the isotopic focus is not homogeneous. Some parts of it are more active
than others. This pattern may change from one scan to the other. The borders of the
focus are often poorly defined with minor variations in the different scans. When the
intensity of the lesion uptake is not too low the active area has a morphology suggesting
that of a vascular territory.

2. *Topographic pattern of foci*

Generally speaking the malacic lesion presupposes a larger cortical involvement.
Consequently on the frontal views it is often triangular or wedge shaped with its
base oriented towards the cortex. The topographic "vascular" pattern of the lesion
is the most valuable diagnostic feature for the differentiation of the ischemic lesion
from others mainly gliomas, hemorrhages, abcesses, etc. In the present series it has

been possible to identify the following topographic types of lesions.

A. Middle cerebral artery territory

(1) Low frontal or orbitofrontal infarcts: 2 cases
(2) Ascending frontal gyrus infarcts: 8 cases
    (a) Frontal operculum: 5 cases
    (b) Parietal operculum: 5 cases
    (c) Frontoparietal operculum: 3 cases
(4) Rolandoparietal infarcts: 7 cases
(5) Parieto-occipital: 3 cases
(6) Extensive suprasylvian infarcts including the operculum and rolandoparietal areas but leaving free the anterior frontal area: 2 cases
(7) Infrasylvian infarcts, extending upon the convexity of the temporal lobe
(1 case) or concerning mainly its posterior upper part (posterior temporal
artery): 4 cases
(8) Subcortical infarcts have been seen mainly associated with extensive
cortical lesions, insular area and adjoining subcortical structures: 4 cases

                  B. Anterior cerebral artery territory 4 cases
                  C. Posterior cerebral artery territory 8 cases
                  D. Cerebellum: Superior cerebellar artery 1 case

                              Total 58 (73.8%)

This table shows that in almost 74% of the positive cases the lesion has a "vascular" morphology.

3. *Clinical correlations*

(a) Severe neurologic deficits are generally associated with dense and large isotopic foci. The topography and dimensions of the latter and their changes within the same scan series and on repeat studies are useful tools for the reevaluation of the neurologic symptomatology of the various vascular accidents. One should stress the point that small subcortical lesions may be poorly or not visualized on the scans. Thus the absence of a radioisotopic focus, when it is associated with severe neurologic signs, has a bad prognostic value.

(b) The mild sylvian clinical syndromes have negative scans or show small and low energy foci. Their evolution is rapidly regressive. Thus the absence of an isotopic focus when associated with mild clinical symtomatology points towards a favorable prognosis.

(c) The transient ischemic episodes are negative from the isotopic point of view, but embolic episodes may not be negative as stated by others (Ojeman *et al.*, 1964).

4. *Arteriographic correlations*

The arteriographic diagnosis of circulatory impairment was made when at least one of the following findings was present:

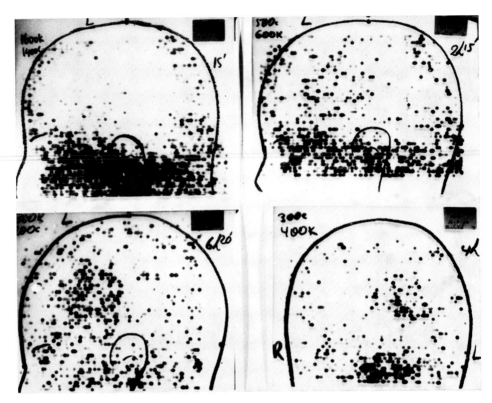

Fig. 4. Intracerebral hematoma (deep subcortical type).

(a) Complete occlusion of the stem or a branch of an artery.

(b) Slowing of circulation in a given cortical area.

(c) Existence of an avascular area associated or not with visualization of recurrent collateral circulation.

(d) Early filling of a draining vein and/or existence of a "blush" in the area suspected to be clinically and/or scintigraphically involved.

Our arteriographic data appear in the following table:

	Cases	%	
Negative arteriogram	30	36,6	
Impairment of middle cer.art. circulation	39	47,56	
Carotid occlusion	6	7.3	57%
Occlusion of post.cer.art.	2	2.44	
Carotid stenosis at the neck	5	6	

Total 82

Thus in the present series 57% of the cases showed definite distal arteriographic signs of circulatory impairment of the brain and 6% had a carotid stenosis at the neck while 37% were arteriographically negative.

The close correlation of arteriographic and isotopic findings permits a closer understanding of the hazards concerning the location, shape and extension of the malacic lesion in each case.

B. Intracerebral hemorrhage group

Our material includes 40 cases of intracerebral hemorrhages and/or hematomas, 8 cases were secondary to a vascular malformation (angiomas, arteriovenous aneurysms or arterial aneurysms); 1 case was the onset episode of a malignant glioma; 31 cases were primitive intracerebral hemorrhages in hypertensive or normotensive patients.

Radioisotopic pattern of intracerebral hemorrhage

(a) Time characteristics. Approximately 40% of the patients were initially scanned during the first week, 30% between the 10th and 20th day and the others the 20th and 30th day after the onset of their lesion. The shortest interval was 48 hours.

The abnormal uptake seems to appear very soon within the first 2 days, but it reaches its full development around the 10th day.

This progression was documented by the fact that the best outlined foci were seen after the first week following the onset of the lesion.

A similar delayed appearance was observed in the infarction group. Nevertheless the hematomas are a little sooner to show up.

(b) Intensity of uptake. Generally the hemorrhagic lesions show a low to moderate increase of concentration, not exceeding at the most 3 to 4 times the uptake of the normal brain parenchyma. In serial scanning they are found to be better stained from the 3rd to the 6th hour following the injection of radioactive Hg or ^{99m}Tc.

The differential uptake is parallelly reaching its highest values at the same time intervals.

In many cases of ^{197}Hg studies the best visualization occurred later, on the 24 hours scan. This points to a retention process taking place within the hematoma. It is worthwhile to point out that the clearance of isotope from the lesion is much delayed when compared to that of normal brain tissue or that of circulating blood.

(c) Morphology of the abnormal area. The hyperactive focus is not homogeneous, its limits may not be well outlined in all directions. Its periphery may appear more active than its center. These findings are in accordance with the fact that the hematoma tissue is mainly the site of increased concentration and not the clot itself (Ojeman *et al.*, 1965; Yamamoto *et al.*, 1964). Within the following hours the content of the hematoma is getting slightly enriched in isotope. This could probably be explained — once a new bleeding has been excluded — by the diffusion, on a pure physicochemical basis, of the isotope from the hyperactive adjacent tissue towards the clot.

(d) Topographic features. There are mainly two radioisotopic types of hemorrhages.
(i) The deep subcortical ones where the main lesion is located into the white matter

encroaching eventually medially upon the ventricular area and laterally upon the cortex. This type of lesion is easily differentiated from an infarct as the latter is composed mainly of cortical involvement.

(ii) The superficial type where a gyrus and the immediately underlying white matter are interested by the lesion. This type may have an elongated shape following the direction of the involved gyrus. Still by thorough analysis of its shape and topography one does not find an identical pattern to that observed in lesions of known arterial territories.

Briefly the isotopic features of intracerebral hemorrhages are the following: Foci more or less well circumscribed with low to moderate uptake with relatively delayed maximal visualization, located mainly deeply under the cortex.

One should stress the point that with the scans the hemorrhagic lesions are located

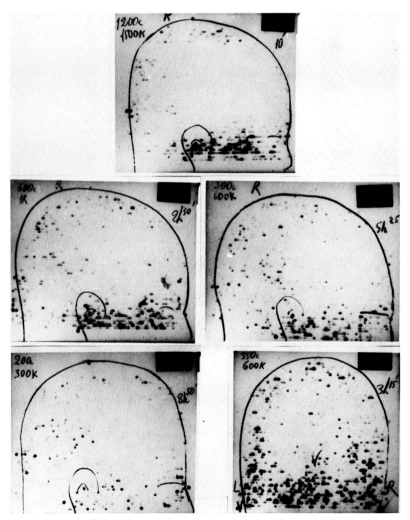

Fig. 5. Intracerebral hematoma (superficial type).

with a high degree of accuracy. The neurosurgeon can easily find them without the additional help of arteriography. In our series 36 out of the 40 cases were positive (90%). On the other hand in 33 of them (82%) the presumptive diagnosis of a hemorrhagic lesion was made on isotopic data.

Hemorrhagic infarct and infarction with edema

In both these conditions the topographic pattern of the lesion favors the infarction etiology and they are easily differentiated from intracerebral hemorrhage.

COMMENTS AND CONCLUSIONS

In our series studied with ^{203}Hg or ^{197}Hg and ^{99m}Tc the overall positive results amount to 79%. In ^{74}As studies this percentage is up to 90% (Ojeman *et al.*, 1964). In 74% of the positive cases the isotopic foci of infarcts have a definite topographic "vascular" pattern which is the main differentiating feature of the lesion. Intracerebral hemorrhages are visualized with isotopes at a high rate (90% in our series of 40 cases). Their hemorrhagic nature is recognized in many cases. Besides their high diagnostic value the scintigraphic studies permit a closer correlation with neurologic, EEG and arteriographic findings and regional cerebral blood flow measurements.

REFERENCES

1 PLANIOL, THÉRÈSE (1966) Gamma-encephalography after ten years of utilization in neurosurgery. *Progr. Neurol. Surg.*, **1**, 94–147.
2 OECONOMOS, D., PROSSALENTIS, A. AND LEVENTIS, A. (1965) Brain scanning with ^{203}Hg and histology of intracranial expanding lesions. *Proc. IIIrd Intern. Congr. Neurosurg., Copenhagen.*
3 GROSS, C., GONSETTE, R., VLAHOVITCH, B. AND GARY-BOBO, J. (1960) La perméabilité des vaisseaux cérébraux. *Acta Neurol. Belg.*, **60**, 481.
4 SOLOWAY, A. H., DE ROUGEMENT, J. G. AND SWEET, W. H. (1960) The re-establishment in dogs of the blood-brain barrier to tri-isopropanolamine borate. *Neurochirurgia*, **3**, 1, 1960.
5 OJEMAN, D. G., ARONOW, S. A. AND SWEET, W. H. (1964) Scanning with positron emitting radio-isotopes in occlusive vascular diseases. *Arch. Neurol.*, **10**, 218–228.
6 OJEMAN, D. G., ARONOW, S. A. AND SWEET, W. H. (1965) Scanning with positron-emitting radio-isotopes: aneurysms, arteriovenous malformations and intracerebral hemorrhages. *J. Neurosurg.*, 489–498.
7 OVERTON, M. C., RAYNIS, T. P. AND SNODGRASS, S. R. (1965) Brain Scans in nonneoplastic intracranial lesions. *J. Am. Med. Assoc.*, **191**, 431–436.
8 WAXMAN, H. J., ZIEGLER, D. K. AND RUBIN, S. (1965) Brain scans in diagnosis of cerebrovascular disease. *J. Amer. Med. Assoc.*, **192**, 453–456.
9 QUINN, J. L. III, CIRIC, I. AND HANSER, W. N. (1965) Analysis of 96 abnormal scans using technetium 99m pertechnetate. *J. Am. Med. Assoc.*, **194**, 157–160.
10 RHOTON, A. L., KLINKERFUSS, G. H., LILLY, D. R. AND TER-POGOSSIAN, M. M. (1966) Brain scanning in ischaemic cerebrovascular diseases. *Arch. Neurol.*, **14**, 506–511.
11 YAMAMOTO, Y. L., FEINDEL, W. AND ZANELLI, J. (1964) Comparative study of radioactive chlormerodrin (neohydrin) tagged with mercury 197 or mercury 203 for brain scanning. *Neurology*, **14**, 815–820.

Echo-encephalography and Cerebral Circulation

M. DE VLIEGER

Municipal Hospital Dijkzigt, Rotterdam (The Netherlands)

Echo-encephalography finds application in the diagnosis of space occupying lesions. These can cause displacement of the midline structures, which displacement is visualized in the echo-encephalogram by a shift of the midline-echo. Reports on series of echo-encephalograms were given by de Vlieger *et al.* (1959), Jeffersson (1959, 1962), Lithander (1961), Jeppsson (1961), Taylor *et al.* (1961), Ford *et al.* (1963), Schiefer *et al.* (1963), Sugar *et al.* (1964), Planiol *et al.* (1964), Greebe (1964), Barrows *et al.* (1965), Kurze *et al.* (1965), Brinker *et al.* (1965), Mikol *et al.* (1965), Klingler (1965) and Achar *et al.* (1966). According to these investigators the reliability of this method is 84–100%.

Echo-encephalography has three interesting aspects in the cerebro-vascular disorders. (1) The place of the midline-echo and other echoes in an echo-encephalogram. (2) The latency time between the echo-pulsations and the QRS complex. (3) The abnormal dicrotism of the echopulsation curves in arterio-venous aneurysms.

In echo-encephalography pulsed ultrasound is transmitted into the skull by a piëzo-electric crystal. The reflected ultrasound pulses are picked up by the same crystal, converted in electrical signals and recorded on an oscilloscope. Reflections can be obtained among others from the inner surface of the opposite side of the skull, from the structures in the midline and from the walls of the lateral ventricles. Reflections from the skull nearest to the transmitting crystal coincide on the scope with the transmitting pulse. The echoes, as displayed on an echoscope demonstrate vertical pulsations. In his first paper on echo-encephalography Leksell (1955) has already described pulsations synchronous with the heartbeat. We recorded these pulsations by connecting the ultrasonic equipment to a recording system through a gating system (de Vlieger *et al.* 1959; ter Braak *et al.*, 1961, 1965; Jeppsson, 1964; de Vlieger *et al.*, 1965). This gating system suppresses all energy except that originating in the reflecting plane or region to be examined. The most common form of the pulsations, thus recorded, is more or less a sawtooth-curve. The sawtooth-shape of these curves is rather similar to that of the carotid pulsations.

Jeppsson (1964) and ter Braak *et al.* (1965) used the rise time of the rising phase of such a curve as a criterion, investigating the pressure of cerebral spinal fluid. These echo-pulsations turned out to correlate with the pressure of the cerebro-spinal fluid. Freund (1965) stated that some of the echoes are caused by the pulsations of the cerebral arteries. To his opinion the echo-pulsations of thrombotic arteries have a lower amplitude than those of normal arteries.

1. The midline echo in cerebro-vascular lesions

The cerebro-vascular disorders were divided into two groups: (a) The intracerebral haemorrhages and infarctions; (b) The haemorrhages into the subarachnoid space.

Within the first group a comparison was made between intracerebral haemorrhages, infarctions by cerebral embolism and non-embolic (thrombotic) cerebral infarctions. Within the second group subarachnoid haemorrhages without an aneurysm were compared with those from an aneurysm and from an arterio-venous aneurysm.

In accordance with Barrows *et al.* (1965) and Achar *et al.* (1966) a shift of at least 3 mm was taken as a significant displacement of the midline structures.

(a) Cerebral haemorrhages and infarctions. The diagnoses were made by clinicians, who did not make the echo-encephalograms. The echo-encephalograms were made by neurologists working in the neurophysiological department. Cerebral haemorrhages were diagnosed, when there was blood or xanthochromia of the cerebro-spinal fluid in acute unconscious, hypertensive patients. The infarction by embolism was diagnosed, when there was a potential source as in atrial fibrillation. The other cases were classified as non-embolic cerebral infarction. This classification is in accordance with that of Achar *et al.* (1966).

432 patients were examined in this way. Of 49 patients with a cerebral haemorrhage 33 (64%) showed a shift of the midline-echo. In cases of cerebral embolism we found

TABLE I

ECHO-ENCEPHALOGRAPHY IN RELATION TO CEREBRAL HAEMORRHAGES AND INFARCTIONS WITH A CONTROL GROUP OF CEREBRAL TUMOURS

Diagnosis	*Number of patients*	*Percentage of patients with a displaced mid-line-echo*
Cerebral haemorrhage	49	64% (33)
Cerebral embolic infarctions	52	19% (10)
Non-embolic cerebral infarctions	331	18% (58)
Cerebral tumours	142	87% (124)

a displacement in 10 (19%) out of 52 patients and in non-embolic cerebral infarction in 58 (18%) out of 331 patients (Table I). Because differentiation between embolic or non-embolic infarction and brain tumour can be difficult, a control group of 144 cerebral tumours was investigated. Of these patients 124 (87%) showed a shift of the midline-echo. It turned out that according to the chi-square test (correction of Yates) there is a relation between diagnosis and percentages of displaced midline echoes. Conform to Table I in cerebral haemorrhages and embolic infarctions is $\chi^2 = 13.9$ ($P < 0.001$), in cerebral haemorrhages and non-embolic infarctions is $\chi^2 = 37.5$

TABLE II

EEG	Number of patients	Displacement
(a) ECHO-ENCEPHALOGRAPHY OF CEREBRAL HAEMORRHAGES IN RELATION TO EEG ABNORMALITIES		
Normal	0	0
General slowing	2	0
General slowing with focal activity	26	58% (15)
(b) ECHO-ENCEPHALOGRAPHY OF CEREBRAL-EMBOLIC INFARCTIONS IN RELATION TO EEG ABNORMALITIES		
Normal	9	0
General slowing	4	0
General slowing with focal activity	32	19% (6)
(c) ECHO-ENCEPHALOGRAPHY OF CEREBRAL NON-EMBOLIC INFARCTIONS IN RELATION TO EEG ABNORMALITIES		
Normal	29	0
General slowing	45	2% (1)
General slowing with focal activity	206	21% (44)

$(P < 0.001)$, in cerebral tumours and embolic infarctions is $\chi^2 = 77.7$ $(P < 0.001)$ and in cerebral tumours and non-embolic infarctions is $\chi^2 = 205.3$ $(P < 0.001)$. In order to obtain some idea about the magnitude of the cerebro-vascular lesions, the echo-encephalograms were compared with the EEG's. The EEG's were divided into three groups: normal, showing generalised slow activity and generalised slow activity combined with focal activity (Table IIa, b and c).

Only patients having an abnormal EEG showed a shift of the midline-echo, especially those demonstrating focal activity. Not all of the patients had an EEG because some were too ill and died soon after admission.

Table III shows that the prognosis of patients demonstrating a shift of the midline-echo is worse than that of those without a shift. More than half of the patients with a cerebral haemorrhage and showing displacement of the midline-echo died.

The greatest difference in prognosis between a shifted or a median midline-echo was in patients having an embolic infarction.

(b) Subarachnoid haemorrhages. In Table IV patients having no demonstrable aneurysm are compared with those showing an aneurysm or an arterio-venous aneurysm on angiography. It is evident, that there is no difference between the patients with (15%) and without (14%) a demonstrable aneurysm in the percentages showing a displacement of the midline structures.

In patients having an arterio-venous aneurysm the percentage showing a displacement is greater (29%).

As anticipated the greatest number of patients showing a displaced midline-echo

TABLE III

PERCENTAGE OF PATIENTS WITH A DISPLACED AND A MEDIAN MIDLINE - ECHO, WHO
LATER DIED FROM THEIR CEREBRAL HAEMORRHAGE, EMBOLIC OR NON-EMBOLIC INFARCTION

Diagnosis	Displacement	No displacement
Cerebral haemorrhage	58% (19/33)	31% (5/ 16)
Cerebral embolic infarction	40% (4/10)	12% (5/ 42)
Cerebral non-embolic infarction	45% (27/58)	21% (58/273)

TABLE IV

ECHO-ENCEPHALOGRAPHY IN RELATION TO SUBARACHNOID HAEMORRHAGES WITH AND
WITHOUT AN ARTERIAL ANEURYSM OR FROM AN ARTERIOVENOUS ANEURYSM

Diagnosis	Number of patients	Percentage of patients with a displaced midline–echo
Subarachn. haem. no art. aneurysm demonstrated	104	14% (15)
Subarachn. haem. with art. aneurysm	60	15% (9)
Art. venous aneurysm	17	29% (5)

TABLE V

EEG	Number of patients	Displacement
(a) ECHO - ENCEPHALOGRAPHY OF SUBARACHNOID HAEMORRHAGES WITHOUT AN ARTERIAL ANEURYSM IN RELATION TO EEG ABNORMALITIES		
Normal	17	0
General slowing	23	4% (1)
General slowing with focal activity	38	16% (6)
(b) ECHO-ENCEPHALOGRAPHY OF SUBARACHNOID HAEMORRHAGES WITH AN ARTERIAL ANEURYSM IN RELATION TO EEG ABNORMALITIES		
Normal	10	10% (1)
General slowing	13	8% (1)
General slowing with focal activity	25	28% (7)
(c) ECHO-ENCEPHALOGRAPHY OF ARTERIO-VENOUS ANEURYSMS WITH A SUB- ARACHNOID HAEMORRHAGE IN RELATION TO EEG ABNORMALITIES		
Normal	1	0
General slowing	1	0
General slowing with focal activity	9	44% (4)

TABLE VI

PERCENTAGE OF PATIENTS WITH A DISPLACED AND MEDIAN MIDLINE-ECHO, WHO LATER
DIED FROM A SUBARACHNOID HAEMORRHAGE

Diagnosis	Displacement	No displacement
Subarachn. haem. without art. aneurysm	53% (8/15)	11% (10/89)
Subarachn. haem. with art. aneurysm	33% (3/ 9)	12% (6/51)
Art. venous aneurysm.	20% (1/ 5)	25% (3/12)

is to be found among those having focal activity in the EEG, while the prognosis of these cases is significantly worse. The arterio-venous aneurysms do not show this tendency, though one has to take into account that their numbers are small.

2. Latency time between the echo-pulsation and the QRS complex

Several methods can be used to demonstrate these pulsations. Amplitude changes can be recorded by photography with long exposure time of one isolated echo on the screen, or by filming these changes (Freund, 1965; Tanaka *et al.*, 1965).

As already has been mentioned, we prefer to use a gating system, which suppresses all energy except that originating in the reflection plane or region to be examined (de Vlieger *et al.*, 1959, 1965; ter Braak *et al.*, 1961, 1965; Wallace *et al.*, 1966).

Only some preliminary results are presented here to give an idea of the value of this method of investigation. To calculate the latency time, we measured the interval between the peak of the R-deflection of the ECG and the point at half the height of the rising phase on the echo-pulsation curve (Fig. 1). This point was chosen because

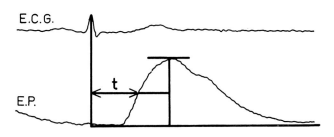

Fig. 1. Measurement of the latency time between R-deflection of the ECG and a point at half the height of the rising phase on the echo-pulsation curve (E.P.).

it proved much more difficult to estimate the exact beginning of the rising phase of the pulsation or of its peak. According to de Vlieger *et al.* the latency times vary tenths of milliseconds in normal subjects. In a diagram in which the latency times are represented at the exact place of the reflected echo, they show a certain symmetry for both hemispheres. The points seem to give an outline of the vascular tree.

This may be due to the fact that several reflecting planes do not pulsate synchro-nously. Some findings suggest that under pathological circumstances the variability of the latency times is larger than in normal subjects. In 5 normal subjects the latency times varied from 180–270 msec. In 3 cases having an arterio-venous aneurysm the latency times varied from 160–325, 110–215 and 150–290 msec. In a patient with an intersection of the right carotid artery they varied as in normals 160–250 msec. In a case of thrombosis of the left carotid artery the latency times varied from 150–220 msec and for comparison in a patient with a frontal tumor from 180–320 msec. Under pathological circumstances especially in patients with an arterio-venous aneurysm, the diagrams gave an asymmetric outline. Apparently an obstruction of one of the main arteries does not influence the latency times significantly.

3. Echo-pulsations in arterio-venous aneurysms

The echo-pulsation curves of patients having an arterio-venous aneurysm sometimes show abnormal dicrotism. Among 17 patients with an arterio-venous aneurysm we found 12 to have such an abnormal dicrotism.

COMMENT

It is important to know how accurate echo-encephalography is; White et al. (1965) compared the results of a qualified and neurologically oriented physician and an unskilled one. The physician was correct in 95% of cases, but the technician obtained false positive results in about 12% of a healthy population of 1008 persons. They believe the method suggests an accuracy, which is not warranted.

In the present investigation nine neurologists made the echo-encephalograms. To estimate the accuracy of the method, we compared the echo-encephalograms at 251 patients with their angiograms and with the findings at autopsy. There was agreement in 228 (91%) patients. Knowledge at a hemiplegia could of course have influenced the results of the echo-encephalography. Of 104 patients with a non-embolic infarction and a hemiplegia 17 (16%) showed a shift of the midline echo. Of the total 331 patients with non-embolic cerebral infarction whether they had a hemiplegia or not 85 (18%) showed a displaced midline-echo.

It is possible to obtain echoes from an intracerebral haematoma (ter Braak et al., 1959; Nagai et al., 1964; Kikuchi et al., 1964; Kazner et al., 1965). I am convinced however, that predicting from an A-scan echo-encephalogram whether the echoes are caused by an intracerebral haematoma or not, will lead to many errors.

In this paper we report preliminary results of our investigation of echo-pulsations. Ter Braak and de Vlieger mentioned already the abnormal dicrotism of the echo-pulsation in patients having an arteriovenous aneurysm. They also found a difference in latency time in 11 out of 19 cases with a supratentorial tumour between carotid pulse and echo-pulsation time at the normal and pathological side. On the patholog-ical side the latency time was longer than normal. This led to our investigation of the latency times of normal subjects and of patients having a cerebro-vascular disorder. Freund (1965) studied the echo-pulsations of several cerebral vessels and found that the echo-pulsations were either lacking or shortened at the side of the obstructed carotid. We have not been able to repeat this observation. However the number of cases we studied was limited. The measuring of the echo-pulsations offers a problem because of several factors: *e.g.* the proper contact between the probe and the skull, the direction and the diameter of the sound beam, the sensitivity of the apparatus etc. It could be very well however, that some pulsations are only slight or altogether lacking in carotid artery thrombosis. Or some pulsating echoes are caused by arteries, while others originate in brain tissue itself. In our opinion however, it is extremely difficult to locate the echo-pulsations from the arteries in every echo-encephalogram, especially under pathological circumstances.

REFERENCES

ACHAR, V. S., COE, R. P. K., AND MARSHALL, J., (1966); Echoencephalography in the differential diagnosis haemorrhage and infarction. *Lancet*, i, 161–164.

BARROWS, H. S., DYCK, P., AND KURZE, T., (1965); The diagnostic applications of ultrasound in neurological disease. *Neurology*, **15**, 361–365.

BRAAK, J. W. G. TER., GRANDIA, W. A. M., AND VLIEGER, M. DE, (1959); 'Echo-encephalography' as an aid in the diagnosis of subdural and extradural haematomas, in: A. Biemond (Ed.), *Recent Neurological Research*, pp. 37–46. Elsevier, Amsterdam.

—, CREZÉE, P., GRANDIA, W. A. M., AND VLIEGER, M. DE, (1961); The significance of some reflections in 'Echo-encephalography'. *Acta Neurochirurgica*, **9**, 382–397.

—, AND VLIEGER, M. DE, (1965); Cerebral pulsations in echo-encephalography. *Acta Neurochirurgica*, **12**, 678–694.

BRINKER, J. W. B., KING, D. L., AND TAVERAS, J. M., (1965); Echo-encephalography. *Am. J. Roentgenol.*, **93**, 781–790.

FORD, R., AND AMBROSE, J., (1963); Echo-encephalography. *Brain*, **86**, 189–196.

FREUND, H. J., (1965); Ultraschall Registrierung der Pulsation einzelner intrakranieller Arterien zur Diagnostik von Gefässverschlüssen. *Arch. Psychiat. Z. ges. Neurol.*, **207**, 247–253.

GREEBE, H. M., (1964); De waarde van de echo-encephalografie als klinische en poliklinische methode van onderzoek. *Ned. Tijds. Geneesk.*, **108**, 10–13.

JEFFERSON, A., (1959); Some experiences with echo-encephalography. *J. Neurol. psych.*, **22**, 83–84.

—, (1962); Clinical experiences with echo-encephalography. *Acta Neurochir.*, **10**, 392–409.

JEPPSSON, S., (1961); Echo-encephalography. *Acta Chir. Scand.*, **125**, *Suppl. 272*, 1–151.

—, (1964); Echo-encephalography V. *Acta Chir. Scand.*, **128**, 218–224.

KAZNER, E., KUNZE, St., AND SCHIEFER, W., (1965); Die Bedeutung der Echo-encephalographie für die Erkennung epiduraler Hämatome. *Langenbecks Arch. Klin. Chir.*, **310**, 267–291.

KIKUCHI, S., ITO, K., AND ABE, Y., (1963); *Diagnosis of apoplexy by ultrasonic pulses. Proc. 4th Meeting Japan Soc. Ultrason. Med., 53–56. Tokyo, Juntendo University.*

KLINGLER, D., (1965); Die diametrale bitemporale Echoencephalographie im A-skope unter Abstimmung auf die ideale Medianebene. *Clin. Neurophysiol. E.E.G.-E.M.G. 6th Intern. Congr. E.E.G. Clin. Neurophysiol., Vienna*, pp. 579–600.

KURZE, Th., DYCK, AND BARROWS, H. S., (1965); Neurosurgical evaluation of ultrasonic encephalograph. *J. Neurosurg.*, **22**, 437–440.

LEKSSELL, L., (1955); Echo-encephalography. *Acta Chir. Scand.*, **110**, 301–315.

LITHANDER, B., (1961); Clinical and experimental studies in echo-encephalography. *Acta Psych. Neurol. Scand.*, **36**, *Suppl. 159*, 1–52.

MIKOL, F., AND HAZEMANN, P., (1965); E.E.G. et écho-encéphalographie. *Clin. Neurophysiol. E.E.G.-E.M.G. 6th. Intern. Congr. E.E.G. Clin. Neurophysiol., Vienna*, pp. 593–595.

NAGAI, H., SAKURAI, K., HAYASKI, M., FURUSE, M., OKAMUSA, K., SHINTANI, A., AND KOBAYASHI, T., (1963); Echo-encephalogram following experimental intracerebral haemorrhage and cerebral infarction — Relationship between echo-encephalography and histological findings. *Proc. 4th Meeting Japan. Soc. Ultrason. Med., 50–53. Tokyo, Juntendo University.*

PLANIOL, T., MIKOL, F., CHARPENTIER, J., AND BUISSON, J., (1964); L'écho-encéphalographie. *Rev. Neurol.*, **110**, 489–505.

SCHIEFER, W., KAZNER, E., AND BRÜCKNER, H., (1963); Die Echoenzephalographie, ihre Anwendungsweise und klinischen Ergebnisse. *Forts. Neurol., Psychiat.*, **31**, 457–491.

SUGAR, O., AND UEMATSU, S., (1964); The use of ultrasounds in the diagnosis of intracranial lesions. *Surg. Clinics N. Am.*, **44**, 55–64.

TANAKA, K., ITO, K., AND WAGAI, T., (1965); The localization of brain tumor by ultrasonic techniques. A clinical review of 111 cases. *J. Neurosurg.*, **23**, 135–147.

TAYLOR, J. C., NEWELL, J. A., AND KARVOUNIS, (1961); Ultrasonics in the diagnosis of intracranial space occupying lesions. *Lancet*, **i**, 1197–1199.

VLIEGER, M. DE, AND RIDDER, H. J., (1959); Use of echo-encephalography. *Neurology*, **9**, 216–223.

—, DENIER VAN DER GON, J. J., LUGT, P. J. M. VAN DER, AND MOLIN, C. E., (1965); Pulsations in echo-encephalography. *Clin. Neurophysiol. E.E.G.-E.M.G. 6th Intern. Congr. E.E.G. Clin. Neurophysiol., Vienna*, pp. 591–592.

WALACE, W. K., AVANT, Jr., W. S., MCKINNEY, W. M., AND THURSTONE, F. L., (1966); Ultrasonic techniques for measuring intracranial pulsations. *Neurology*, **16**, 380–383.

WHITE, D. M., CHESEBROUGH, J. M., AND BLANCHARD, J. B., (1965); Studies in ultrasonic echo-encephalography. *Neurol.*, **15**, 81–86.

Pallencephalography

J. J. BARCIA-GOYANES AND J. L. BARCIA-SALORIO

Valencia (Spain)

Pallencephalography (PEG) is a method which consists in recording changes in intracranial pressure through the cranium and other intact coverings by means of a microphone placed on the surface of the scalp. Its name (from $\pi\alpha\lambda\lambda\omega =$ I shake, the same root which gives pallaesthesia) indicates that its register covers a wide range of frequencies and includes not only the cerebral pulse, recorded previously through burr holes, fontanelles or bone defects, but also the more rapid frequencies, such as murmurs or bruits recorded previously by means of conventional phonography, and intermediate frequencies not registered until the present time.

This method has been devised, developed and applied by the authors since 1953 in more than 3,000 cases of neuropsychiatric or neurosurgical patients, finding an ample scope of usefulness, from the diagnosis and localization of surgical processes such as haematomata and tumours, to changes in cerebral circulation and even in the study of certain psychoses.

The slower variations of pressure registered in the endocranium–leaving aside aperiodic ones produced by impletive processes–were known ever since ancient times (Galenus, Oribasius, Celsus, Baglivi, Haller, etc.) because they produce movements in the cerebral mass and meninges, in the course of a trepanation or through fontanelles or bone defects.

These movements, known as cerebral pulse, include two different types independent of each other, differentiated by Leyden (1866): those synchronized with the breathing and those synchronized with the periferic arterial pulse. Later works confirmed this discovery (Salathe, Fredericq, Giaccomini, Mosso, etc.) and since then two types of waves have been distinguished: the respiratory and the circulatory.

The fundamental problem in Pallencephalography lies in the posibility of capturing these waves through the cranium as there is no doubt that it is certainly possible to capture the highest frequencies, being always pathological, known to surgery as cephalic souffles (or thrills, bruits, etc.) and which were studied by many authors (Hamburger; McKenzie; Wadie and Mockton; Cohen and Miller; Dalsgaard and Nielsen; Cushing and Bailey) or registered with phonocardiographic apparatuses by Olivecrona and Ladenheim.

The brain, like any organ, possesses volumetric variations due to the changes in its blood-content along the cardiac cycle. If an arm is placed in a plethysmograph, the afore-mentioned volumetric variations appear. They disappear or diminish if the apparatus is closed completely and is filled with a liquid such as water. Nevertheless, in these circumstances the brachial pulse continues to exist, but what occurs is that the cardiac energy is now transformed into changes of pressure rather than changes of volume.

The same occurs in the cranium, because when a bone defect or fontanelle exists, the box possesses great distensibility (Hurthle's Dehnungsfähigkeit) at this point and the volumetric variations are greater than those in pressure. On the contrary, within the closed cranium, which is very rigid, the variations in pressure are greater than those in volume, or displacements of mass (Massenverschiebungen). This attribute of the cranium is of special interest to us, because it is that which is going to allow us to record variations in pressure: the object of Pallencephalography. This attribute allows the passage of rapid or audible vibrations through the cranium, permitting the auscultation of endocranial souffles from the exterior, or the passage of ultrasonic waves (Echoencephalogram of Leksell). In a similar way, it will allow the passage of infrasonic waves. Schwarzacher (1924) demonstrated how the pressure, which is produced in the exterior of the cranium in a closed traumatism passes in the form of waves to the interior, as Kocher (1910) and later Payr, Hauptmann, Sauerbruch, etc. had already sustained. Finally Walker (1944) with Hamilton's manometer and Gurdjian, Webster and Lissner (1945) with their technique were able to see and measure the bone deformation which allows the passage of pressure (inbending and outbending) at the moment of the blow.

The authors have demonstrated how endocranial pressures may, although very greatly diminished, spread from within the cranium to the exterior. This damping depends on the frequency of the pressure waves and, while in the audible frequency

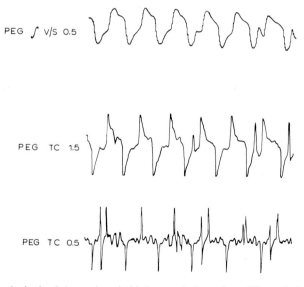

PEG ∫ v/s 0.5

PEG TC 1.5

PEG TC 0.5

Fig. 1. PEG record obtained (second and third curves) through a differentiating amplifier with 1.5 and 0.5 time-constant respectively. In the first curve we can see the cerebral pulse obtained through integration.

it is negligible, in the frequency of 30 c/s it is of —40 db, and in the frequency of 50 c/s it is of —60 db. The basic wave of the cerebral pulse, of a frequency of around 80 c/min (i.e. 0.9 c/s), is practically damped.

As the cerebral pulse, in the same way as the arterial pulse, is composed of a variable range of frequencies, the cranium behaves like a selective filter, damping the frequencies more which differ from its own, which is a frequency of around 200 c/s according to Walker (1944) and 700 c/s according to Gurdjian (1945).

METHOD

The method developed by the authors consists of a piezoelectric microphone for low frequencies, placed on a special support which, in the first place enables it to be connected to standard point of the cranium always under the same pressure, and in the second place enables it to be connected to a column of 150 kg weight in order to eliminate ballistocardiogram movements. Gutierrez-Mahoney and Cuevas (1964) have introduced a modification to eliminate the support and to place the microphone manually under a constant pressure, avoiding the patient any trouble. Samsó and Vila-Badó (1957) used contact microphones for the first time simultaneously, instead of one alone which is placed successively at each point, as in our original procedure. This has the advantage of more speed and convenience but has the disadvantage that the output of the microphone is proportional to the derivate of the pressure, and, if the head is not fixed, the balistocardiogram may interfere. Finally B. Weeks, Toole and R. Robinson (1965) used similar microphones.

The amplifier used by us as well as by our colleagues has been that used in electro-encephalography, because a big gain is needed for the considerable damping of the bone upon the cerebral pulse to which we have referred before. As the EEG is designed for the amplification of very low frequencies, it is ideal for the amplification of the cerebral pulse through the cranium, because it partly compensates for its distortion-effect. Nevertheless, it has the disadvantage of being a differentiating amplifier and

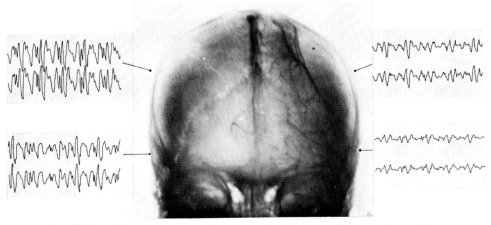

Fig. 2. PEG in subdural haematomata. We can see the flattening of the records on the haematoma.

therefore its output is proportional to the differential of the microphone output. The PEG record is therefore the cerebral pulse lineally distorted through the cranium and differentiated by the amplifier. Thus the typical record resembles the profile of the cerebral pulse very little. The authors have connected circuits and integrating amplifiers so that a graphic record of the cerebral pulse is obtained.

PATHOLOGICAL PEG

The cerebral pulse is involved in intracranial pathological processes. Riechert and Heines (1950) saw how, with the increase of intracranial pressure, the pulse rate diminished or disappeared, a fact verified by Gerlach (1950). Noto (1935) studied the cerebral pulse in brain tumours, finding a flattening of the former with very rounded waves. Later Colombati confirmed the discovery and Gerlach himself found the said changes in the neighbourhood of the tumour, which contrasted with the normality of the pulse in the healthy hemisphere.

In PEG we find the same changes found through burr holes, but in this case through the intact cranium. In generalised hypertension e.g. in closed hydrocephalus, cerebral oedema, pseudotumours, etc. there exists a diminution of the wave-length, which appear rounded and with lower frequency in all the explored points of the cranium. In tumours, the points neighbouring them contrast with the symmetrical ones of the healthy side, the process being able to be localized perfectly. In gliomata, the typical register is very flat and of very low frequency, especially when they have arterio-venous fistulas. On the contrary, in meningiomata rapid frequencies of 30 c/s appear which are useful for their specific diagnosis. This specification of the tumour type is due to the different vascularization of each tumour. While in gliomata there is an increase in the speed of the circulation, in meningiomata there is a delay.

Where the method is shown to be of great use is in the diagnosis of closed trauma-tisms of the skull. Both extradural haematomata and subdural ones produce an abolition or great diminution of the cerebral pulse where they are found producing a great diminution in the breadth of the waves of the PEG, which allows its diagnosis with great rapidity and certainty (100% in our statistics). These results in the diagnosis of tumours have been confirmed by Gutierrez-Mahoney and Cuevas (1964) and Weeks and Toole (1965).

PEG IN HAEMODYNAMIC CHANGES

Burdach (1822) and Bichat and Richerand (1823) thought that the cerebral pulse was a passive movement of the brain due to the basal arteries, but Hurthle (1927) argued that the latter represent a very small volume in comparison with those of the rest of the brain. The changes in pressure which form the cerebral pulse are a result of the cyclic dilatation of the cerebral arteries, as if the brain were placed in a plethysmograph and also, as we have been able to demonstrate with PEG, there exists a delay between the record at one point of the skull and at another, following the path of the main arteries.

The fact that by means of PEG we have the outline of the arterial cerebral pulse, allows us to apply the laws of hydrodynamics created by Ludwig's kymograph regarding the arteries of the rest of the body and which were without application for the cerebral arteries.

One of the most interesting problems in the study of a determined circulation is to discover its regulation.

The concept of vascular resistance, deduced from Poiseuille's law (1799–1869) assuming a continuous regimen in which the outflow depends lineally on the diameter of the blood-vessel is of doubtful application to the brain. An increase in the bore of its blood-vessels, necessary to adjustment, implies an increase in cerebral volume ("congestion cérébrale" de Brachet (1830)) with consequent endocranial hypertension. The Monro, Kellie and Abercrombie's law (1783) although partially belied by the displaceability of the third element, C.S.F., is still partially valid. On the other

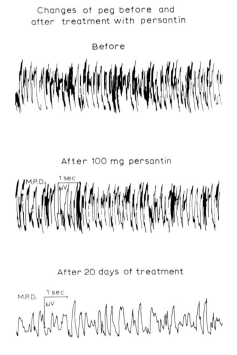

Fig. 3. PEG in a commotional syndrome with a clear fast-waves component. After a treatment with Persantin we can see the waves become slower.

hand, the fact that the outflow of the cerebral arteries oscillates, as we can see from the cerebral pulse and the PEG records, has obliged us to confront the problem of cerebral haemodynamics in accordance with the theory of the alternating current introduced in haemodynamics by Womersley (1955) and McDonald (1957). According to these authors, rather than vascular resistance, we must speak of arterial impedance. The vasomotor activity during the vasoconstriction caused by noradrenaline p.g.

increases impedance in the artery for low frequencies with a considerable increase in its reflection coefficient, but nevertheless diminishes the impedance for high frequencies. The vasodilation has the inverse effect, diminishing impedance for low frequency components. This is shown in PEG by the fact that, when a vasoconstriction exists, there often a clear predominance of high frequencies appears, which often converts the tracing into that of a souffle and which in the clinic can be heard by the patient as tinnitus.

The increase of O_2 by hyperventilation produces this phenomenon. On the contrary, the increase of CO_2 or papaverine and the derivatives of pyrimido-pyrimidin produce a disappearance of the rapid components and the further reappearance of the slow components.

The increase and predominance of the rapid vibrations appear in certain states of the cerebral artery which, not presenting any lesion, makes it necessary to conclude that we are dealing with pure haemodynamic alterations through change of their vasomotor activity, a typical finding in the endogenous depressions, Morgagni-Stewart-Morel syndrom, Barré-Liéou syndrome, Ménière disease and post-commotional syndrom. The treatment with the afore-mentioned vasodilators normalises the PEG record, simultaneously with the clinical remission. We think that all this must be based on changes in arterial impedance and that in the afore-mentioned pathological processes an alteration of the artery would exist with a loss of circulatory energy in the form of acoustic energy which would be the cause of certain symptoms, such as tinnitus, dizziness, etc. The control through impedance without any great change of the arterial bore would explain the small change in the diameter of the cerebral arteries up to a point.

The morphological arterial alterations also follow this law. The arteriovenous fistulas, in which the arterial impedance is very low caused by disappearance of capillary resistance, a great predominance of low frequency waves exists, and when the defect is very great, as the regime becomes continuous, cerebral pulsations and PEG waves disappear. After the operation pulsations come back with the removal of the fistula and the record becomes normal. In aneurysms we have found an increase in the rapid components in the neighbourhood of the altered artery, especially when a strong spasm exists.

The method also serves to diagnose thromboses, embolisms, etc. and it is very useful in the study of cerebral arteriosclerosis. The loss of the arterial contraction and of the damping effect (Windkessel) produces certain records with very broad diastolic waves with no tendency to disappear. These records correspond to normotensvee patients in advanced middle age and who have had several crises of cerebral vascular claudication. Another group of arteriosclerotic patients is formed of younger individuals, who are hypertensive and have tinnitus, dizziness, headache and depressive syndromes. They show a record very rich in rapid vibrations, indicating an increase in arterial impedance with a high index of reflection in the circulatory waves produced by a narrowing of arterial bore.

REFERENCES

COHEN, J. H. AND MILLER, P. (1956) Eyeball bruits. *N. Engl. J. Med.*, 255–459.

COLOMBATI, S. (1950) Caratteri del polso cerebrari nei tumori endocranici. *Neuropsichiatr.*, 328–352.

GERLACH, J. (1952) Zerebraler Grenzdruck und Hirnpuls. *Acta Neurochirurg.*, **11**, 120–158.

GURDJIAN, E. S. AND LISSNER, H. R. (1945) Deformation of skull injury; study with "stresscoat" technic. *S.G. & O.*, **81**, 679–687.

GUTIERREZ-MAHONEY AND CUEVAS (1965) La Palencefalografia: Un nuevo método para la exploracion del cerebro. *Rev. Esp. O.N.O. y Neurocirurg.*, 138.

HAMBURGER, L. P. (1931) Head murmurs. *Am. J. Med. Sci.*, **181**, 756.

HAUPTMANN (1913) Untersuchungen über das Wesen des Hirndrucks. *Z. Neur.*, 14.

LEYDEN, W. (1866) Beiträge und Untersuchungen zur Physiologie und Patologie des Gehirns. *Virchow's Archiv*, **37**, 511–599.

MCDONALD, D. A. (1960) *Blood flow in arteries*. Mon. of Physiol. Soc., Edward Arnold, London.

MCKENZIE, I. (1956) The intracranial bruit. *Brain*, 78.

OLIVECRONA AND LADENHEIN (1957) *Congenital arteriovenous aneurysms of the carotid and vertebral arterial system*. Springer Verl.

PAYR, E. (1921) *Der frische Schädelschuss*. In: Handbuch der ärtzlichen Erfahrungen im Weltkrieg, Bd. I.

RIECHERT, T. AND HEINES, K. D. (1950) Ueber zwei Untersuchungsmethoden zur Beurteilung der Hirndurchblutung. *Nervenartz*, **21**, 9–16.

SAUERBRUCH, F. (1909) Beitrag zur Pathologie der Commotio und Compressio cerebri nach Schädeltrauma. *Mschr. Psychiatr.*, **26**, 140.

SCHWARZACHER (1924) Ueber traumatische Markblutungen des Gehirns. *Jb. Psychiatr.*, **43**, 113.

WADIEN, H. AND MOCKTON, G. (1957) Intracranial bruit in health and disease. *Brain*, **80**, 492.

WALKER, A. E., KOLBROS, I. I. AND CASE, T. J. (1944) The physiological basis of concussion. *J. Neurosurg.*, **1**, 103.

WEEKS, D. B., TOOL, J. F. AND ROBINSON, R. (1966) Pallencephalography. *Neurology (Minneap.)*, **16**, 153–160.

Thermography[*]

A. WACKENHEIM

Professeur Agrégé d'Electroradiologie à la Faculté de Médecine de Strasbourg, Strasbourg (France)

Since the work of Wood (1965) it cannot be disputed that thermography has secured a place of its own among complementary examinations in nervous pathology. On the basis of works currently published and personal experience, five main categories of indications may be distinguished:

(1) Unilateral vascular deficits. The existence of a fronto-orbital homolateral cool area in cases of thrombosis of the internal carotid artery, has paved the way to thermography in nervous pathology. Several authors have come across this cool area, which is now a classical feature. It calls for a few comments:

(a) it makes it possible to follow the evolution of the vascular deficit, especially in cases of stenosis in the region of the carotid artery siphon.

(b) in about one third of cases this cool area turns into a warm area, following an increase in the blood flow resulting from a facio-ophthalmic anastomosis.

(c) in nervous pathology the fronto-orbital cool area becomes of paramount im-

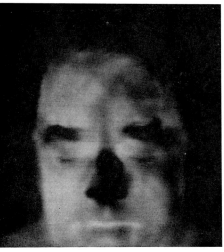

Fig. 1. Right fronto-orbitary cool area in a case of vertebrobasilary insufficiency. This thermogramme justifies a rightsided carotis angiography.

* Work carried out by the Neurology Clinic (Prof. F. Thiebaut) and the Radiology Clinic (Prof. Ch. Gros) of Strasbourg University Hospital Center.

References p. 230

portance, when clinical symptomatology is complex as is often the case with diffuse arteriopathy. Thus, a fronto-orbital cooling off may accompany a clinical symptomatology of vertebral basilar insufficiency, and justify, at the outset, an angiography of the carotid artery (Fig. 1). This thermographic examination, therefore, becomes of considerable value, especially in the case of out-patients.

(d) our present experience leads to some reservations as to the absolute value of the cool area. The important fact is the presence of a thermic asymmetry of the face. It is usually the coolest side wich proves to be pathological. More generally, however, it is the asymmetry which amounts to a symptom. Here, we meet once more one of the fundamental principles of neuro-radiological reasoning: comparison as between left and right in the interpretation of indirect signs.

(2) The blood diversions of the external carotid artery give rise to a facial cool area which mainly affects the lower part of the face. This is so in all cases of "steal", typical of which is the carotid cavernous fistula with an increased internal carotid flow. Post-operation thermography makes it possible to verify the correction of the external carotid "steal".

(3) Recordable inflammatory and tumoral processes which raise diagnostic problems in regard to nature, malignity and operability lend themselves to thermographic exploration. The anterior cervico-facial region is easy to explore. The type of tumor is the carotid glomus. This is not so in the region of the skull and neck where pilosity acts as a screen.

(4) As we have seen, multifocal, more or less stenosing diffuse cerebro-vascular diseases result in a thermographic asymmetry of the face, the reaction of which to the in-

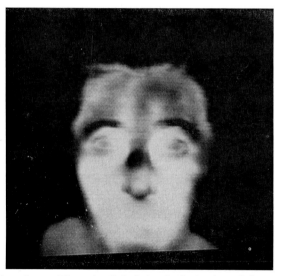

Fig. 2. Right frontal cool area. The only clinical sign is diminution of the carotidal pulse homolateral. In this case also, a right carotidal angiography will be performed first.

jection of therapeutical vaso-dilators is worth studying. It is astounding to note the variability of the responses with regard both to the time which elapses before the thermographic answer appears, as compared with the time of injection, and to the duration and intensity of the obtained warming up. In certain cases a cooling off period is recorded after the warming up period. Prescription of long-continued treatment with vaso-dilators should be preceded by thermographic tests. These would make it possible to choose the most effective product. In this group of cerebro-vascular diseases, thermography makes it possible to strengthen an angiographic indication. This is the case with all subjects with a slight symptom which were not angiographed in the past (Fig. 2).

(5) Thermography affords to the surgeon the possibility of observing the correction of thermic asymmetries in the after-effects of operations on stenoses of the vessels of the neck.

Over and above these five categories of diseases of the nervous system, thermo-

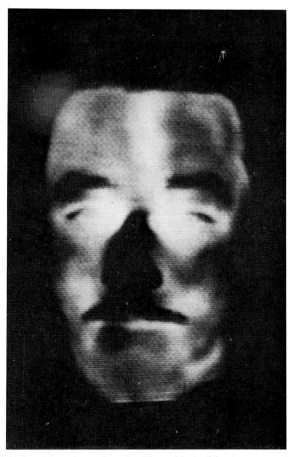

Fig. 3. Right frontal cool area by a healthy subject without any symptomatology.

graphy may prove usefull in the quest for the clinically imprecise sensitive medullar levels, in the study of the neuro-vegetative disturbances accompanying peripheral and central paralyses of the members.

The main advantage of thermography lies in its harmless nature which prevents any incident or accident and, therefore, allows frequent and ambulatory repetitions of the examination. Whatever the technic used, account must be taken all along of the mechanism of the thermographic picture's formation. It is the picture of a function: thermogenesis. An initial thermogramme has a certain information value. However, in medical practice, the most important services will be rendered by the check thermogrammes, thanks to the information they provide concerning thermic distribution.

Finally, to stress the caution and critical sense which the integration of thermographic information calls for, a picture is shown of a cool frontal area in a perfectly healthy subject (Fig. 3). In such cases, the local causes likely to have changed the emission of infrared rays (cutaneous diseases, unilateral respiratory disorders . . .) should be looked for.

REFERENCES

GROS, Ch., ET WACKENHEIM, A., (1966); Thermographie. *J. Radiol. Electroradiol. Méd. Nucl.*, **47**, 178–179.
—, —, ET VROUSOS, C., (1967); La thermographie dans les affections du système nerveux. *J. Radiol Electroradiol. Méd. Nucl.*, **48**, 45–47.
HEINZ, E. R., GOLBERG, H. I., and TAVERAS, J. M., (1964); Experiences with thermography in neurologic patients. *Ann. New York Acad. Sci.*, **121**, 177–189.
WOOD, E. H., (1965); Thermography in the diagnosis of the cerebrovascular disease. *Radiology*, **85**, 270–283.
WOOD, E. H., (1967); Thermography. In: Toray (Ed.), *Diagnostico Neuroradiologico* (Sole Llenas et Wackenheim), pp. 672–681. Barcelona.

Intracarotid and Intravertebral Injection of Drugs **

L. PERRIA, G. ROSADINI and G. F. ROSSI

*Clinica Neurochirurgica dell'Università, Genova, and Impresa di Elettrofisiologia del C.N.R., Italy**

This report deals with some of the practical utilizations in neurosurgery of the intra-carotid and intravertebral injection of drugs. The direct injection of drugs into one of the main arteries supplying the encephalon has been largely utilized in experimental neurophysiology. Used for the first time in man by Wada in 1949, the technique has been subsequently employed for diagnostic purposes by several authors. The drugs to be injected must obviously satisfy the two following requirements: (1) they shall not produce any damage to the arterial walls and central nervous system, (2) they shall cross the blood-brain barrier. So far, the drugs used in man are amobarbital sodium (see references in Alemà' *et al.*, 1966; Andrioli *et al.*, 1966; Rosadini *et al.*, 1966b; Rossi and Rosadini, 1967), cardiazol (Bennet, 1953; Gloor *et al.*, 1964) and megimide (Werman *et al.*, 1959a, b; Corletto *et al.*, 1967), i.e. drugs having respectively depressing and exciting action on the central nervous system neurons. According to the type of drug employed, the method permits of selectively putting out of function or of increasing the excitability of the cerebral structures belonging to the territory of distribution of one or the other of the two internal carotid arteries or of the vertebro-basilar circulation. We shall briefly report here our personal experience in some fields of neurosurgical interest. On the whole, the technique has been applied on more than 200 patients. The details of the technique have been previously described (Rosadini *et al.*, 1966b; Corletto *et al.*, 1967).

SEARCH FOR THE SIDE OF CEREBRAL DOMINANCE FOR SPEECH

The identification of the side of speech representation is a relevant problem in neuro-surgery. Its importance is particularly evident when one has to operate on the temporal lobe in absence of gross brain pathology, as for instance in temporal epileptic patients. It is well known that handedness is not necessarily related to the side of speech dominance. The intracarotid injection of amobarbital sodium provides an efficient means for the identification of the latter. The injection of about 100 to 200 mg of the drug into one internal carotid artery produces the temporary suppression of all functional properties of the ipsilateral hemisphere. As originally reported by Wada (1949) and sub-

* Direttore: Prof. L. Perria.
** Part of the personal researches reported here have been supported by the Consiglio Nazionale delle Ricerche (Impresa di Elettrofisiologia) and by the Air Force Office of Scientific Research through the European Office of Aerospace Research, OAR, United States Air Force (Contract AF 61-052-901).

sequently by others (Wada and Kirikae, 1949; Terzian and Cecotto, 1959; Wada and Rasmussen, 1960; Alemà' and Donnini, 1960; Da Pian *et al.*, 1961; Perria *et al.*, 1961; Rosadini and Rossi, 1961; Terzian, 1964; Branch *et al.*, 1964; Serafetinides *et al.* 1965; Rosadini *et al.*, 1966b; Rossi and Rosadini, 1967) the occurrence of speech disturbances indicates that speech is represented in the barbiturized hemisphere (to be considered the "dominant" one; Fig. 1); persistence of speech indicates that the

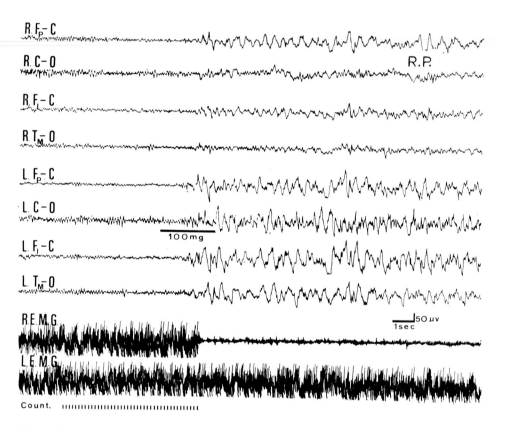

Fig. 1. Effect of left intracarotid injection of 100 mg of amobarbital sodium on the EEG, motor power and speech. Slow high amplitude waves appear on the left EEG recordings (and to some extent on the contralateral frontal regions); right hemiparesis and aphasia occur. R: right; L: left; Fp: frontopolar; C: central; O: occipital; Tm: midtemporal EEG recordings. R: right; L: left; EMG: electromyographic recordings from the deltoid muscles. Count: the patient is counting numbers.

barbiturized hemisphere is the "non-dominant" one. Our experience on this field is based on 95 patients. The observations made allow us to confirm the reliability of the method, as judged by the confrontation of the results of its application with those of surgery. In addition, they have led to the following remarks, which may have practical interest; (1) left speech dominance is present in a high percentage (28.6%) of the left-handed subjects; (2) right speech dominance is present in a small percentage (1.4%) of the right-handers; (3) bilateral representation of speech can occur in the same subject (3 cases out of 95).

SEARCH FOR THE RELATIVE IMPORTANCE AND INTERDEPENDENCE OF BILAT-
ERAL EPILEPTOGENIC ZONES

The existence of bilateral epileptogenic zones is often regarded as a contraindication to neurosurgery. However, the right judgement on the possibilities of surgical therapy can be grounded only on the knowledge of the relative importance and interdependence of the two zones. The intracarotid amobarbital test may efficiently contribute to such a knowledge, as indicated by the first results of the School of Montreal (Rovit et al., 1960, 1961; Gloor et al., 1964; Coceani, et al., 1966) and by our own results (Corletto et al., 1966; Andrioli et al., 1966; Rosadini et al., 1966, 1967).

According to our experience, the effect produced by the intracarotid barbiturate on the epileptic discharges of the ipsilateral and of the contralateral hemisphere in patients with bilateral non-synchronous epileptic activity can be different in the different subjects. It is likely that these differences are to a great extent related to the spatial location of the epileptogenic zones and to the reciprocal influences between the epileptogenic zones of the two hemispheres. In our opinion, based on the results of the bilateral application of the amobarbital test in 74 epileptic patients of the type considered, useful indications to surgery are provided in the following cases; (1) the barbiturization of

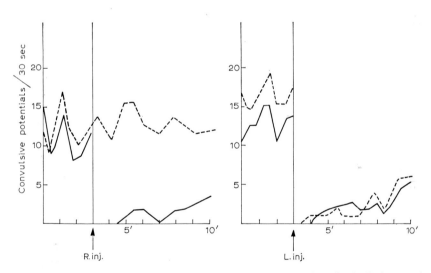

Fig. 2. Effect of right and left amobarbital intracarotid injection (100 mg) on the epileptic discharges of the two hemispheres. Right injection is followed by the sudden drop of the convulsive potentials recorded from the ipsilateral hemisphere, while the contralateral ones are unaffected. Left injection produces a bilateral marked reduction of the epileptic activity. The left hemisphere is considered, therefore, the dominant one for epilepsy. — Right hemisphere; - - Left hemisphere.

the hemisphere A suppresses the epileptic activity of both hemispheres, while the barbiturization of the hemisphere B is without effect or affects only ipsilateral epileptic discharges; the latters are likely to be dependent on (or facilitated by) the contralateral hemisphere (A) (Fig. 2); surgery may be performed on the hemisphere A. (2). Both the barbiturizations of the hemispheres A and B affect the ipsilateral epileptic

activity, leaving unaltered (or increasing) the contralateral one; independent epileptogenic zones (or epileptogenic zones having reciprocal inhibitory influences) appear to
be located in the two hemispheres; surgery is contraindicated.

Useful additional information can be obtained in the same subjects by the intracarotid injection of a convulsant drug. So far, Cardiazol (Gloor *et al.*, 1964) and
Megimide (Corletto *et al.*, 1967) have been used. A lower convulsant threshold to the
intracarotid Cardiazol or Megimide in one side than in the other may indicate that the
low threshold hemisphere is the "dominant" one for epilepsy.

SEARCH FOR THE ROLE OF SUBCORTICAL STRUCTURES IN THE GENESIS OF EPILEPSY OF "CENTRENCEPHALIC" TYPE

Stimulated by the results obtained by the application of the amobarbital test in patients
with bilateral non-synchronous epileptic discharges, we made an attempt to study
patients suffering from epilepsy of the socalled "centrencephalic" type, eletroencephal-
ographically characterized by bilateral synchronous convulsive activity (see also
Gloor *et al.*, 1964). Intracarotid amobarbital injections were bilaterally performed in
six patients. In all cases a bilateral suppression or marked reduction of the epileptic
activity was produced, both when the right and the left hemispheres were barbiturized.
This effect, though difficult to be interpreted, seems to indicate that in the cases
examined the bilateral epileptic activity was not dependent on (or "secondary" to) an
epileptogenic zone located in one of the two hemispheres.

In five patients amobarbital was injected into the vertebro-basilar circulation. In all
of them, when the injection was made on a background of epileptic activity, the latter
was not modified by the barbiturate. On the other hand, by injecting the drug when no
epileptic activity was present in the electroencephalogram, typical discharge of 3 c/sec
bilateral spike-and-wave complexes occurred (Rosadini *et al.*, 1967). This effect was
interperd as a "liberation" of the epileptogenic area from restraining influences coming from the barbiturized territory, namely from structures of midbrain and/or pons
and medulla oblongata. The epileptogenic area appears to be located in front of this
territory, i.e. not belonging to the brain stem; however, its precise location is not indicated by these results.

SEARCH FOR THE ROLE OF CORTICAL AND BRAIN STEM STRUCTURES IN THE MECHANISMS OF DYSKINETIC MANIFESTATIONS

An attempt to utilize the intracarotid and intravertebral amobarbital test for the study
of the possible mechanisms of dyskinetic manifestations was initiated by us some years
ago (Alemà' *et al.*, 1961 and 1964). Parkinsonian patients were injected. Both the
intracarotid and the intravertebral amobarbital injections were found to suppress
tremor. The effect was limited to the contralateral side when the drug was administered into the carotid artery (Fig. 3), while it was bilateral in the case of intravertebral
injection. Moreover, it was found that the amount of barbiturate capable of suppressing tremor was far lower than that necessary to produce paresis and to affect the
postural tone. The latter finding was interpreted as an indication that the tremor and
the dystonia of the parkinsonian patients may to a a certain extent depend on different

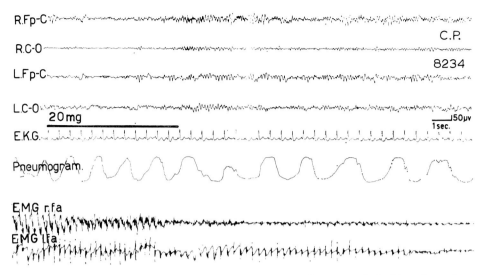

Fig. 3. Effect of left amobarbital intracarotid injection (20 mg) on the tremor of a Parkinsonian patient: suppression of the contralateral tremor (EMG r.fa) and persistence of the ipsilateral one (EMG l.fa) with a dose of barbiturate too low to produce slow waves on the EEG and impairment of motor power.

neural systems or mechanisms. Moreover, knowing that the depressing effect of the barbiturate is due to its action on the neuron somata (or "synapsis") and not on the axons, the results of the intravertebral amobarbital indicate that parkinsonian tremor can be abolished without affecting the pyramidal system. The comparison of these findings with those obtained by the application of the test on patients suffering from other dyskinetic manifestations (now in progress) might provide useful informations on the neural mechanisms underlying the latters and therefore on the limits and possibilities of their surgical therapy.

The aim of the present report was that of providing evidence for the practical utilization of the intracarotid and intravertebral injection of drugs. We hope that the few examples reported were sufficient to illustrate the possible use of the method in clinical fields of neurosurgical interest. We feel that the method can be safely employed and that the use of other drugs, besides the ones so far utilized, may provide in the future even more information.

REFERENCES

ALEMA', G. AND DONNINI, G. (1960) Sulle modificazioni cliniche ed elettroencefalografiche da introduzione intracarotidea di iso-amil-etil-barbiturato di sodio nell'uomo. *Boll. Soc. ital. Biol. sper.* **36**, 900–904.

ALEMA', G., PERRIA, L., ROSADINI, G., ROSSI, G. F. AND ZATTONI, J. (1966) Functional deactivation of the brain stem and level of consciousness in man. *J. Neurosurg.*, **24**, 629–639.

ALEMA', G., ROSADINI, G. AND ROSSI, G. F. (1961) Prime esperienze sugli effetti della introduzione intracarotidea di amytal sodico nelle sindromi parkinsoniane. *Boll. Soc. ital. Biol. sper.*, **37**, 1036–1037.

ALEMA', G., ROSADINI, G., ROSSI, G. F. AND ZATTONI, J. (1964) Effetti dell'introduzione intravertebrale di amobarbital sodio sul tremore parkinsoniano. *Boll. Soc. ital. Biol. sper.*, **40**, 841–842.

ANDRIOLI, G., ANGELERI, F., BERGONZI, P., CANTORE, P., FERRONI, A., GENTILOMO, A., MINGRINO, S., RICCI, G. B., ROSADINI, G. AND ROSSI, G. F. (1966) Inquadramento diagnostico dell'epilettico in neurochirurgia. *Min. Neurochir.*, **10**, 49–144.

BENNET, F. E. (1953) Intracarotid and intravertertebral metrazol in petit mal epilepsy. *Neurology*, **3**, 668–673.

BRANCH, C., MILNER, B. AND RASMUSSEN, T. (1964) Intracarotid sodium amytal for the lateralization of cerebral speech dominance. *J. Neurosurg.*, **21**, 399–405.

COCEANI, F., LIBMAN, I. AND GLOOR, P. (1966) The effect of intracarotid amobarbital injections upon experimentally induced epileptiform activity. *EEG clin. Neurophysiol.*, **20**, 542–558.

CORLETTO, F., GENTILOMO, A., ROSADINI, G. AND ROSSI, G. F. (1966) Effetti dell'iniezione intracarotidea di amobarbital sodico sull'attività epilettica elettroencefalografica nell'uomo. I° - Attività bilaterali e sincrone; II° — Attività diffuse e asincrone; III° – Attività focali. *Boll. Soc. ital. Biol. sper.*, **23**, 1694–1703.

CORLETTO, F., ROSADINI, G. AND ROSSI, G. F. (1967) Megimide intracarotideo per lo studio della soglia convulsiva emisferica. *Riv. di Neurol.*, in press.

DA PIAN, R., BRICOLO, A., DALLE ORE, G. AND PERBELLINI, D. (1961) Amytal sodico intracarotideo. *Giorn. Psichiat. Neuropatol.*, **89**, 885–912.

GLOOR, P., RASMUSSEN, T., GARRETSON, N. H. AND MAROUN, F. (1964) Fractioned intracarotid Metrazol injection. A new diagnostic methods in electroencephalography. *EEG clin. Neurophysiol.*, **17**, 322–327.

PERRIA, L., ROSADINI, G. AND ROSSI, G. F. (1961) Determination of side of cerebral dominance with amobarbital. *Arch. of Neurol.*, **4**, 173–181.

ROSADINI, G., GENTILOMO, A., PERRIA, L. AND ROSSI, G. F. (1967) Recherches sur les effects de l'injection intracarotidienne et intravertébrale d'amytal sur les décharges convulsives EEG. *Neurochirurgie*, **13**, 537–546.

ROSADINI, G., GENTILOMO, A. AND ROSSI, G. F. (1966a) Studio dei rapporti di interdipendenza di attività epilettiche focali bilaterali mediante amytal intracarotideo. *Min. Neurochir.*, **10**, 309–312.

ROSADINI, G., RIVANO, C., ROSSI, G. F., DAVINI, V. AND ROSA, M. (1966b) Ricerche e considerazioni sulla dominanza e specializzazione emisferica nell'uomo. *Min. Neurochir.*, **10**, 237–249.

ROSADINI, G. AND ROSSI, G. F. (1961) Ricerche sugli effetti elettroencefalografici, neurologici e psichici della somministrazione intracarotidea de amytal sodico nell'uomo. *Acta Neurochir.*, **9**, 234–250.

ROSSI, G. F. AND ROSADINI, G. (1967) Experimental analysis of cerebral dominance in man. In: *Brain Mechanisms underlying Speech and Language.* Grune & Stratton, New York.

ROVIT, R. L., GLOOR, P. AND RASMUSSEN, T. (1960) Effect of intracarotid injection of sodium amytal on epileptic form EEG discharges: a clinical study. *Trans. Amer. Neurol. Ass.*, 161–165.

ROVIT, R. L., GLOOR, P. AND RASMUSSEN, T (1960) Intracarotid amobarbital in epileptic patients *Arch. of Neurol.*, **5**, 606–626.

SERAFETINIDES, E. A., HOARE, R. D. AND DRIVER, M. V. (1965) Intracarotid sodium amylo-barbital and cerebral dominance for speech and consciousness. *Brain*, **88**, 107–130.

TERZIAN, H. (1964) Behavioral and EEG effects of intracarotid sodium amytal injection. *Acta Neurochir.*, **12**, 230–239.

TERZIAN, H. AND CECOTTO, C. (1959) Su un nuovo metodo per la determinazione e lo studio della dominanza emisferica. *Giornale Psichiat. Neuropatol.*, **57**, 889–923.

WADA, J. (1949) A new method for the determination of the side of cerebral speech dominance. A preliminary report on the intracarotid injection of sodium amytal in man. *Med. Biol., Tokyo*, **14**, 221–222.

WADA, J. AND KIRIKAE, T. (1949) Neurological contribution to the induced unilateral paralysis of human cerebral hemisphere; special emphasis on the experimentally induced aphasia. *Acta Med. Hokkaid.*, **24**, 1–10.

WADA, J. AND RASMUSSEN, T. (1960) Intracarotid injection of sodium amytal for the lateralization of cerebral speech dominance. *J. Neurosurg.*, **17**, 266–282.

WERMANN, R., ANDERSON, P. AND CHRISTOFF, N. (1959) Electroencephalographic changes with intracarotid megimide and amytal in man. *EEG clin. Neurophysiol.*, **11**, 267–274.

WERMANN, R., CHRISTOFF, N. AND ANDERSON, P. J. (1959) Neurological changes with intracarotid amytal and megimide in man. *J. Neurol. Neurosurg. Psychiat.*, **22**, 333–337.

Vertebro-basilar Stenoses and Thromboses

M. DAVID, R. MESSIMY, D. DILENGE, L. HARISPE AND J. METZGER

Clinique Neurochirurgicale de la Pitié-Salpêtrière, 75 Paris (France)

Arising from the anatomical and clinical studies of the last twenty years and the valuable contribution of cerebral angiography, it has been possible to construct a precise symptomatology of the vertebro-basilar stenoses and thromboses.

The aim of this work has been to use the authors' personal experience to extract the principal trends apparent in the study of vertebro-basilar pathology.

The frequency of atheromatous lesions at different stages along the vertebro-basilar axis and associated carotid lesions account for the complexity of the facts.

Schematically one can distinguish between: 1. Vertebro-basilar insufficiency; 2. Pathology of the basilar artery; and 3. Pathology of the vertebral artery.

VERTEBRO-BASILAR INSUFFICIENCY

Following the studies of Kubik and Adams and of Biemond, Denny-Brown introduced the term vertebro-basilar insufficiency, the existence of which has since been confirmed by numerous studies including those of Millikan and Siekert, Meyer, Sheehan and Bauer, Williams and Wilson and most recently, by Schott *et al.*

We have extracted from 50 cases of vertebro-basilar stenosis or thrombosis, 12 cases characteristic of gross vertebro-basilar insufficiency; this was most common in men over 40 years, and was always associated with brain stem signs and sometimes with occipital lobe or cerebellar signs.

The mode of onset was variable, and could be: visual disturbance, posterior headache, vertigo, hemiplegia, paraesthesia, monoplegia, or even trigeminal neuralgia in one case.

Duration of evolution was variable and unpredictable; from several days to several weeks, and occasionally even years: 7 and 10 years in two cases.

The transitory nature of these disturbances seem to us to be essential, as does the production of symptoms by hyperextension of the head with lateral displacement.

Their intermittent character, a varying hemiplegia or homonymous hemianopia are, equally, very suggestive.

Ancillary investigations provide information of varying value:

EEGs were obtained in 12 of our cases; it was normal 3 times, but in one case there was a discrete posterior focus of slow waves.

We have not used provocation tests such as swing tables or carotid compression systematically.

Gamma encephalography showed discrete posterior foci in two cases.

We would lay particular stress on the use of vertebral angiography.

Angiographic exploration of the vertebro-basilar circulation has few contraindications nowadays. In agreement with Loeb and Meyer, we believe that it should never be carried out in the following cases: *when there is a severe neurological deficit* which may be associated with a thrombosis of the basilar artery, *when the clinical syndrome* seems to respond favourably to medical treatment, *when there is significant arterial hypertension*, and finally *in the presence of a recent myocardial lesion*. In our cases, following these criteria, there were no important complications and, in general, we can confirm that the clinical picture is never aggravated by this procedure. It should not be forgotten, however, that this is a delicate technique which should only be carried out with all necessary precautions.

With regard to the exploration of the vertebral artery, we prefer to carry it out by means of catheterizing the brachial artery, pushing the catheter into the subclavian artery as near as possible to the origin of the vertebral artery. In two cases, the introduction of the catheter was blocked at the level of the distal segment of the subclavian artery and, unfortunately, despite several attempts, we could not obtain opacification of the vertebral artery; one such opacification was obtained at a second attempt by introducing the catheter via the femoral route and by injection of the contrast medium

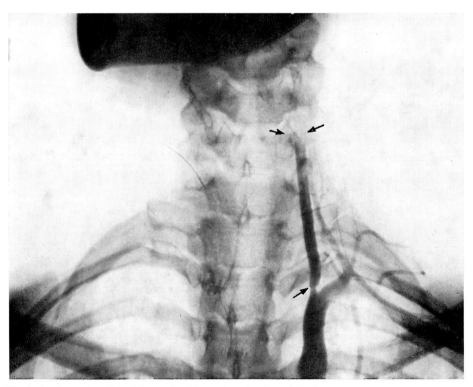

Fig. 1. Angiography of the left vertebral by catheterization of the femoral artery. Ostial stenosis (↑) associated with a thrombosis of the vertebral artery.
The contrast medium is obstructed at the level of C6 (↓↓). The obstruction remains unchanged in all arteriograms in the series.

at the level of the aortic arch. This method of opacifying the vessels of the neck by an injection at the level of the aortic arch can be used with profit, thanks to the technique of subtraction, and seemed to us particularly useful in the case where it was equally necessary to examine the initial segment of the primitive left carotid artery. Six ml of CONTRIX 28 by injection is sufficient to obtain good opacification of the vertebral artery after catheterization of the brachial artery, and the injection can if necessary be repeated several times. In the case of injection at the level of the aortic arch, at least 30 ml of a 60% contrast medium are needed to obtain a good result; we try in this case to avoid repeating the injection.

If, on the other hand, the clinical picture does not exclude the possibility of a tumour, or if one suspects a lesion of the basilar trunk or an intracranial branch, we prefer direct percutaneous puncture under general anaesthesia to start with.

Of the 12 cases of vertebro-basilar insufficiency, we carried out 6 vertebral arterio-grams which in each case demonstrated an anomaly: basilar stenosis twice, stenosis of the cervical segment of the vertebral twice, an abnormally tortuous artery once, and ostial stenosis and obliteration at C5-C6 confirmed in all the serial films once (Fig. 1).

The symptomatology of these vertebro-basilar insufficiencies was related to ischaemia in the occipital, cerebellar and lateral medullary territories, supplied by narrow terminal arteries. As proposed by Williams and Wilson, it is probable that certain cases of deafness and certain vestibular syndromes, unilateral or bilateral, occurring unexpectedly and acutely in elderly subjects are due to partial vertebro-basilar occlusions.

THE PATHOLOGY OF THE BASILAR ARTERY

Since the fundamental work of Kubik and Adams on occlusion of the basilar artery, numerous studies have appeared. We shall therefore only deal with some points of detail.

The syndrome of the whole basilar

We have observed 5 cases associated with signs of peduncular and pontine involvement; cerebellar signs; one hemianopia. Evolution was in each case rapid, with coma, quadriplegia, hypertonicity and death. Anatomical verification always demonstrated extensive ponto-peduncular, cerebellar and occipital lesions with, in four cases, more-or-less complete occlusion of the basilar artery, and once an embolus in the basilar trunk, verified histologically.

The pontine syndromes are classical.

The peduncular syndromes appeared to us more unusual, not only the paramedian peduncular syndromes, but especially the median peduncular syndromes, associated with major disturbances of consciousness and bilateral IIIrd nerve involvement.

Thrombosis of the anterior group of the retro-mamillary peduncle, which mainly supplies the thalamus, was responsible for a specific clinical syndrome of which dementia is the essential sign (Castaigne *et al.*). On the other hand thrombosis of the posterior group supplying the peduncular reticular substance, mainly causes a disturbance of consciousness varying from a quasi-lethargic hypersomnolence to akinetic mutism.

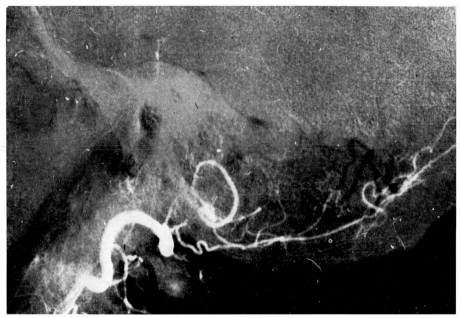

Fig. 2. Direct approach vertebral angiography. The intracranial vertebral and the basilar trunk are very irregular, only the terminal portion being clearly outlined. This is an almost complete thrombosis of these two vessels, verified at autopsy, with an histological picture of secondary recanalization. The same type of lesion was discovered at the level of the initial segment of the posterior inferior cerebellar artery which, on the angiogram, appears less distinct and irregular in calibre.

With regard to one personal case of akinetic mutism, we have already gone over the points in favour of this being due to a partial involvement of the reticular substance.

In a man aged 41, with arterial disease following a vertebro-basilar accident, akinetic mutism associated with decerebrate rigidity was observed.

Arteriography showed a segmental thrombosis of the *posterior inferior cerebellar artery at its origin, an almost complete thrombosis of the basilar trunk with only a very thin line of contrast passing the obstruction* (Fig. 2).

Anatomical verification demonstrated a total thrombosis of the right vertebral, a stenosis of the left vertebral and the initial portion of the posterior inferior cerebellar artery, *and an almost complete thrombosis of the basilar trunk with an histological picture showing secondary recanalization. Finally, there was softening of the peduncular tegmentum with two foci of symmetrical superior cerebellar softening.*

Observations proving correct exploration of basilar thrombosis are rare in the literature. Besides the case cited, we have twice accidentally discovered permanent stenoses of the basilar trunk 1 cm from its anterior end in patients who presented with a meningeal haemorrhage, a picture which would be difficult to interpret as being associated with spasm, because it was constant in all respects in all the films taken. There was no evidence elsewhere of any vascular malformation (Figs. 3A and 3B).

Extrinsic basilar stenoses have a symptomatology mixed with that of the underlying causal lesion. We have observed this in three cases of posterior fossa tumours.

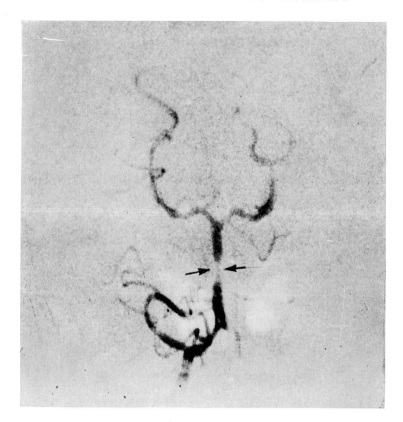

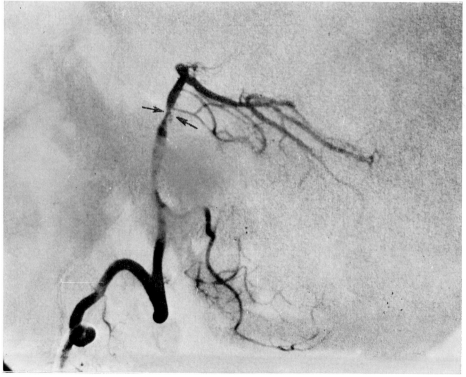

Figs. 3A and 3B. Reduction in calibre clearly shown at the level of the basilar trunk. The morphology of this segment is noteworthy, and its persistence in different series of angiograms favours an organic stenosis.

We can cite as an example, a meningioma of the free border of the cerebral tento rium, encircling the posterior cerebral artery to the point of completely obstructing it, as was demonstrated by vertebral angiography.

Basilar stenoses with recovery

We observed a case of a woman of 26 who, after a period of vertebro-basilar insuffi-ciency, suffered a spasmodic tetraplegia with multiple cranial nerve palsies. Arterio-graphy showed a segmental block in the basilar trunk. In spite of important sequelae, this young patient started to walk again after several years confinement to bed.

Vertebro-carotid lesions

These have been isolated by Hutchinson and Yates, and seem common; we have observed five cases. The second, which was particularly spectacular, consisted of bilateral carotid thromboses confirmed by arteriography; a complete thrombosis of the right vertebral, the single left vertebral artery maintaining the blood supply to the whole of the brain.

PATHOLOGY OF THE VERTEBRAL ARTERY

Although it is sometimes difficult to dissociate the pathologies of the vertebral artery and the basilar artery, one can with Schott make distinctions within the limits of the pathology of the vertebral artery: a bulbar area, a medullary area, the subclavian steal syndrome and finally the latent stenoses or thromboses of the vertebral artery.

Localized bulbar syndromes

We will only mention the bulbar or retro-olivary softening of Dejerine, correspond-ing to the descriptions of Wallenberg. We have observed 12 cases recently.

The discussion concerning the artery at fault is not settled, the frequency of anatom-ical variations, the constant multiplicity of the lesions defying all systematization.

The important point remains the constant involvement of the vertebral artery. Despite the importance of the clinical signs of neurological deficit, vertebral arterio-graphy does not show occlusive lesions when it is carried out.

We can mention one very recent case where arteriography demonstrated the com-plete absence of opacification of the left vertebral in the course of this syndrome (Fig. 4).

In our series, we wish only to emphasize the clinical picture: the frequency of vertigo at the onset along with vestibular signs; the frequency of formes frustes; the invariably favourable outcome; and the possibility of onset marked by malaise with definite hypothermia at 35° or below, as observed in two of our cases. We have not found these facts mentioned in the literature.

At the autopsy of one case dying with the clinical picture of acute bulbar syndrome, we observed an extension of the lesion to the opposite side, in accordance with the opinion of Guillain and Alajouanine.

Vertebro-medullary syndromes following occlusion of the vertebral seem rare. They appear in the form of a Preobrajansky syndrome or a Brown-Sequard syndrome.

Boudin and co-workers have recently reported 3 cases presenting syndromes of hemisection of the cervical cord either associated or not with a brain-stem syndrome.

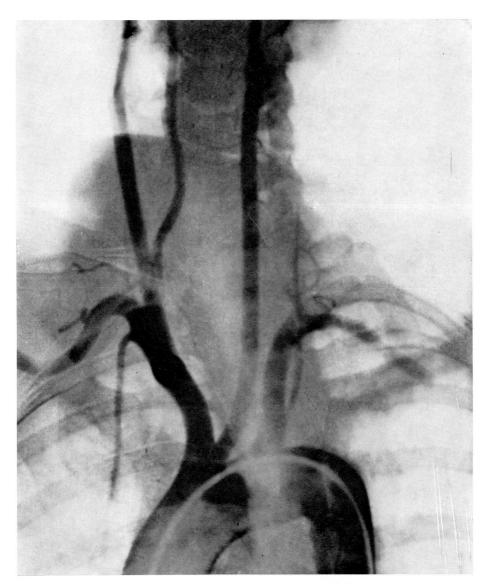

Fig. 4. Wallenberg's syndrome. Failure of injection of the thrombosed left vertebral artery. Note also that the primitive origin of the left carotid artery is at the level of the right innominate artery.

In each case the arteriographs showed partial or complete thrombotic lesions of the initial part of the left vertebral artery.

The subclavian steal syndrome has only been known since 1960. The paretic weakness and the signs of circulatory insufficiency of the left upper limb constantly associated with cerebral manifestations of vertebro-basilar insufficiency are very suggestive. We are indebted to Professor agrégé Garnier for the observations we have made with him.

Aortography showed complete thrombosis of the left subclavian, of which only the stump was visible, while elsewhere there was only a right carotid stenosis. Angiographical and physiopathological studies have confirmed that occlusion of the subclavian above the origin of the cerebral could produce a reversal of blood flow by siphon action from one vertebral to the other, from the basilar trunk to the vertebral and from the external carotid to the vertebral.

The matter of latent stenoses or thromboses of the vertebral artery remains obscure; we have recently observed five cases.

Fisher *et al.* have recently recorded 178 systematic autopsies; 5 cases of vertebral occlusion in the neck seem to have been latent.

Certain aetiologies are very specific:

(a) Cervical spondylosis

There is much interest in the role of cervical spondylosis in the genesis of the vertebral stenoses. Certain authors attach only secondary importance to this pathogenesis rather emphasizing deformation due to movement.

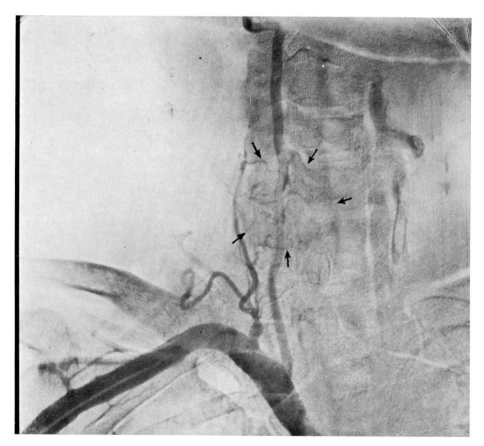

Fig. 5. Bony metastases at the level of C5/C6 (↓↓) discovered during vertebral angiography by catheterization of the brachial artery. Besides the presence of new vessel formation, note the irregular opacification of the stenosed segment of the artery which is encircled by the tumour.

Stenosis, however, frequently exists, and arteriography can demonstrate it even at the stage of the smallest lesions.

In addition, it should not be forgotten that certain stenoses may remain undetected if seriographs are not taken with rotation of the head and neck.

Cervical spondylosis was found in 25% of 180 stenoses studied by two of us in collaboration with Professor J. S. Meyer. Of course the role of cervical spondylosis ought to be assessed, taking into account the anatomical configuration and the state of the vessel walls.

(b) Trauma

Traumatic lesions of the vertebral artery are rare but are well recognised, whether by unrecognised fracture-dislocation, by osteopathic manipulation, or by direct trauma to the cervical portion of the artery.

(c) We have observed two cases of vertebral stenosis due to pressure from tumours:

In one case it was a chordoma at C1-C2; and in one case of metastases at C6-C7, subtraction arteriography clearly showed the artery enveloped by the tumour, the difference of tonality and the irregular character (Fig. 5).

Several points concerning treatment deserve emphasis:

Medical treatment ought always to be used, whether or not it is associated with a surgical procedure.

(a) Besides prophylactic treatments or those aimed at the aetiology (atherosclerosis diabetes, syphilis), it is necessary to stress present interest in:

Papaverine

Hydergine which ameliorates cerebral ischaemia and reduces capillary resistance. Three types of drug merit discussion:

anticoagulants are only advisable following intermittent manifestations of vertebro-basilar insufficiency.

the efficiency of *thrombolytics* used recently is not yet proven.

Rheomacrodex (L.M.W.D.) seems very effective and free from risk.

Surgery of the vertebro-basilar system is limited by unpropitious anatomical dispositions, particularly the inaccessibility and small calibre of the vessels.

Other than sympathectomy by stellectomy and section of the vertebral nerve, three techniques are now in use:

—Removal of the obstruction is rarely practised at this level because the thrombus generally extends the whole length of the vertebral as far as the basilar trunk.

—Endarterectomy and arterioplasty with a patch.

—Subclavian-vertebral anastomosis.

In conclusion, it is necessary to repeat that arthritic compressions can benefit by the surgical treatment of cervical disc and joint disease by an anterior cervical approach.

(b) It is difficult to decide on indications. The last two important works are that of De Bakey *et al.* and of M. Wertheimer *et al.*

The essential clinical criterion is the state of consciousness, and any disterbance of this considerably worsens the prognosis.

In association with the clinical picture, the angiographic criteria permit a discussion of the operative technique.

Finally, the surgical exploration will decide the attitude to be adopted.

The results published by De Bakey are the most important to our knowledge, and emphasize the fact that even if the operative mortality in cases of vertebro-basilar insufficiency is greater than in those with carotid stenosis, the long term recovery picture does seem better.

Collateral Circulation in Occlusive Vascular Lesions of the Brain

The role of the middle meningeal artery in the collateral circulation in compensating for occlusions of the internal carotid artery or its branches

EDUARDO TOLOSA

Barcelona (Spain)

The subject of this report is of such scope that it is not even possible to summarize it within the limits of time and space which have been given us. For this reason, we have decided to limit ourselves to discussing one concrete point of this question: *the role of the middle meningeal artery in the collateral circulation in compensating for occlusions of the internal carotid artery or its branches.*

For this purpose we have examined one series of 20 cases of occlusion of the internal carotid and 9 cases of occlusion of the middle cerebral artery. In the first group, we found that only in three cases was the collateral circulation between the external and internal carotid arteries effected almost exclusively through the middle meningeal artery. In the second group, it was possible to discover only a single example in which the middle meningeal took part in the revascularization of the middle cerebral artery.

CASE 1

A female patient of 49, suffering from a right parasellar tumour (probably a meningioma) of 3 years evolution, and clinically characterized by partial paralysis of the III nerve, paralysis of IV and VI nerves, pains in the area of the first branch of the V nerve and lessening of the right corneal reflex.

The angiographic examination shows a right parasellar tumour, the size of a cherry, which incorporates the intracavernous portion of the carotid siphon, completely (or almost completely) blocking the artery at the level of siphon knee. Thanks to the collateral circulation through the middle meningeal and ophthalmic arteries, the blood flow was restored at the level of the supraclinoid carotid and middle cerebral territory (Fig. 1). The left carotid showed both anterior cerebral arteries in this way completing the revascularization of the right hemisphere. The angiographic examination of the vertebral-basilar system shows that these take no part in this.

The detailed examination of the angiograms show that the collateral circulation of the ophthalmic artery comes almost exclusively through the middle meningeal artery (Fig. 2) one of whose branches passes from the cranial cavity to the orbit to continue on with a branch of the ophthalmic artery, and finally joining up with this.

The left carotid arteriography with compression of the right carotid artery showed

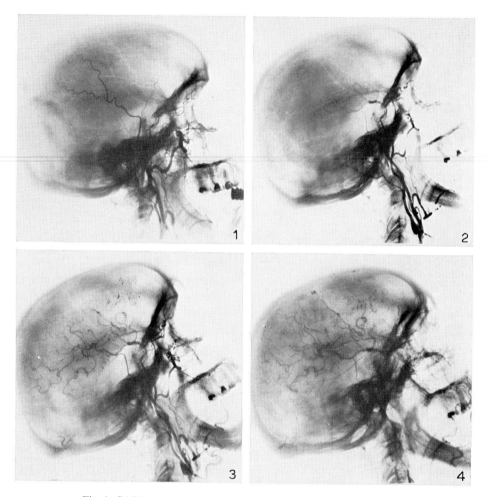

Fig. 1. CASE 1. 4 consecutive phases of a right carotid arteriogram.

in the right side, that the anterior cerebral artery was well filled while the middle cerebral, poorly. In the phlebographic picture, at 4 ″, a bilateral filling was obtained which was, however, considerably weaker on the right. These results indicate only a certain degree of efficiency of the anterior communicating artery.

The arteriogram of the right carotid artery with compression of the left one showed, on the right side, the filling of middle and anterior cerebral arteries and, on the left, a trace of visualization of the anterior cerebral and of the inital portion of the middle cerebral artery. The compression of the left carotid was well tolerated.

We questioned which branch of the ophthalmic artery anastomoses with the middle meningeal. On the basis of the data presented by Dilenge, David and Fischgold, in their monograph on The Ophthalmic Artery, we are inclined to believe that it is precisely a question of the lacrimal artery, for these authors indicate that the anterior branch of the middle meningeal gives out branches which enter the orbit

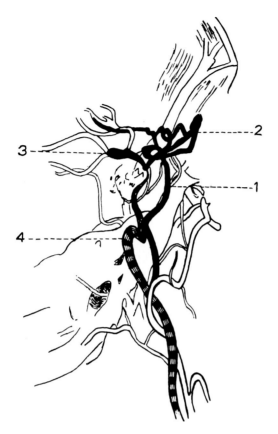

Fig. 2. CASE 1. Schematic tracing of a right carotid arteriogram. Filling of the supraclinoid portion of the carotid siphon through the middle meningeal and ophthalmic arteries. 1: Middle meningeal artery. 2: Ophthalmic artery. 3: Supraclinoid portion of the carotid siphon. 4: Internal carotid artery.

through the superior orbital fissure and are able to anastomose with the lacrimal branch. In regard to anomalies, cases have been described in which the lacrimal artery starts in the middle meningeal.

Another possible hypothesis is that communication with the ophthalmic artery is carried out by anastomosis of the middle meningeal artery with the anterior meningeal, and that the ophthalmic artery is reached through one of the ethmoidal arteries. In our case, we opt for the first hypothesis, as, in the sagittal arteriograms, we see the twistings of the anastomotic branch reach the ophthalmic artery from outside, which favours the hypothesis suggesting the lacrimal branch as responsible.

Considering the overall results of the angiographic examination we see that although there existed an obstruction at the level of the right carotid siphon, the irrigation of the corresponding hemisphere is assured by a double compensation mechanism: First, collateral circulation originating from the right external carotid, by way of the middle meningeal-ophthalmic; second, collateral circulation originating from the left internal carotid through the anterior communicating artery.

The case was surgically explored by exposing the opto-chiasmatic territory through a right transfrontal access. The lesion occupied the parasellar area, the supra-clinoid carotid was laterally displaced, the optic nerve raised. It was decided then, not to excise the tumour which would have meant the sacrifice of the optic nerve and the creation of a permanent syndrome of the cavernous sinus. There existed, in addition, the risk of injury to the ophthalmic artery and of interrupting the collateral circulation destined for the irrigation of the right hemisphere, given the uncertainty of the anterior communicating artery being able to compensate completely for the circulatory deficit created.

CASE 2

A female patient of 52 was first examined in March 1966. In June 1965, she complained of paraesthesias in the right arm. In February 1966, she suffered a stroke with aphasia and right hemiplegia. EEG: slow activity in left temporal leads.

The left carotid angiogram shows an occlusion of the internal carotid in the neck, 2 centimeters away from the bifurcation of the common carotid, and a strong filling of the external carotid, especially of the middle meningeal, whose size far exceeds that of the internal maxillary. A branch of the middle meningeal artery enters the orbit and anastomoses with the ophthalmic artery after describing some tortuosities. Through the ophthalmic artery the supraclinoid portion of the siphon, and although weakly, the anterior cerebral and the pericallosal arteries revascularize. A very fine upward branch, the deep anterior temporal, appears to participate in the revascularization of the ophthalmic artery, although in a negligible manner (if a comparison is made between the sizes of this artery and the middle meningeal).

The right carotid angiogram shows, in this case, a partial occlusion of the internal carotid, 2 centimeters from the bifurcation of the common carotid artery. A thin thread of the contrast follows along the internal carotid artery to the siphon but the latter's flow comes principally from the ophthalmic artery, whose size equals that of the siphon. Access to the ophthalmic artery occurs through the middle meningeal artery and through the deep anterior temporal and lacrimal arteries. Finally a small part of the collateral circulation follows the route: external maxillary-angular-superior palpebral branch of the ophthalmic artery. Past the siphon, an almost normal visualization is obtained of the anterior and middle cerebral arteries.

In the sagittal angiographs only a visualization of the right hemisphere was achieved.

In this case, with bilateral occlusive lesions of the internal carotid artery, the collateral circulation stems from, on both sides, the external carotid, it being unable to compensate the left hemisphere through the anterior communicating artery or the vertebral-basilar system.

The clearly insufficient collateral circulation of the left side takes place almost entirely by means of the middle meningeal artery. On the right side, on the other hand, the middle meningeal artery is only one of the anastomotic channels (between the external and internal carotid arteries) followed by the collateral circulation.

The aphasia and right hemiplegia shown by the patient proves that the lesion of the left internal carotid artery is not, or was not, compensated for by the collateral circulation. This contrasts with the lack of focal symptoms referable to the right hemisphere but here it is necessary to take into account, among other facts, that the occlusion of the right internal carotid artery is not complete.

CASE 3

Male patient of 57. Three weeks before admission, after complaining of paraesthesia in the right lower limb, he suffered a stroke with right hemiplegia and aphasia. Little regression of focal symptoms occurred.

The left carotid angiograph showed an occlusion of the internal carotid at the bifurcation of the common carotid artery. There was a trace of collateral circulation through the middle meningeal, one of whose branches appears to reach the siphon directly, without taking the indirect route of the ophthalmic artery.

In the first film (1″), the proximal portion of the branches of the external carotid are filled. In the second film (2″), the branches of the middle meningeal and the ophthalmic arteries are filled, the latter possibly through the anterior branch of the middle meningeal. In a further film (3″), the carotid siphon opacifies being reached separately by both the ophthalmic artery and a branch of the middle meningeal. In the last film (4″), the contrast appears in the pars insularis of the middle cerebral artery, the supraclinoid carotid being still visualized.

In this case, there was collateral circulation only in a rudimentary form through the external carotid, but this was carried out almost completely by means of the middle meningeal. One part of the circulation followed the ophthalmic artery but another appeared to be carried out through anastomotic branches going directly onto the internal carotid and perhaps onto frontal branches of the middle cerebral, through the rete mirabilia.

It was not possible in this case, to show a revascularization of the left hemisphere through the anterior communicating artery or the vertebral-basilar system.

Finally, the collateral circulation through the middle meningeal may contribute to the compensating for the obstruction of one branch of the internal carotid as, for example, the middle cerebral artery. It is clear that in this case, the blood flow, stemming from the meningeal, cannot use the ophthalmic to reach the ischaemic territory but it does follow the path of the rete mirabilia.

This is a case that especially illustrates these facts, the only example of this type that has been found in a series of 9 observations of occlusive lesions of the middle cerebral artery.

CASE 4

A female patient of 19, admitted 19 August 1966 with a syndrome of intracranial hypertension, the sequel of a tuberculous meningitis. No focal symptoms from the cerebral hemispheres.

An encephalographic examination showed the presence of an extensive left temporal lesion with displacement toward the right of the ventricle complex and a narrowing of the left lateral ventricle (especially of segment 3).

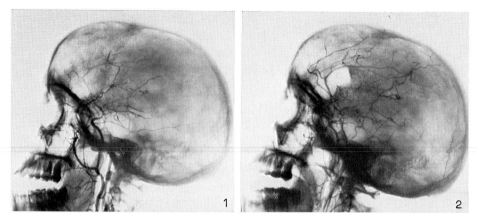

Fig. 3. CASE 4. Left carotid arteriogram. Revascularization of the middle cerebral artery through the middle meningeal artery and rete mirabile.

The sagittal angiograph of the left common carotid showed, paradoxically, that the anterior cerebral was to be found situated on the middle line and that the middle cerebral artery was obstructed and reduced to a fine branch. Its territory was discovered to be revascularized through the external carotid, more exactly through the middle meningeal, a fact which was confirmed by the lateral angiograph.

The lateral angiographic series showed that the revascularization of the middle cerebral region was initially effected by means of the middle meningeal and the rete mirabilia (Fig. 3); in later stages it could be seen that branches stemmed from the posterior cerebral artery and the posterior choroidal, from the anterior cerebral and even from the anterior choroidal, contribute also to the collateral circulation. It seems however, that the collateral circulation destined to compensate, in this case, for the obstruction of the middle cerebral comes initially from the middle meningeal and therefore from the external carotid.

The clinical and angiographic examinations showed that the circulation in the region of the left carotid was on the whole slowed as the deep veins did not appear until 7″–8″.

The angiographic and clinical demonstration that the obstruction of the middle cerebral artery was compensated for in a satisfactory manner, was an excellent guide to later surgical procedures.

Surgery on 24/11/66, was carried out through a left fronto-temporal craniectomy. Dura adhered to the cortex at the level of the Sylvian fissure. Enlarged frontal con-volutions. Excision of an area of the frontal cortex, 5 cm by 4 cm and exposure of a large multilocular abscess, deeply located inside the Sylvian fissure, without direct contact with the dura. Its external wall was found to be joined to the already obstructed middle cerebral branches, and their cutting, during the excision of the lesion, did not give place to any heamorrhage. Only on dissecting the infero-internal portion of the abscess did important bleeding take place, which necessitated the clipping of the large arterial branches coming from the initial portion of the middle cerebral. The abscess occupied the position of a meningioma of the Sylvian fissure. The operating area was continually irrigated with chloramphenicol and streptomycin. Hermetic suture of the dura.

Histologic examination: Tuberculous granuloma.

A postoperative roentgenograph showed the position of the clips placed on the branches of the middle cerebral.

Two months later, a further left carotid angiogram showed that the collateral circulation compensating for the obstruction of the middle cerebral stemmed from the anterior and posterior cerebrals and from the anterior choroidal arteries but not from the middle meningeal, for this vessel, and the rete mirabilia which were there connected, had been interrupted in cutting through the dura and in turning it back for the exposure of the lesion. The vertebral arteriograph showed the left posterior cerebral participating in the revascularization of the middle cerebral.

We see, in this case, that the collateral circulation through the middle meningeal artery and the rete mirabilia plays an important part in the revascularization of the middle cerebral artery. This role however, is not decisive, for, when the anastomotic route was interrupted by the operation, the revascularization was maintained through other anastomoses and no postoperative focal defects ensued.

The pictures to which we have referred present certain similarities with those of the external carotid in cases of convexity meningiomata in which it is realized that the vascularization of the tumour stems, at least in part, from the middle meningeal artery.

One cannot, nevertheless, compare the two cases. In the case of the meningiomata, the tumour is implanted in the dura, its irrigation coming therefore directly from the meningeal arteries while, on the contrary, in our case, the lesion was not in direct contact with the dura and was found to be completely submerged beneath the cerebral cortex, in the depths of the Sylvian fissure. Under these circumstances the arrival of the contrast medium at the lesion implies the revascularization of the middle cerebral territory by means of the meningeal.

COMMENTS

The cases that we have described, chosen from among a series of twenty occlusions of the internal carotid and nine cases of occlusion of the middle cerebral, show that in a certain percentage, the middle meningeal plays an important role in the complex anastomotic system which connects the external and internal carotid arteries, a system which can contribute to the collateral circulation if a blockage of the internal carotid or one of its branches takes place.

These facts confirm angiographically the data already presented by anatomic studies on the existing anastomotic connections between the ophthalmic and middle meningeal arteries. Various authors (Adachi, Tiedeman and Dubrevil) have observed cases in which the ophthalmic artery originates in the middle meningeal. Hayreh and Dass have shown cases in which the ophthalmic comes from both the middle meningeal artery and the carotid siphon.

The connections between the middle meningeal and collateral branches of the ophthalmic (lacrimal, anterior and posterior ethmoidal) have also been anatomically confirmed.

The same may be stated in regard to direct anatomoses (without a diversion through the ophthalmic artery) between the middle meningeal and the cerebral vessels. Some anatomists, among whom can be quoted Testut and Batson, have described the existence of small arterial channels extending between the dural branches of the meningeal arteries and the superficial arteries of the brain (rete mirabilia).

Our cases 3 and 4 pose, from the angiographic point of view, this interesting problem, already discussed in the papers of Denny-Brown, Soler Llenas, Mount and Taveras.

The importance of the collateral circulation via the middle meningeal is less in case 3 in comparison with the efficiency that it seems to possess in case 4. However, even in this last case, it does not play an exclusive role in the revascularization of the territory of the middle cerebral.

We see therefore that the middle meningeal represents only one of the numerous anastomotic routes which bring into communication the territories of the internal and external carotids and that it only plays an important part in the collateral circulation in a limited number of occlusions of the internal carotid.

Even in the cases where angiographic examination emphasizes the importance of the middle meningeal (as in cases 1 and 4) we see that its role in the collateral circulation is by no means exclusive.

In cases 2 and 3, there has not been observed any regression of the focal neurological defects, which indicates that the collateral circulation through the middle meningeal was hardly satisfactory in these cases, even if (case 2, left side) it appeared to be highly developed.

Surgical Considerations in Extracranial Occlusive Lesions

M. VINK and H. W. DICKE

Department of Surgery, Leyden University Hospital, Leyden (The Netherlands)

INCIDENCE AND PATHOLOGY

The criteria for selection of a patient with symptomatic cerebral arterial insufficiency as a candidate for surgical therapy differ in various institutes. For this reason it is difficult to interpret the data on incidence provided by large statistics. Roughly speaking, in about 50% of the patients with symptoms of deficient cerebral circulation the cause is an extracranial occlusive lesion, which is often segmental and multifocal. Consequently, most of the patients in this category are potential candidates for reconstructive arterial surgery.

Atherosclerosis is the most common cause of the obstructing process. However, emboli, septic thrombosis, trauma, X-ray damage of the vascular wall, outside pressure *e.g.* from chemodectoma, etc. etc. should be remembered as possible etiologic factors in exceptional cases.

Atherosclerotic lesions, though symptomatic of a generalized disease of the vascular wall, are often segmental. Characteristic locations are:

1. the bifurcation of the common carotid and the origin of the internal carotid artery.
2. the origin of the vertebral artery from the subclavian artery.
3. the origin of the branches of the aortic arch, i.c. the innominate, the left common carotid and the left subclavian artery.
4. the origin of the right subclavian and common carotid from the innominate artery.
5. combinations of two or more of the just mentioned types, for multifocal lesions are frequent.

SYMPTOMATOLOGY

The symptomatology differs according to the main type of the occlusion:

1. The carotid type. Recurrent dizziness or instability, contralateral numbness or even paralysis of one limb, transient ipsilateral blurring of vision, deterioration of the ability to do mental work.
2. The vertebrobasilar type. Transient periods of vertigo, weakness of the limbs, visual disturbances (of both eyes), and cerebellar ataxia.
3. A combination of 1. and 2. in the aortic-arch-branches' syndrome, and the special type with reversed blood flow in the vertebral artery producing the "steal syndrome".

References p. 258

The diagnosis of intermittent, progressing or complete cerebrovascular insufficiency is a clinical one and does not per se correspond with the arteriographic findings.

In most of the patients with brachiocephalic disease physical examination is diagnostically rewarding (diminished pulse or loss of pulse, systolic bruit or thrill). EEG studies with intermittent compression of the common carotid artery, ophthalmodynamometry and thermometry provide useful information. However Crawford *et al.* (1966) state that approximately 35 % of these patients has no localizing physical signs.

The diagnosis should be confirmed by arteriography. In so-called clear-cut cases of carotid bifurcation lesions a bilateral percutaneous carotid arteriography might provide sufficient information, but we prefer a four-vesse langiography. However, in our clinic four-vessel angiography is not performed in patients who for other reasons (cardiac, pulmonary, etc.) are no suitable candidates for major surgery anyway: one should remember the average 3–5 per cent of neurological complications following angiography.

INDICATIONS FOR OPERATION AND SELECTION

We would like to stress that arteriographic evidence of a stenosis or occlusion of an extracranial artery does not mean that the patient is a candidate for surgery, unless his symptoms are reasonably explained by the demonstrated lesion. Therefore, the selection for operation is based on the clinical picture *and* the arteriographic findings. Surgical treatment is indicated in:

1. Patients with transient attacks of cerebral vascular insufficiency caused by:
   a. a stenotic lesion in one or more cervical arteries;
   b. an occluding lesion in the branches of the aortic arch;
   c. an obstructing lesion in the subclavian artery proximal to the origin of the vertebral artery (steal syndrome);
   d. kinking of a cervical artery.
2. Patients with a progressing stroke and minor neurological deficit on the base of an extracranial arterial stenosis.
3. Patients with a completed stroke caused by extracranial arterial obstruction to prevent recurrence or worsening of the condition.
4. Patients with an asymptomatic but significant obstruction who have to be submitted to a major intrathoracic or abdominal operation, with the chance of hypotension and deterioration of the cerebral function, as a prophylactic intervention.

CONTRAINDICATIONS

1. The generally accepted contraindications for major surgery.
2. Acute stroke.
3. Complete obstruction of the internal carotid artery.

4. Significant intracerebral stenosing or occluding lesions on the ipsilateral side of an extracranial arterial obstruction.
5. An asymptomatic extracranial obstruction of a major artery.

SURGICAL TECHNIQUE

In the past decade major surgical principles in reconstructive arterial surgery have been stabilized to a large extent.

The most favored methods are:

1. Endarterectomy, eventually combined with a patch graft angioplasty. This procedure is specifically suitable for lesions of the carotid bifurcation and in the internal carotid and vertebral artery area.
2. Resection of the diseased segment and insertion of a venous or heteroplastic prosthesis.
3. Bypass procedures are employed in lesions of branches of the aortic arch; especially if there are multiple segmental lesions. The application of this technique depends on the extent and location of the lesion and the condition of the patient (intra- versus extrathoracic approach).

ANESTHESIA

Local anesthesia may be used in surgery of the cervical carotid bifurcation. In all other types of surgery, i.c. of the branches of the aortic arch, inhalation anesthesia with controled respiration is mandatory.

Some authors prefer the use of hypothermia and hyperpressure chamber to prolong the safe period of occlusion, but we abandoned this method in favor of the temporary intra-arterial shunt.

Hypotension should be prevented by all appropriate measures. In patients treated with antihypertensive drugs medication either should be stopped several days before the planned operation or be replaced by short-acting ones.

Some authors favor the Trendelenburg position to promote maximal arterialization.

COMMENT

According to a survey of the international literature, surgical technique has become standardized. Variations, dependent on personal experience and skill are worth studying, but they are not essential to the present problem.

Indications and contraindications still may give rise to a highly controversial discussion, however, with on one side those who favor a conservative approach and adhere to a treatment with anticoagulants, and on the opposite side the surgeon who operates even on a patient with an acute stroke (Hardy, 1963; Hunter, 1965; DeBakey, 1965).

The best candidates for operation are patients with intermittent attacks of cerebral arterial insufficiency who are neurologically intact. Second best are the patients with progressive neurologic deficits and those with a stable neurologic deficit. The latter do not benefit by the operation as far as the neurologic deficit is concerned, but a new attack may be prevented.

The principles of the postoperative treatment, i.c. the use of anticoagulants and antihypertensive drugs have not yet been settled. In our clinic we prescribe lifelong anticoagulant therapy from a prophylactic point of view.

Hypertension over 200 mm Hg is treated with antihypertensive drugs. This regimen has been used for the last 7 years and, at least in our hands, proved to be satisfactory, as shown by tables I and II.

TABLE I

OPERATIVE RESULTS OF PATIENTS WITH TRANSIENT ISCHEMIC ATTACKS AT THE MO MENT OF DISCHARGE FROM HOSPITAL

Number of patients	died		worse		no change		improved		asympto- matic		improved in total	
	no.	%	no.	%	no.	%	no.	%	no.	%	no.	%
31	2	6	1	3	—	—	7	23	21	68	28	91

TABLE II

FOLLOW-UP DATA OF THE PATIENTS WITH TRANSIENT ISCHEMIC ATTACKS

Number of patients	died		worse		no change		improved		asympto- matic		improved in total	
	no.	%	no.	%	no.	%	no.	%	no.	%	no.	%
29	—	—	1	3	2	7	11	38	15	52	26	90

ACKNOWLEDGMENT

We wish to thank R. J. A. M. van Dongen, M. D., head of the Department of Surgery, Hospital "De Goddelijke Voorzienigheid", Sittard and J. R. von Ronnen, M. D., head of the Department of Radiology, Leyden University Hospital for permission to use the slides shown in this presentation.

REFERENCES

CRAWFORD, E. S. (1966) Surgical treatment of occlusive cerebrovascular disease. *Surg. Clin. N. Amer.*, **46**, 873.
DEBAKEY, M. E. (1965) Cerebral arterial insufficiency: one to eleven years results following arterial reconstructive operation. *Ann. Surg.*, **161**, 921.
HARDY, J. D. (1963) On the reversibility of strokes; case of carotid artery repair with prompt recovery after hemiplegia and coma for two days. *Ann. Surg.*, **158**, 1035.
HUNTER, J. A. (1965) Emergency operation for acute cerebral ischemia due to carotid artery obstruction: review of 26 cases. *Ann. Surg.*, **162**, 901.

Reconstructive Surgery on the Branches of the Aortic Arch

L. HEJHAL and P. FIRT

Institute for Clinical and Experimental Surgery, Prague (Czechoslovakia)

Reconstructions on arteries supplying the brain have acquired an important place in vascular surgery.

In our institute we performed on these arteries a total of 257 reconstructive operations. In this paper, however, we evaluate only the results of operations performed until December 1965 because since then a sufficient period of time has elapsed for an adequate follow-up. Until then 133 reconstructions were made in the cervical region and 60 in the mediastinal. Preoperatively 135 patients had permanent or transient symptoms, 58 were without complaints (Table I).

TABLE I

SURGERY OF THE BRANCHES OF THE AORTIC ARCH

Location of lesion	No of cases	Symptomatic		Asymptomatic	
		No.	%	No.	%
Cervical segments	133	77		56	(42)
			(58)		
Intrathoracic segments	60	58	(97)	2	(3)
Total	193	135	(70)	58	(30)

Today stenoses causing transient symptoms are generally accepted as the main and indisputable operative indication. In our group transient symptoms of the cervical involvement were present in 62 patients and in 48 with changes in the mediastinal area. Postoperatively (follow-up controls on the average after 3 years but at least 1 year postoperatively) 98 patients were without complaints, 9 improved, only in 2 the condition was the same. The operative mortality rate was 2 patients (Table II).

In severe but asymptomatic stenoses the opinion on the problem of the advisability of the operation is not so unanimous. However, provided that the angiographic finding is of marked degree, we believe that here the operation is almost just as vital. A severe stenosis entails the danger of further growth of pathological changes with the possibility of embolization or total occlusion of the artery. To postpone the operation until neurological symptoms develop or until onset of the total occlusion would represent a substantial danger for the patient. A follow-up of 56 preventively operated

TABLE II

RESULTS OF ARTERIAL RECONSTRUCTION

Before operation	No. of cases	Without symptoms	After operation		
			Improved	Unchanged	Deaths
Asymptomatic	58	58	0	0	0
Transient cerebral ischemia	110	98	9	2	1
Persistent neurol. symptoms	25	9	4	11	1
Total	193	165 (85.4%)	13 (6.7%)	13 (6.7%)	2 (1.1%)

patients showed slight transient complaints in only 1 patient. By contrast, in a group of 26 unoperated patients (they disagreed with the operation or postponed it for various reasons) during 2 years 3 died of cerebral ischemic stroke and 2 suffered a hemiplegia.

As for complete occlusions, we think that only operations in the acute phase have a chance of real success. Since time is the decisive factor, the results directly depend on a good organization and competent management. If progress is to be achieved, special units similar to the one which is just being built in our institute, are indispensible. The value of operations of chronical occlusions remain, in our opinion, doubtful. When analyzing the results of all operations for occlusions of the internal carotid artery, we should bear in mind the tendency of many patients towards a spontaneous recovery. It is also incorrect to include into the successful cases those improved patients in whom reconstruction in the proper meaning of the word was impossible.

The operation is usually performed under general anesthesia. Always the pressure gradient as well as the peripheral pressure is measured after clamping the segment where blood flow is to be interrupted during the operation. If its value is higher than one third of the patient's arterial blood pressure we operate without using a shunt. However, if it is lower we use an internal shunt. When using this method we were never confronted with a peroperative ischemic cerebral complication.

For the reconstruction in the cervical segments of the carotid artery and the internal carotid artery we always prefer endarterectomy and close the opening in the artery with simple continuous suture or with patch graft. A mere widening by a patch without removing the sclerotic plaque is, in our opinion, incorrect.

In stenoses at the bifurcation of the anonimous artery, at the subclavian artery and at the origin of the vertebral artery we usually employ endarterectomy with patch graft. In occlusion of the bifurcation of the anonimous artery we resect the occluded segment and replace it by a bifurcation prosthesis. In all occlusions or severe stenoses extending to the aortic arch, we overbridge the affected segment with a bypass, the central end of which is joined end-to-side to the ascending aorta. We employ the bypass also in all patients with the Takayashu type of arteritis. Here the central end is joined to the ascending aorta and the peripheral, if possible, at a sufficient distance from the involved arterial segment.

Finally, we would like to emphasize that intrathoracic involvements are relatively frequent and represent a very suitable field for reconstructive procedures. The operative mortality rate is surprisingly low. In our group not a single patient died as consequence of the operation and in 93 % full success was achieved.

We believe that the future of surgical procedures on arteries supplying the brain lies in early operations performed prior to the onset of irreversible damage to the cerebral tissue *i.e.* prior to the onset of a total occlusion of the artery.

Microangeional Surgery and its Techniques

R. M. PEARDON DONAGHY and GAZI YASARGIL

*Laboratories of the University of Vermont and the Mary Fletcher Hospital,
Burlington, Vermont (U.S.A.)*

The term Microangeional Surgery was coined in the laboratories of the University of Vermont to denote surgery upon blood vessels less than 4 millimeters in outside diameter. Most of the work actually performed in these laboratories has been on vessels less than 2 millimeters in outside diameter. The term microangeional surgery has been used in preference to small vessel surgery, because the latter is a purely English term, and hence scarcely appropriate for techniques which have universal application. It has been used in preference to "neuro-vascular surgery" because it is applicable to vessels in any part of the anatomy and because the term "neuro-vascular" like the term "micro-vascular" is a bastard term, half Latin and half Greek.

Personal interest in microangeional surgery began in 1959 when we were confronted with small vessel occlusions intracranially which we could not correct.

It was necessary to work out a surgical technique in the laboratory which would allow the clearing and repair of 0.5-2 mm vessels and still maintain patency.

We have accomplished this in the rabbit with a patency rate of 64%. Patency rate in the dog is even better but dog series is much smaller and hence less valid statistically.

Failures were found to be due to one of the following:

1. Narrowing of the lumen at the suture line.
2. Foreign material exposed to the lumen.
3. Infection.
4. Spasm.
5. Immediate local thrombosis.
6. Inaccurate suture placement due to poor visibility.
7. Too long a period of occlusion.

These problems were met in the followings ways:

PROBLEM	REMEDY
1. Narrowing	Application of a vein patch.
2. Foreign material exposed to lumen (Fig. 1)	Patch-vessel-patch technique.
3. Infection	Technique improvement.
4. Spasm	Intra- and extravascular procaine.
5. Local thrombosis	Intravascular heparin.

References p. 266–267

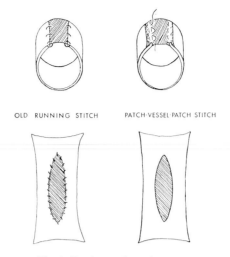

OLD RUNNING STITCH   PATCH-VESSEL-PATCH STITCH

Fig. 1. Patch-vessel-patch suture.

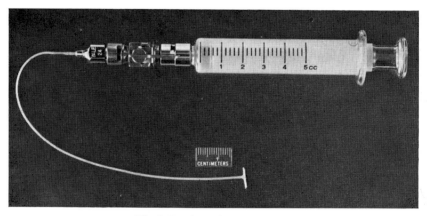

Fig. 2. T-tube to fit 2-mm vessel.

6. Inaccurate suture placement   Adoption of Jacobson's technique for use of the dissecting microscope.

7. Too long a period of occlusion   The use of a T-tube by-pass (Fig. 2).

This T-tube has a number of advantages:

1. Flow can be restored within a few minutes.
2. Flow can be constantly monitored visually.
3. Flow may be checked in either direction separately.
4. A pathway for intravascular injection of any desired drug is maintained.
5. The long limb of the T-tube may be used as a handle to facilitate vessel rotation without trauma to the vessel wall.

By use of these techniques it has been possible to perform intimectomy on the cortical vessels of dogs with a patency rate of 85%. For the basilar artery patency rate was 90%. Anastomosis of the superficial temporal artery to the internal carotid

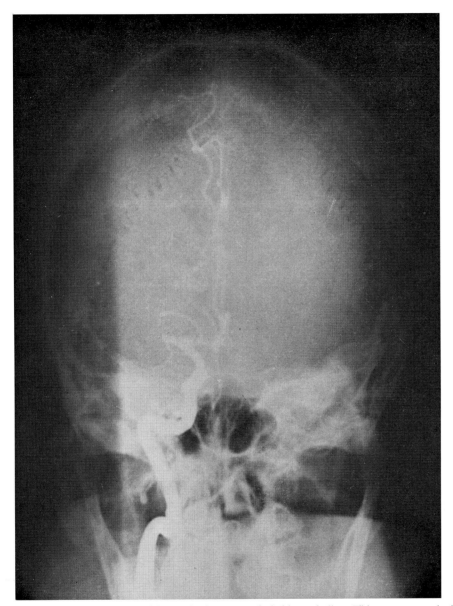

Fig. 3. Pre-operative view of middle cerebral artery occluded by embolism. This case operated with J. H. Jacobson.

artery or a branch of the middle cerebral artery have had a maintained patency of 55 %.

In humans seven middle cerebral artery occlusions have been removed. There have been three deaths but two of these were operated late when there was edema and hemiplegia and one died of a cause which could not be ascribed to the procedure. Two vessels remained open and one had a small embolus to a more distant site.

Only one of these patients was operated with the completed technique and this vessel remained open. Unfortunately one patient with an open vessel died 48 hours after

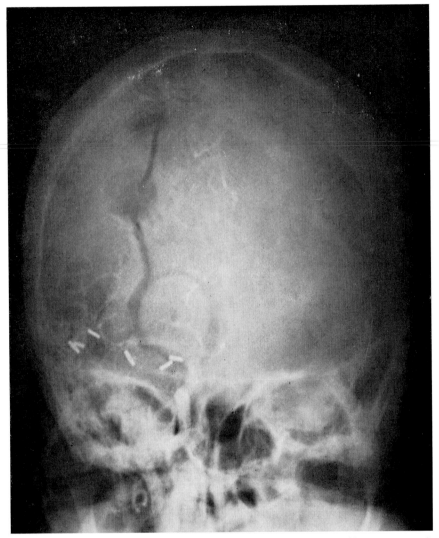

Fig. 4. View of patent middle cerebral artery 48 hours following surgery. This case operated with
J. H. Jacobson.

surgery of a complication of angiography and the other patient with an open vessel
also died of edema as the procedure had been done too late and opened flow into an
area of infarction.

REFERENCES

CRAWFORD, STANLEY E., BEALL, ARTHUR C., ELLIS, JR., PAUL R. AND DEBAKEY, MICHAEL E.
(1960) A technique permitting operation upon small arteries. *Surgical Forum*, **X**.
JACOBSON, J. H. AND SUAREZ, E. L. (1960) Microsurgery in Anastomosis of Small Vessels. *Surgical
Forum*, **II**, 243–245.
JACOBSON, J. H., WALLMAN, L. J., SCHUMACHER, G. A., FLANAGAN, M. E. AND DONAGHY, R. M. P.
(1962) Microsurgery as an Aid to Middle Cerebral Artery Endarterectomy, *J. Neurosurg.*,

19, 108–115.

DONAGHY, R. M. P. (1967) Patch and By-Pass in Micro-Angeional Surgery. *Proc. First Intern. Microvascular Conf. Burlington, Vermont*, October 6–7, 1966 (in press).

YASARGIL, GAZI (1967) Experimental Intracranial-Extracranial Shunts and Patching and Grafting on Brain Arteries of Dog. *Proc. First Intern. Microvascular Conf. Burlington, Vermont*, October 6–7, 1966 (in press).

The Natural History of Patients with Intracranial Aneurysm after Rupture

ALAN E. RICHARDSON

Department of Neurosurgery, Atkinson Morley's Hospital, Wimbledon (England)

We must firstly consider the implications of the title of this paper.

1. Natural History. This I will consider as the result of treatment by strict bed rest together with other supportive measures, but, excluding any therapy more specifically designed to reduce the risk of further haemorrhage. Unless otherwise stated the results are those measured six months after the presenting ictus.

2. Of Patients. The data concerns patients in a trial in progress since 1958 in which treatment is randomly allocated. Excluded from this trial were patients with life threatening haematomas, inoperable lesions, or who died before angiography.

3. With Aneurysms. All cases had aneurysms proven by angiography. In some cases of multiple aneurysms it was not possible either radiologically or clinically to be certain as to which lesion had ruptured. These patients were only included if the lesions could be treated by a single surgical procedure, either common carotid ligation or intracranial operation.

4. After Rupture. All patients suffered subarachnoid haemorrhages within the eight weeks preceding admission as evidenced by clinical features and L. P. findings. The majority of patients were in fact admitted within 48 hours of the ictus.

Patients suffering haemorrhage from an aneurysm are a heterogeneous group, so for any comparative purpose, one must introduce prognostic factors. Of these the most important, we have found, is conscious level.

The natural prognosis is clearly very dependent on conscious level following the ictus. In most of the cases in stupor or deep coma, death resulted from the brain damage already sustained whereas in the alert and drowsy group, death if it occurred, was usually a result of recurrent haemorrhage. These latter are the cases potentially suitable for treatment so I would like to confine my further consideration only to this non-comatose group. Time will not allow of a complete review of all the factors involved in prognosis so I will merely consider some typical examples.

Age has little influence on natural history except that patients under the age of 40 particularly if the blood pressure is normal have a much better outlook than their older or hypertensive counterparts.

Sex similarly has little influence on prognosis except that the sex distribution of the various aneurysms is different.

The site of the aneurysm is important (Table II).

TABLE I

CONSCIOUS LEVEL AND PROGNOSIS

	Number of patients	Mortality	%
Alert	198	59	29%
Drowsy	178	100	55%
Stuporose	38	27	71%
Comatose	21	19	90%

TABLE II

SITE OF ANEURYSM

	Number of patients	Mortality No.	%
Anterior cerebral/anterior communicating	150	62	41%
Middle cerebral	103	40	38%
Posterior communicating	41	15	37%
Multiple	38	20	52%
Basilar/vertebral	44	22	50%

The presence of an aneurysm of the vertebral/basilar system or of multiple aneurysms clearly worsens the natural history. In multiple lesions it should be stressed that it is extremely rare for more than one of the aneurysms to rupture. The time interval from the ictus is of paramount importance as is shown by the following graph which shows the subsequent mortality with the passage of time, at two major sites (Fig. 1).

Whilst this shows a somewhat similar pattern for the two sites and indicates that the maximum risk of rebleeding occurs in the first two weeks and thereafter rapidly declines, it also illustrates that the rebleeding patterns are not identical. Thus the incidence of late recurrent haemorrhage in posterior communicating aneurysms is much higher than for anterior communicating aneurysms. The widely differing prognosis of individual cases based on these and other factors make it difficult to assess the risk in any given case and particularly difficult to assess the value of treatment in *selected* cases. I and my co-workers have endeavoured to solve this problem by a mathematical evaluation of prognostic factors for any given aneurysmal site. If I may take as an example the aneurysms of the anterior communicating complex (Richardson *et al.*, 1964) — we studied in detail 103 cases from the trial and selected 20 prognostic factors. Simple evaluation reduced these to 12 and these were later reduced to 8 factors which were relatively independent (indicated by ++).

Using the technique of discriminant function analysis it was possible to assign mathematical values to the 8 factors which were age, sex, blood pressure, conscious level, shape of aneurysm, direction of aneurysm and time elapsed from the haemorrhage.

The resulting figure could then be plotted on a previously constructed graph which would then show the predicted mortality (Fig. 2).

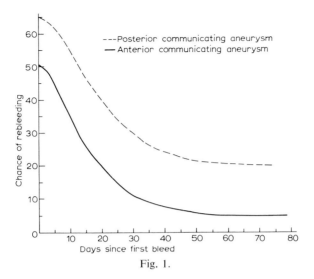

Fig. 1.

TABLE III

PROGNOSTIC FACTORS

(+)   Age.   (+) Sex.
(++)   Conscious level - fully alert.
                        - drowsy.
                        - very drowsy.
(++)   Blood pressure - diastolic.
                        - systolic.
(++)   Direction of aneurysm.
(++)   Length/breadth ratio of the aneurysm.
        Area/orifice ratio of the aneurysm.
        Absolute size of the aneurysm.
        Locularity.
        Presence of vascular spasm.
        Filling characteristics of aneurysm.
(++)   Time elapsed from original rupture in days.

We should now instance one or two cases of anterior communicating aneurysms to show the widely differing *natural* prognosis depending on the prognostic factors derived. If we work out the score for a typical "good risk" surgical case *i.e.* a normotensive alert male with a downward pointing sausage-shaped aneurysm at about 14 days after the haemorrhage we find this to be about 10. When this is plotted on the graph the patient is seen to fall into the group whose untreated mortality rate is of the order of 5%. On the other hand a 50 year old, very drowsy, hypertensive woman with an upward pointing spherical aneurysm seen at the sixth day following her haemorrhage, would have a score of about 78 and this would place her in the group whose expected untreated mortality would be of the order of 90%. Thus in the first case a surgical mortality of 5% would afford little advantage whereas in the second a surgical mortality rate of 50% or 60% would be quite acceptable. One possible

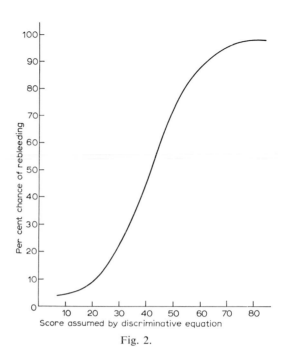

Fig. 2.

TABLE IV

WEIGHTINGS FOR PROGNOSTIC FACTORS

	(i)	To	0.9 if female, 0 if male
add	(ii)		$0.18 \times$ systolic B.P. in mm Hg
&	(iii)		$0.26 \times$ diastolic B.P. in mm Hg
&	(iv)		0 if alert, 11.6 if drowsy, 20.6 if very drowsy
&	(v)		0 if downwards, 10.2 if forwards, 15.6 if forwards and upwards, 24.6 if directly upwards.
& subtract	(vi)		11.9 $\times$ ratio of length to breadth of aneurysm
&	(vii)		0.98 $\times$ number of days since haemorrhage
&	(viii)		0.174 $\times$ the patient's age in years

objection to this method of assessment would be that it is as yet incompletely tested. This objection must be accepted to some extent, though it has been tested on a random group of conservatively treated cases from another centre and shown to have an overall error rate of 16%. It should however be stressed that the main inaccuracies occurred in patients with intermediate scores *i.e.* 30–50, whereas the inaccuracy at the extreme ends of the graph was negligible.

We have worked out a similar technique for aneurysms of the internal carotid artery at or near the origin of the posterior communicating artery (Richardson *et al.*, 1966), and have found the prognostic factors to be somewhat different. Thus in this aneurysm, age, blood pressure, shape and direction of aneurysm and to some extent conscious level are unimportant whereas sex, the presence of vascular spasm and/or

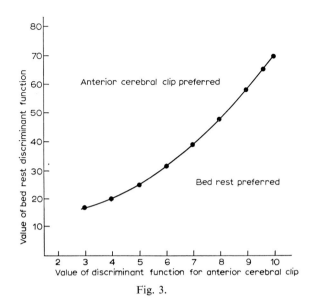

Fig. 3.

haematoma and the size of the lesion are very important and have a direct bearing on the natural history.

Fig. 3 is a preliminary conception of a method for assessing alternative treatments in anterior communicating aneurysms. A discriminant analysis was performed on 94 such patients treated by the relatively standard operation of proximal anterior cerebral artery ligation (Richardson *et al.*, 1966). The combination of this and the scoring system for bed rest cases might enable one to determine which is more appropriate in any given case. Clearly it is possible to apply this to any other method of treatment provided sufficient experience of the method is available for analysis in order to derive the discriminative equation.

I have only been able to touch on some of the prognostic factors in natural history but I hope I have made clear the following points.

1. The natural history is extremely heterogeneous and so the prognosis of the group cannot be applied to the individual.
2. The use of prognostic factors helps in this problem but the important factors may be different for the varying aneurysm sites.
3. The use of a mathematical technique to assess the influence of all the factors in any particular case is being further explored. Preliminary results are encouraging.

REFERENCES

RICHARDSON, A., J. JOHN AND P. PAYNE (1964) Assessment of the Natural History of Anterior Communicating Aneurysm. *J. Neurosurg.*, **21**, 266.

—, —, —, (1966) Prediction of morbidity and mortality in Anterior Communicating Aneurysms treated by proximal Anterior Cerebral ligation. *J. Neurosurg.*, **25**, 280.

—, —, AND D. YASHAN (1966) Prognostic factors in the untreated course of posterior communicating aneurysms. *Arch. Neurol.*, **14**, 172.

Anatomical Research on the Intracranial Arterial Aneurysms

M. SACHS, C. C. CABEZAS, J. T. POSADA AND MARCEL DAVID

Clinique Neurochirurgicale du Groupe Hospitalier Pitié-Salpêtrière,
75 Paris (France)

This anatomical research deals with the macroscopic dissection of 104 circles of Willis, in which 126 aneurysms were discovered. All patients had died after aneurysmal rupture; 42 had been operated upon. 46 aneurysms were found on the anterior communicating artery (ACoA), 42 on the internal carotid artery (ICA) and 30 on the middle cerebral artery (MCA). Most of the patients were female and 40 to 70 years old. 15 % of the cases had multiple aneurysms.

1. The ACoA Aneurysms

A. Two-thirds were located entirely on the ACoA, either on its whole length, or on a part of it: one-third originated from this vessel and the initial segment of a pericallosal artery. Only one case was found on both parts of the ACoA and the distal segment of an anterior cerebral artery (ACA). These variations of origin can be of importance from the surgical point of view.

B. The lateral portions of the sac, when directed upwards, were related sometimes very tightly to the pericallosal arteries on both sides, but anatomical dissection was always possible postmortem.

C. Heubner's arteries, in patients with these aneurysms, were located more distally than usual, *i.e.* at the level of the ACoA.

D. If the aneurysm was lateralized on the ACoA, it was usually ipsilateral to the largest or unique ACA (Fig. 1).

E. When the ACoA was found to be multiple or scale-like (9 cases), the aneurysms were located in 7 cases on the superior branch and directed upwards (Fig. 2).

F. The average size of these 46 aneurysms was 8 mm, the average neck only 3 mm. Most of these aneurysms showed no false sac.

G. 20 % of the cases had major abnormalities of the hexagone, this percentage being roughly the same as Alpers and Berry's (1963).

2. The ICA Aneurysms

A. The origin on the ICA was extremely variable, since the aneurysm was located from the juxta-clinoidian part to the bifurcation. Nevertheless, most of the malfor-

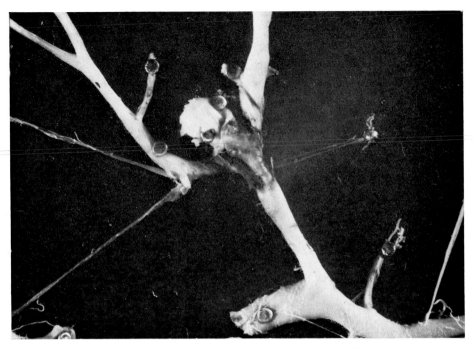

Fig. 1. ACoA aneurysm lateralized on the ACoA. The malformation is also located on the origin of the left pericallosal artery. The aneurysm originates ipsilateral to the largest ACA.

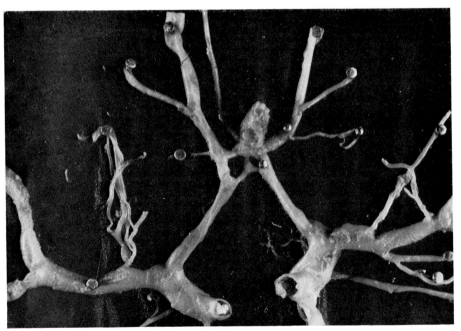

Fig. 2. ACoA aneurysm located on the superior branch of a scale-like AcoA. The two Heubner's arteries originate from the initial segment of the pericallosal arteries.

mations have been encountered between the anterior choroidian artery and the posterior communicating artery (PCoA). Ten out of the 42 ICA aneurysms were located
on both the ICA and the PCoA, and fell into the so-called group of PCoA aneurysms.
Among these 126 aneurysms none located completely on the PCoA were encountered.

B. Two-thirds of the PCoA ipsilateral to the aneurysms were very small.

C. The average size of these aneurysms was 10 mm, thus significantly larger than
the ACoA group. But the average width of the neck was the same (3 mm). Only very
large aneurysms, often with a false sac, were tightly related to the ACA or the MCA,
especially if located on the ICA bifurcation.

3. The MCA Aneurysms

A. It is now a very classical fact to notice that the aneurysms are always located
at the bifurcation or division of the MCA in secondary branches, usually on the
first 20 or 30 mm of its trunk (Sachs, 1966).

B. The relations with secondary branches depend upon the width of the stalk.
Narrow ones often allow an easy dissection of the sac except when secondary branches stick to the fundus of the sac. A certain number of aneurysms was located both
on the bifurcation and the origin of a secondary branch.

C. No ratio was found between MCA aneurysms and size of the arterial trunk. A
very small number of major abnormalities of the circle of Willis has been encountered
in these 30 cases of MCA aneurysms.

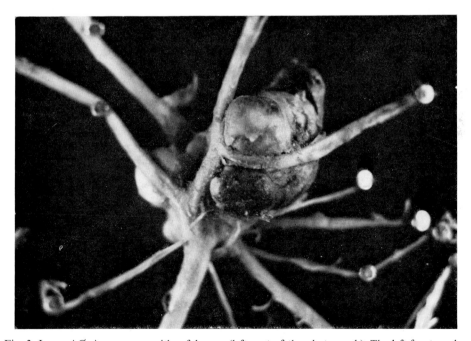

Fig. 3. Large ACoA aneurysm with a false sac (left part of the photograph). The left fronto-polar
branch sticks to the sac and can easily be thought arising from the sac. Careful anatomical dissection
was performed postmortem.

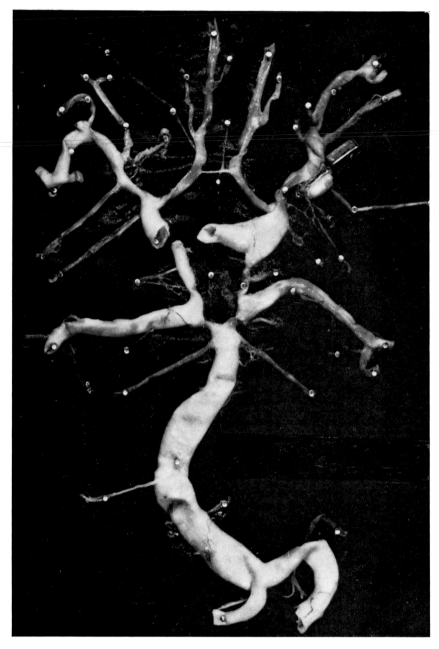

Fig. 4. MCA aneurysm with a Mayfield clip on its neck. Notice both generalized and localized atheroma. Very thin ACoA.

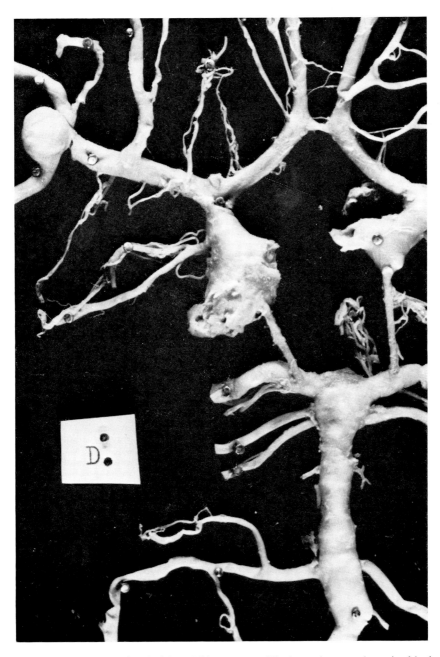

Fig. 5. MCA aneurysm associated with an ICA aneurysm. The latter, larger and proximal had ruptured. Notice atheroma, especially on the basilar trunk.

D. Size of the sac and width of the neck are very comparable to those of ACoA aneurysms. False sacs are rare.

4. *Site of the Aneurysms*

Whatever the site of the aneurysms, certain facts must be kept in mind:

(a) No collateral branches have been macroscopically identified, arising from the sac. Crompton (1966) and Stehbens (1962, 1963a and b) have made the same observations. Thus, if a small or secondary branch is thought to arise from the sac either by angiography or at the time of surgery, one must consider this as an artefact (Fig. 3), and never as a contraindication for proper and cautious dissection of the sac.

(b) Nearly all the ruptures were located at the apex of the sac (Crawford, 1959; Crompton, 1966). If not, it was usually at the junction of the real and false sac, or at the level of a very weak, bulging region. These modifications of the aneurysmal sac are very close to the atheromatous arterial ones.

(c) Since a very high percentage of major abnormalities of the circle of Willis has been encountered in the 104 cases studied, one must be very careful before certifying that vascular spasm is responsible for such a thin artery as seen on the angiograms. Often what is supposed to be spasm, revealed itself to be a very small vessel from the anatomical point of view. Spasm has to disappear after death.

(d) 42 patients had been operated upon. We have tried to understand these deaths but we found very few clips or silks badly fitted, very few major vessels interrupted or major post-operative internal carotid thrombosis. Thus we have thought that, taking into account the general and neurological status of the patient before operation, deaths could perhaps be explained by the haemodynamic changes that could occur in the post-operative course, if major abnormalities of the hexagone were associated.

(e) 28% of the cases showed an important atheroma, both generalized or localized to the aneurysmal sac (Fig. 4).

5. *Conclusions*

From this macroscopic study certain conclusions can be drawn:

(a) Angiograms cannot always give a precise knowledge of the neck, size, shape and relations of the aneurysms. Even when a vessel seems to arise from the sac, only a careful dissection, not always possible or desirable, will give you the correct response.

(b) If aneurysms are multiple, and no sufficient clinical data can be gathered to assess which one has ruptured, it is usually the largest and the most proximal (Fig. 5). Jain (1963) and Crompton (1966) have also made this observation.

(c) It is most important, if possible, to obtain a clear view of the entire circle of Willis before operation. If an ACA or a PCoA is not visualized, spasm must not automatically be assumed responsible. This vessel can be simply missing. It is then easy to understand of what importance such a fact may be.

REFERENCES

ALPERS, B. J., AND BERRY, R. G., (1963); Circle of Willis in cerebral vascular disorders. The anatomical structures. *Arch. Neurol. Chicago*, **8**, 398.

CRAWFORD, T., (1959); Some observations on the pathogenesis and natural history of intracranial aneurysms. *J. Neurol. Neurosurg. Psychiat.*, **22**, 259.

CROMPTON, M. R., (1966); Mechanisms of growth and rupture in cerebral berry aneurysms. *Brit. Med. J.*, **1**, 1138.

JAIN, K. K., (1963); Mechanisms of rupture of intracranial saccular aneurysms. *Surgery*, **54**, 347.

SACHS, M., (1966); Les anévrysmes de l'artère sylvienne (The aneurysms of the middle cerebral artery). A propos de 75 observations (About 75 cases). *Ann. Chir. Sem. Hôp. Paris*, **20**, no 15/16–17/18, 998.

STEHBENS, W. E., (1962); Hypertension and cerebral aneurysms. *Med. J. Aust.*, **49**, 8.

—, (1963a); Histopathology of cerebral aneurysms. *Arch. Neurol. Chicago*, **8**, 272.

—, (1963b); Aneurysm and anatomical variation of the cerebral arteries. *Arch. Path.*, **75**, 45.

The Pathology of Intracranial Aneurysms

JULES C. GOVAERT AND A. EARL WALKER

University of Ghent (Belgium)

Several theories have been proposed to account for the development of cerebral aneur-ysms. The most generally accepted thesis relating these vascular conditions to congen-ital abnormalities such as persistent embryonic vessels or defects in the wall of the artery is not entirely adequate. Although these congenital abnormalities occur not infrequently in the brains of children dying from causes unrelated to the nervous system, aneurysms are indeed rare. Moreover, a number of characteristics of aneurysms are not explicable by this hypothesis. The late onset of symptoms is difficult to recon-cile with the early development of difficulties occurring in most congenital abnormal-ities of the vascular system. The frequency curve of the age at which symptoms arise from angiomatous malformations of the brain has a peak 10 years earlier than that of

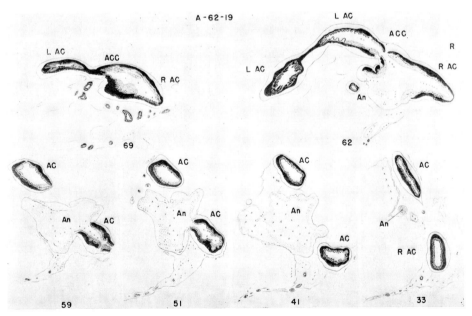

Fig. 1. (A-62-19) Sketches of representative serial sections of an aneurysm arising from the junction of the right anterior cerebral and anterior communicating arteries of a 37 year old colored man. Note the atheromatous plaque on the medial aspect of the wall of the right anterior cerebral artery just proximal to the aneurysm. The internal elastic layer (represented by the many ink lines) is split and fragmented at the aneurysmal margin. However, a few elastic slivers are seen in the wall of the sac in sections 52, 59 and 51. In the distal segments of the anterior cerebral arteries the vessel walls appear normal.

aneurysms. Finally, it is difficult to demonstrate aberrant vestigial vessels associated with aneurysms.

METHODOLOGY

This study is based upon an examination of the cerebral vessels related to cerebral aneurysms occurring in 25 patients. These dilatations were primarily located as follows:

Anterior communicating artery —	5 cases
Anterior cerebral artery —	4 cases
Middle cerebral artery —	3 cases
Internal carotid artery —	5 cases
Posterior communicating artery —	7 cases
Basilar artery —	1 case
Total	25 cases

Because the specimens were removed at post-mortem from patients dying after a rupture or attempt at surgical repair of the aneurysm, the series is not representative of intracranial aneurysms, but is composed of the more lethal ones.

A varying amount of the circle of Willis and adjacent aneurysm was embedded in celloidin, cut serially and adjacent representative sections stained with H & E, Mallory's PTAH, and for elastic tissue by Verhoeff's, Van Gieson's or Weigert's

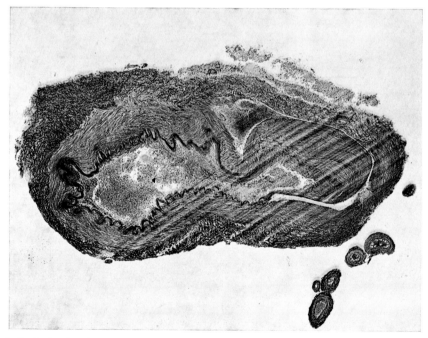

Fig. 2. (A-62-1). The atheromatous plaque in the right internal carotid artery proximal to an aneurysm at the take-off of the posterior communicating artery. The intima and elastica except for the involved segment appears relatively normal (Verhoeff, × 40).

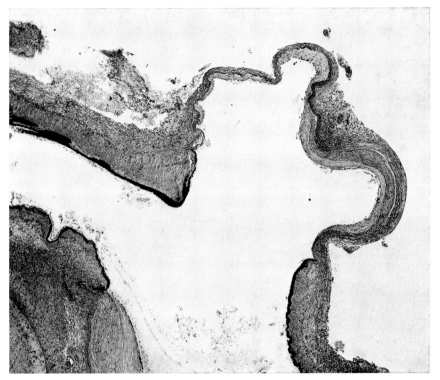

Fig. 3. (A-63-5). A section through the mouth of an aneurysm to show the abrupt termination of the normal structures of the arterial wall and the thinned out fibrous wall of the aneurysmal sac in the right middle cerebral artery at its trifurcation in a 35 year old white man.

methods. Photomicrographs or drawings were used to demonstrate alterations. In each case special attention was given to the anatomical components of the vessel wall adjoining the aneurysm.

PATHOLOGICAL ANATOMY

Characteristically one side of the wall of the vessel just proximal to the aneurysm contained an atheromatous plaque which merged with the rostral margin of the aneurysmal wall (Fig. 1). Although the plaques were usually well developed and frequently as thick as the vessel wall adjacent to the aneurysm, in other sections proximal to bifurcation of an artery small subintimal pads of connective tissue with little or no evidence of degeneration were often found. These were considered to be the precursors of the larger plaques. This plaque not infrequently appeared adjacent to a normal arterial wall and abruptly passed to a dilated segment of the vessel containing a laminated subintimal thickening (Fig. 2). At the junction with the aneurysm, the elastic layer may abruptly cease as it turns over the fragmented end of the muscular tunic (Fig. 1, Section 62) or it extends in fragments along the aneurysmal sac. The elastica interna of the parent vessel presented abnormalities such as: (1) thinning or splitting of the fibrils, some of which penetrated the muscularis mediae, (2) fragmentation of the

peripheral layer with apparent widening of the elastica, (3) narrowing and straighten-
ing of the elastic layer with varying degrees of degeneration characterized by thin
isolated and poorly stained fibers, or (4) total absence of a segment between normal

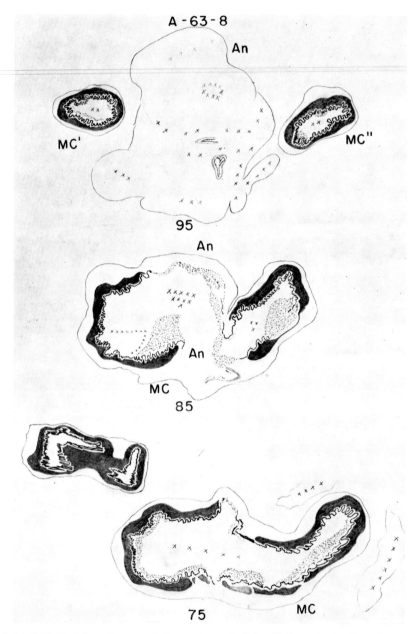

Fig. 4. (A-63-8). Sketches of representative sections of a left middle cerebral trifurcation aneurysm
which shows the atheromatous condition of the parent vessel (section 75); just proximal to the aneurysm
the structural development of the dilatation (section 85) and the relatively normal appearance of the
arteries distal to the aneurysm (section 95).

appearing elastica interna. In many instances, the muscularis mediae at the margin of the aneurysm had degenerative alterations such as loss of nuclei, hyalinization, etc. (Fig. 3).

The aneurysmal wall was composed of several different types of tissue:

(1) a thin layer of fibrous connective tissue with a poorly developed intima and no evidence of elastica muscularis. The fibrous sac seemed to be continuous with the adventitial layer of the parent vessel; (2) an attenuated arterial wall with, in places, fragments of intima, elastica, muscularis, and adventitia (Figs. 4 and 5). The intimal layer in places appeared normal but frequently had subintimal proliferations in various states of degeneration. The elastic layer usually was markedly attenuated or absent—rarely was a normal wavy elastic layer present. This wall was composed of a well developed muscular layer in places but in other areas the muscle fibers were absent or scarce. The adventitia served as the outer lamina of the aneurysmal sac; (3) multi-layered capsule composed of fibrous lamina with interposed hemorrhagic strips usually about a central core of degenerated fibrous tissue, calcification, cholesterol crystals, foam cells, loose hyalinized connective tissue and hemosiderin deposits.

Frequently the atheromatous changes were located about the site of penetrance of vasa vasorum near the bifurcation of the parent artery. These were sites of predilection for degenerative changes in the subintimal tissues.

It is noteworthy that distal to the aneurysm, the arterial walls were of normal structure (Fig. 5).

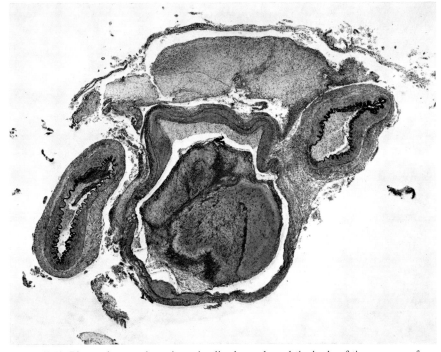

Fig. 5. (A-63-8). Photomicrograph to show the distal vessels and the body of the aneurysm from the case illustrated in Fig. 4. (Verhoeff, × 20).

DISCUSSION

Although congenital abnormalities of the arteries may be responsible for initiating degenerative changes at certain sites, it seems probable that the latter are the causative factors in the production of aneurysmal dilatations. It seems likely that the formation of subintimal pads or plaques proximal to the bifurcation of the major intracranial vessels causes an impedance to the flow in the vessel and a turbulence of the stream just distal to the plaque.

In addition, the intimal lesions being situated at the stoma of vasa vasorum impair the nutrition of the distal vessel wall causing further degenerative changes which weaken the vessel wall so that the abnormal turbulence produces an out-pouching. This further impairs the blood supply to the vessel wall and so the aneurysm enlarges. The preferential site of the atheromatous plaque is probably due to hemorrhagic in-filtration of the vessel wall at the site of vasa vasorum with subsequent degenerative changes in the media and adventitia.

Cerebral Circulation Times in Subarachnoid Haemorrhage

ALEX R. TAYLOR AND VIJAY K. KAK

Department of Neurological Surgery, Royal Victoria Hospital, Belfast (N. Ireland)

INTRODUCTION

Spasm of cerebral vessels is, to surgeons at least, a well recognized hazard. In subarachnoid haemorrhage it would appear to bear some fairly constant time relationship to the ictus, to the angiographic appearances of spasm and to cerebral blood flow (Kagstrom *et al.*, 1965). It may also be related to biochemical changes in the CSF, in particular a lowering of pH (Froman and Smith, 1967) and the appearance of 5-hydroxytryptamine in the region of the basal blood vessels (Buckall, 1966). Connolly (1962) and McKissock *et al.* (1965) have observed that subarachnoid haemorrhage patients with spasm seen angiographically have a poorer operative prognosis, and a larger percentage of ischaemic lesions. It seems likely that both the spasm and the infarction are associated with a diminished total or regional cerebral blood flow.

This paper describes the result of cerebral circulation studies on 90 patients with subarachnoid haemorrhage. The cerebral circulation times are related to the arterial spasm seen at angiography and the operative complication rate, morbidity and mortality. It is suggested that serial estimations of cerebral circulation time may be a useful guide to the timing of angiography and surgery in the management of patients with subarachnoid haemorrhage.

SELECTION OF PATIENTS

This study deals with 90 patients admitted to the Royal Victoria Hospital, Belfast over the last four years. This is only 21 per cent of the total admitted with subarachnoid haemorrhage during that period. Only those patients were selected in whom it was considered likely that the results would be informative or helpful. This resulted in the selection of a high percentage of ill or difficult patients. The morbidity and mortality rate is higher than that in the whole series. Age and sex distribution is seen in Table I. It conforms to the usual pattern for such a series.

METHOD

This has been described elsewhere (Oldendorf, 1962; Taylor and Bell, 1966), but will be briefly recapitulated. 50 μC of [^{131}I]Hippuran, dissolved in 2 ml of a blue dye,

References p. 294

TABLE I

AGE AND SEX DISTRIBUTION OF 90 PATIENTS

Sex	Age in years						
	11–20	21–30	31–40	41–50	51–60	61–70	71–80
Males	1	8	8	12	10	3	1
Females	3	4	3	12	15	9	1

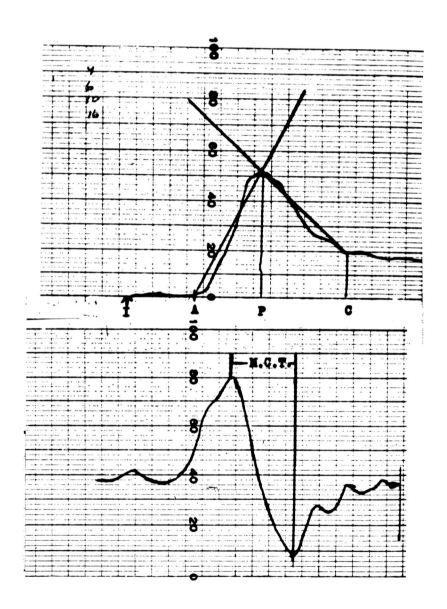

is injected to an anticubital vein. After passage through heart and lungs, the radioactive stream, about 14 sec long, arrives in the head, and its first passage from carotid to jugular vessels is monitored by a collimated sodium iodide crystal placed on the inion and directed at a point 2.5 cm above the nasion. Gamma impulses are received, amplified and passed to a graph recorder moving at 15 cm/min. A primary curve is thus obtained (Fig. 1). The points marked are: A (first appearance in the head) and C (clearance or return to the recirculation base-line). The AC interval is the total transit time (TT) of the injected 2 ml bolus. Below, the first derivative of the curve is simultaneously recorded. This is a rate of change curve, and the distance between the two peaks is the mean circulation time (MCT). This is the most important parameter measured. It is closely related reciprocally to the total cerebral blood flow. In this study we are only concerned with total transit time (TT) and mean circulation time (MCT).

RESULTS

All patients but 10 had conventional angiograms, and all had circulation studies. In considering the relationship of spasm and circulation times to operative morbidity and mortality, two groups — 49 without spasm seen angiographically, and 31 with spasm — have been considered separately. Mean values for 50 normals reported elsewhere are: TT = 18 sec ± 1, MCT = 8 sec ± 1.

Circulation Times and Angiographic Spasm

Table II compares the circulation times of all patients with and all patients without

TABLE II

ANGIOGRAPHIC SPASM AND CIRCULATION TIMES
(Showing mean difference in circulation times between groups with and without spasm seen on angiograms)

	No.	TT	MCT
Without spasm	49	18.53	8.95
With spasm	31	23.16	11.58
No angiogram	10	25.10	11.80
Difference between		4.63	2.63
spasm and no spasm		(25%)	(29%)

spasm. The mean difference in TT is 4.63 sec or 25 per cent. The mean difference in MCT is 2.63 sec or 29 per cent. The mean times for the 49 no-spasm patients lie in the normal range TT 18.5, MCT 8.9. Note also that the patients deemed too ill or too neurologically damaged to have angiograms had circulation times even higher than the group with angiographic spasm.

Circulation Times and Post-operative Complications

Table III deals with 37 patients operated on. Of 13 without spasm, five or 21.7 per

TABLE III

POST-OPERATIVE COMPLICATIONS

(Comparing incidence of post-operative complications with circulation times in 37 patients undergoing surgery)

	Total	Good Result			Complications			Percentage Complicated
		No.	TT	MCT	No.	TT	MCT	
No spasm	23	18	18.33	8.88	5	18.40	9.20	21.7%
With spasm	14	4	21.75	11.00	10	23.20	11.40	71.4%

cent, had some complication: slow return to consciousness, neurological signs not present before operation, respiratory difficulties, transient hypertension, hemiparesis, etc. Of the 14 with spasm, 10 or 71.4 per cent, had some post-operative complication.

There is no significant difference in the circulation times of the complicated and uncomplicated groups, but the same differences as before between the spasm and no-spasm groups.

Circulation Times and Final Results

Results have been divided into four groups: I = completely recovered, II = slightly

TABLE IV

FINAL RESULTS

Group	Without Spasm			With Spasm			Totals
	No.	TT	MCT	No.	TT	MCT	
I	36	18.47	8.80	12	21.83	10.41	48
II	6	18.46	8.83	10	23.60	11.60	16
III	2	18.50	8.00	3	23.00	12.66	5
IV	5	19.00	10.60	6	25.16	13.33	11

I. Recovered; II. Slightly disabled; III. Severely disabled; IV. Died.

disabled, III = severely disabled, IV = died (Table IV). In Group I, 36 of 48 had no spasm and circulation times in the normal range; in groups II, III and IV there are more showing spasm than not. This time, however, there is a steadily rising circulation time, both TT and MCT, from groups I to IV in the spasm group. In other words, the outlook of the individual patient with spasm is better the shorter his circulation time.

DISCUSSION

What emerges from these figures is already known — that it is a bad thing for the patient to have angiographically demonstrable spasm. Equally clearly and not previously described — angiographic spasm is very closely reflected in increased circulation times and increased circulation time itself carries a steadily and proportionately worse prognosis. As estimation of circulation time is simple, safe and repeatable, we have here a paraclinical method which is of great potential help in the handling of patients and the reduction of risk. It is not safe to omit angiography in the early stages because a patient may have a prolonged circulation time from the presence of a surgically removable clot. But, once angiography has been done and the presence of spasm and an increased circulation time established, no further angiography or operation should be considered until the circulation times approach normal for that patient's age.

Two case reports will illustrate in what spheres this information can be useful:

Case 1

A 38 year old man with coarctation of the aorta had a subarachnoid haemorrhage, remained well for a week, then became confused, intermittently unconscious and had increased neck stiffness. Repeated lumbar puncture did not show fresh bleeding, but angiograms showed spasm of both internal carotid arteries and a large basilar aneurysm. Circulation times at that time were: TT–27 sec, MCT–13 sec. He was observed for three weeks, by which time TT was 20 sec, and MCT 10 sec. The larger of the two vertebral arteries was then clipped. Operation was uncomplicated and he remains at full work three years later. We do not consider that he would have tolerated vertebral occlusion in the earlier stages.

Case 2

A 50 year old man bled from a right posterior communicating aneurysm. Three weeks later angiography showed no spasm but the circulation times were: TT–24 sec, MCT–12 sec. In spite of this, right common carotid ligation was done uneventfully. Four years later he has a clumsy "parietal" L. hand with astereognosis. He would appear to be developing a softening at the boundary zone of his R. middle and posterior cerebral territories. Angiography shows no demonstrable coincident lesion such as a tumour.

In a patient without spasm, who had these circulation times, we would now consider it safer to attack such an aneurysm directly, rather than deprive the patient of 25 per cent of his cerebral circulatory reserves.

Our general conclusions from the study described here are that the observation of circulation times is a guide, in particular, to the probable existence of arterial spasm following subarachnoid haemorrhage. Serial observations help the surgeon to decide when it is safest to operate, and tell him post-operatively what effect his direct attack on the aneurysm or proximal artery ligation has had on the cerebral blood flow.

Added to observations already available, this should help to reduce morbidity and mortality in the treatment of subarachnoid haemorrhage.

SUMMARY

Cerebral circulation studies, using a simple isotope method, were carried out on 90 patients following subarachnoid haemorrhage; 80 also had angiographic studies.

References p. 294

It was found that an increase in circulation time was closely related to the occurrence of arterial spasm, and also to the post-operative morbidity and mortality. Serial observations were particularly helpful in indicating the best time for operative intervention.

Two illustrative case reports are quoted showing where cerebral circulation studies have reinforced clinical judgement.

REFERENCES

BUCKALL, M., (1967); *Biochemical aspects of ruptured aneurysms*. Meeting of Society of British Neurological Surgeons.

CONNOLLY, R. C., (1962); Cerebral ischaemia in spontaneous subarachnoid haemorrhage. *Ann. Roy. Coll. Surg. (Eng.)*, **30**, 102.

FROMAN, C., AND SMITH, A. C., (1967); Metabolic acidosis of the cerebrospinal fluid associated with subarachnoid haemorrhage. *Lancet*, **i**, 965.

KAGSTROM, E., GREITZ, T., HANSON, J., AND GALERA, R., (1965); Changes in the cerebral blood flow after subarachnoid haemorrhage. *Excerpta Medica, International Congress Series, No.* **110**, 629.

MCKISSOCK, W., RICHARDSON, A., AND WALSHE, L., (1965); Anterior communicating aneurysms. *Lancet*, **i**, 873.

OLDENDORF, W. H., (1962); Measurement of the mean transit time of cerebral circulation by external direction of an intravenously injected radioisotope. *J. Nucl. Med.*, **3**, 382.

TAYLOR, A. R., AND BELL, T. K., (1966); Slowing of cerebral circulation after concussional head injury, *Lancet*, **ii**, 178.

Aneurysm of the Anterior Communicating Artery

G. NORLÉN

Göteborg (Sweden)

In the foreword to the presentation of the papers from the first meeting of the European Neurosurgical Societies in Zürich, 1959, Krayenbühl wrote: "il n'y a pas de doute que le point noir dans le lot des anévrysmes supraclinoïdiens rompus est le groupe des anévrysmes de la communicante antérieure." Important papers appeared at that meeting and during the past years up to now valuable contributions have been published, influencing our attitude to different problems in connection with aneurysms of this location, but we must admit that many "points noirs" still exist in our knowledge of the behaviour of these lesions and of the best method of treatment. My paper will be limited to a few questions in connection with a presentation of our material and the surgical methods used.

We have accepted the view that surgery is always indicated in cases of a ruptured aneurysm, and it is our task to demonstrate when and under which circumstances surgery can be performed with a minimum of risks. Certain contra-indications do exist and these must be established. The methods used must also be reliable, which means that the risk of a recurrent bleeding must be eliminated.

We all know that in many cases the bleeding from a ruptured aneurysm is of such a degree and so severe that the patient is beyond any kind of useful therapy. However, in most cases the clinical picture indicates therapeutic steps to be taken, the purpose of which might be to eliminate a life-threatening intracranial hypertension or to evacuate a local expanding intracerebral haemorrhage and to eliminate the source of bleeding in order to prevent a recurrent bleeding.

All of us are aware of the potentially increased risks when these patients are operated upon very early after the bleeding. The problem of spasm is still unsolved both concerning its patho-physiology and its treatment. The high frequency of recurrent bleedings and mortality during the first weeks are also well known, and these problems make it difficult to compare the results of treatment from different clinics as the selection of cases might be different. We all agree that the material must be divided in different risk groups, not only based on the clinical condition of the patient but also on the time factor, *i.e.* the time between the bleeding and the operation, in order to evaluate as correct as possible the result of the therapeutic methods. However, in this respect there is no generally accepted uniform classification, which increases the difficulties in the discussion.

However, these are problems which are common to ruptured aneurysms of any location and in this connection only a few questions will be mentioned, which are special for aneurysm of the anterior communicating artery.

In 1953 we drew attention to the different patterns of circulation through the anterior part of the circle of Willis in these cases and its importance for the discussion of different surgical procedures. At that time the angiography with contralateral compression of the carotid artery was perhaps not systematically performed in all cases to give a true picture of the frequency of these different patterns, why it might be of some interest to have this question illustrated in our present material (Table I).

TABLE I

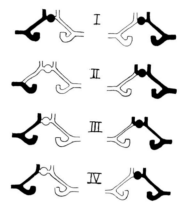

I.	Aneurysm filled from both sides. One or both pericallosal arteries visualized at the same time	40
II.	Aneurysm and both pericallosal arteries filled only from one side. Ant. cerebral artery not visualized from the other side	13
III.	Aneurysm and both pericallosal arteries filled from only one side. Ant. cerebral artery and homolateral pericallosal artery visualized from the other side	18
IV.	Aneurysm and homolateral pericallosal artery only filled from one side. Ant. cerebral artery and pericallosal artery visualized from the other side	7
		78

As expected you can see that the frequency of bilateral visualization of the aneurysms in this material is higher, no doubt depending on a more adequate compression. Some factors influencing the appearance of these different patterns have been discussed by Lepoire, Dilange, David and others. Spasm, the presence of a haematoma, direction and precise origin of the aneurysms, etc., have been discussed in this connection.

At the moment there are only two surgical methods considered by us as adequate, *i.e.* methods which definitely eliminate the risk of a recurrent bleeding, and those are ligating or clipping the stalk of the aneurysms and trapping, which in these aneurysms means ligating the anterior communicating artery on both sides of the stalk or excluding the circulation through this artery by one ligature, which includes the stalk and the artery. Our attitude has been to try to ligate or clip the stalk in all cases, but considering the delicate location of these lesions several aneurysms have been trapped in order to avoid a prolonged and troublesome dissection of the stalk, which might cause untoward side-effects from the procedure. This depends, of course, on the judgement of the technical possibilities at the operation. The exact knowledge of the circulatory pattern is therefore of paramount importance. In cases of type 2, proximal clipping of the anterior cerebral artery, and trapping might carry a considerable risk. In cases of type 4, trapping can be performed without any angiographically demonstrable impairment of the blood flow to the two hemispheres, as already in the preoperative angiogram the anterior communicating artery did not permit a collateral blood flow. However, the compression test might have been inadequate and trapping might interrupt small vessels, which have their origin from the anterior communicating artery itself, and are of clinical importance. In one of our cases, which was trapped, a moderate diabetes insipidus developed on the fourth postoperative day and in another case a permanent hypothermia occurred in connection with electrolyte disturbances.

Table II presents the risk groups that we have used. In the discussion we have to

TABLE II

RISK GROUPS

A.	Patients admitted or operated upon in deep coma.
B.	Patients admitted or operated upon within 3 weeks after their last bleeding, partly or completely recovered from effects of their bleeding.
C.	Patients admitted or operated upon more than 3 weeks but within 8 weeks after their last bleeding.
D.	Patients admitted or operated upon more than 8 weeks after their last bleeding.

consider not only the patient as a surgical risk but also the patient as running the risk of a recurrent bleeding. These two questions are difficult to separate in evaluating our therapeutic possibilities and steps. A revision of our classification will perhaps be necessary when the different groups are big enough to permit reliable conclusions when the cases are analysed concerning the different factors, which might influence mortality and morbidity. There is a tendency in our material that the surgical risks are diminished after the first week and that it is just during this week that unexpected complications might occur, during or after the operation, in most cases related to spasm. This has recently caused us to introduce a new approach in this stage. The patients are given epsilon-aminocaproic acid in order to increase the development of a clot or thrombosis at the point of rupture in order to diminish the risk of a recurrent bleeding. The operation is postponed about a week and until the general condition of the patient has improved. Fig. 1 demonstrates such a clot at the point of rupture of an aneurysm operated 5 days after the bleeding.

In Table III our material is presented according to the different therapeutic procedures used. As can be seen adequate procedures have been possible in 90% of the cases and in 60% stalk ligature was performed.

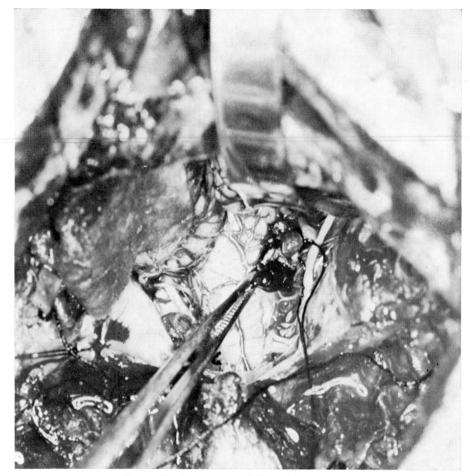

Fig. 1. Blood clot removed from the aneurysm.

TABLE III

ANEURYSMS OF THE ANTERIOR COMMUNICATING ARTERY 1953-1966 (105 CASES)

	A	B	CD	Total
Stalk ligature	3	19	33	55(60%)
Trapping	—	7	21	28
Adequate procedures	3	26	54	83(90%)
Stalk ligature not successful	1	1	—	2
Exploration	—	—	1	1
Wrapping	—	—	6	6
Shunt operation	—	—	1	1
Inadequate procedures	1	1	8	10
No operative treatment	8	1	3	12
Total	12	28	65	105

TABLE IV

ANEURYSMS OF THE ANTERIOR COMMUNICATING ARTERY 1953–1966. (REASON FOR NO OPERATION; 12 CASES)

	No.	Risk group
Angiography not quite convincing	1	B
Pronounced brain atrophia, severe mental deterioration, hemiplegia	3	D
Deep coma moribund	8	A

TABLE V

ANEURYSMS OF THE ANTERIOR COMMUNICATING ARTERY 1953–1966. (OPERATIVE RESULTS; 93 CASES)

	A	B	C	D	Total
Operative mortality	2	2	1		5
Total disability					
from preop. damage		2	1	2	5
„ op. „	1		3	2	6
„ other causes				1	1
Partial disability					
from preop. damage		2	1	2	5
„ op. „		3	7		10
„ other causes					
Full working capacity	1	18	24	18	61
Total	4	27	37	25	93

62

Table IV demonstrates the reason why surgery was not performed in some of our cases.

In Table V our results are presented. As can be seen, 10 of these cases presented already preoperatively a total or partial disability and in one case total disability at the follow-up was a consequence of other causes. This means that full working capacity has been achieved in 74 %. The operative mortality in those cases, operated more than 3 weeks after the bleeding, is only 1.6 %, whereas in group B the operative mortality is 7.4 %. In Table VI the causes of death are presented.

The clinical picture, causing the morbidity in these lesions, presents certain characteristics which are of great interest. In one of our papers from 1953 we observed a few cases which apparently developed a Korsakoff's syndrome after the operation. A methodical psychiatric study was started to analyse the amnestic syndrome in these patients, but for various reasons it could not be concluded. During the last few years, however, it has again been possible for us to attack this problem. We have analysed 33 cases with careful psychological tests preoperatively and at repeated intervals postoperatively. Memory changes as described in Korsakoff's syndrome were seen in

TABLE VI

ANEURYSMS OF THE ANTERIOR COMMUNICATING ARTERY 1953–1964. (CAUSES OF DEATH; 5 CASES)

	Risk group	No.
Operated upon in coma Massive intracerebral haemorrhages	A	2
Prolonged hypertension Multiple intracerebral malacias	B	1
Circulatory insufficiency. Operated upon in hypothermia	B	1
Pulmonary embolism 11 days after successful operative procedure	C	1

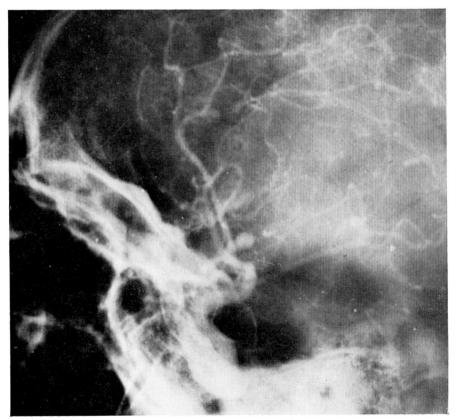

Fig. 2. Aneurysm directed posteriorly.

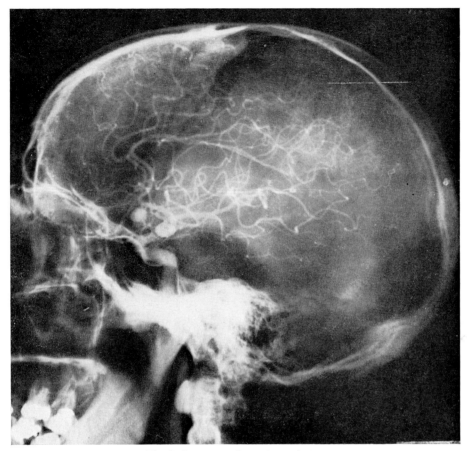

Fig. 3. Aneurysm directed anteriorly.

17 of these cases, but in most of them these troubles disappeared in relatively short time. They might therefore be overlooked if not a careful psychological test is performed early after the operation. However, in 5 cases it became more or less permanent and complicated with a state of confusion as in a true Korsakoff's syndrome.

The appearance of this syndrome is of course a very important complication and we are interested to know, which anatomical structure, the damage of which is responsible for the appearance of this syndrome, and we think that the septal area is the region in question.

We also want to know if this amnestic syndrome appears only under certain anatomical conditions such as anomalies of the circle of Willis, location and size of the aneurysm.

It is also important to know if these syndromes are of such a degree that our indication for surgery will be influenced, and if it is possible to avoid these complications by changing our operative technique.

The precise location of the anterior communicating artery might vary and in some cases it is located more posteriorly than in others. The aneurysm itself might also vary in its direction which is also well known. In some cases it is directed posteriorly (Fig. 2) from the anterior communicating artery and in others anteriorly (Fig. 3). In our material it was a definite predominance for the Korsakoff's syndrome to appear, when the aneurysm was directed posteriorly.

No doubt a Korsakoff's syndrome was also more frequently observed after trapping than after stalk ligature, but as this method was used in those cases, where the anatomy was more complicated and the operative procedure more difficult, it is not quite sure that the method per se is responsible. This question requires more study.

We have not been able to show, that resection of the tip of the frontal lobe increases the occurrence of a postoperative Korsakoff's syndrome and this is in accordance with the experiences of Laine, presented in 1957.

In these series of 93 operated cases of aneurysm of the anterior communicating artery direct intracranial approach was used. Adequate procedures were achieved in 90% of the cases and stalk ligature with preserved circulation through the anterior communicating artery in 60%.

Our experience might justify the conclusion that the operative mortality in patients operated upon more than 3 weeks after the bleeding is low enough to balance the expected mortality from new bleedings if these patients are left alone.

During the first 3 weeks after the bleeding the operative mortality is also comparatively low, if not the patient is operated upon in coma.

The patho-physiology of many factors influencing the operative risk is still unknown and if a pronounced spasm is present, this no doubt carries a considerable risk.

In aneurysm of this location the surgical procedure carries a certain risk concerning morbidity and memory changes might occur. This risk is increased if the aneurysm is directed posteriorly.

Surgical Treatment of Aneurysms of the Anterior Communicating Artery

BENIAMINO GUIDETTI

Department of Neurosurgery, University of Rome
Medical School, Rome (Italy)

The purpose of this report is to present results obtained by the Division of Neurological Surgery at the University of Rome with surgical treatment of aneurysms involving the anterior communicating artery.

The investigation includes 45 consecutive patients operated upon prior to December 1965. In this series are not included a few patients with multiple aneurysms.

The patients in this series were admitted after intervals varying from hours to weeks following an initial hemorrhage or following a recurrent hemorrhage. One patient had 4 attacks of bleeding before operation, two had 3 attacks, 10 had 2 and 32 had just one.

The total number of cases comprised 18 females and 27 males. The ages of the patients ranged from 20 to 64 (patients over 65 were refused operation).

In order to evaluate the operative results, the classification of the present material has been divided into four risk groups, as follows:

Group A: Patients in coma on admission, moribund or approaching that state (4 cases).

Group B: Patients deeply stuporous on admission with eventual major neurologic deficit (5 cases).

Group C: Patients drowsy or confused without significant impairment of brain function (20 cases).

Group D: Patient alert and cooperative with or without signs of blood in subarachnoid space (16 cases).

Bilateral angiographic studies with appropriate compression of the opposite carotid artery in order to demonstrate the cross circulation between the hemispheres were made of all patients. The conventional lateral and anteroposterior views were often supplemented by oblique views. The exact knowledge of the cross circulation between the two halves of the circle of Willis is especially important if an uncontrollable hemorrhage from rupture at operation occurs and trapping contemplated.

In our series of patients it was our general policy to obtain angiographic studies as soon as possible provided the patient was young and in a reasonably good condition. This means bilateral angiographic studies on the day of admission in groups C and D, and delayed angiography in groups A and B and in old patients, except

TABLE I

OPERATIVE RESULTS IN TERMS OF MORTALITY ACCORDING TO THE TYPE OF SURGICAL PRO-
CEDURE EMPLOYED AND THE CLINICAL STATUS AT THE TIME OF THE OPERATION

Pre-operative risk	Total number of cases	Wrapping, number of cases/deaths		Trapping, number of cases/deaths		Neck lig., number of cases/deaths	
A	4	1	1	—	—	3	2
B	5	—	—	3	1	2	1
C	20	1	—	10	2	9	—
D	16	1	—	3	—	12	—
Total	45	3	1	16	3	26	3

TABLE II

OPERATIVE RESULTS IN TERMS OF MORTALITY ACCORDING TO THE CLINICAL STATUS AND
TIME INTERVALS FOLLOWING THE LAST HEMORRHAGE

Pre-operative risk	Time after the last hemorrhage					
	0–7 days		8–21 days		over 8–21 days	
	Cases/Deaths		Cases/Deaths		Cases/Deaths	
A	4	3	—	—	—	—
B	3	2	2	—	—	—
C	6	1	10	1	4	—
D	3	—	5	—	8	—
Total	16	6	17	1	12	—

TABLE III

RESULTS FOLLOWING SURGICAL TREATMENT – RISK GROUPS C AND D (36 CASES)

	Wrapping	Trapping	Neck Lig.	Total
Operative and late mortality	—	2	—	2
Full working capacity	2	6	17	25
Impaired working capacity:				
(a) from preoperative damage	—	2	3	5
(b) from operative damage	—	3	1	4
Total cases	2	13	21	36

if there is a suspicion of a massive intracerebral hemorrhage. In this last group the angiographic studies were delayed several days until the vital signs became stabilized and the state of consciousness improved. The same attitude was adopted for the patients with severe widespread vasospasm on carotid angiography.

In our series of 45 patients operated upon, in only 8 cases was the aneurysm filled from both sides. In 21 cases there was angiographic evidence of a more or less severe vasospasm. Intracerebral hematoma was observed in 6 patients.

Tables I, II and III give the operative results in terms of mortality and morbidity according to the type of procedure employed, the patients' clinical status and the time interval following the last hemorrhage and operation.

DISCUSSION

Many important factors, such as the timing and technique of operation, influence the success or failure of surgery on ruptured aneurysms of the anterior communicating artery. Some of these factors will be commented on in accordance with our experience and reports from literature.

Timing of operation

The primary object in the treatment of patients with ruptured aneurysms is the prevention of recurrent bleeding and the evacuation of a large hematoma if present. The selection of the best timing for the operation depends on the surgeon's estimate of the relative hazards of early intervention versus the risk of further bleeding. In determining the timing for surgery we consider the condition of the patient more important than the interval from the last hemorrhage. So if the patients are young and in good condition (groups C and D) we proceed with the operation as soon as possible and not later than the end of the first week after the bleeding. We believe that, for this group of patients, a delay of the operation for more than a week, as suggested by some, may lead to a fatal recurrent hemorrhage and that the mortality from recurrent hemorrhage might be greater than the loss of patients from increased operative mortality (the incidence of renewed bleeding rises sharply in the second week in every series).

The time interval between the last hemorrhage, the clinical status and operation is indicated in Tables I and II.

If a patient's condition does not show signs of recovery within a reasonable interval after the bleeding, or there is angiographic evidence of severe vasospasm, surgical treatment should be postponed until the patient seems in reasonably good condition and vasospasm is reduced.

Operation is not indicated for very sick patients, except if there is a massive intracerebral hematoma. Of our 4 patients operated upon in coma (group A), 3 died following surgery and the other one became a permanent invalid. Of the 5 patients in the risk group B, 2 died following the operation. Of the 36 patients in risk groups C and D, only two died after the operation. Table III shows the residual disability after the operation.

Hypothermia

Twenty-four patients in risk groups A, B and C, and four in risk group D were operated upon in moderate hypothermia (the temperature was usually close to 28°C).

The use of temporary precautionary intracranial clips on both anterior cerebral arteries has not been a routine practice with our patients. We used the temporary clips in only ten cases, in 4 before and in 6 after an accidental rupture of the aneurysm (both anterior cerebral arteries were clipped continuously for over 10 minutes).

We believe that direct attack upon an intracranial aneurysm has been made safer by the use of hypothermia and intracranial temporary clips. We also believe that hypothermia is particularly indicated in the patients who undergo surgical procedures in the acute phase and in the patients in which a stalk ligature would seem, from angiographic studies, not easy to accomplish. In this last group of patients the temporary clips on both anterior cerebral arteries would enable a careful, unhurried dissection on the neck of the aneurysm and would facilitate the application of a clip or ligature across it.

Operative exposure

In 14 patients an osteoplastic unilateral right craniotomy was performed. In 8 of these cases it was necessary to resect the frontal lobe tip in order to explore the aneurysm. In 31 patients a bifrontal craniotomy flap was turned. This ample operative exposure offers, in our opinion, better access to the anterior communicating artery without sacrificing the tip of the frontal lobe.

Reduction of Brain Volume

The access to the aneurysm was facilitated by intravenous Mannitol or oral or intravenous Glycerol. In a few cases spinal drainage helped to obtain an excellent exposure.

Controlled Hypotension

In 9 patients the blood pressure was lowered with "Arfonad" at the time of exposure of the aneurysm (the systolic pressure was lowered to approximately 60 mm Hg).

Hypotension, by reducing the pressure in the aneurysm's sac, permits a better exposure of the neck and its closure. It is contraindicated if a trapping is contemplated.

Intentional rupture of aneurysm

We have used opening of the aneurysm in 10 patients. In these cases the aneurysm was deliberately opened and the blood and the collapsed sac held in the suction tip until a correct dissection was accomplished. A silver clip or ligature was afterwards placed at its neck.

After this experience, some of the indications for proceeding to the opening of an aneurysm deliberately are in our opinion: (1) a sac so large that it cannot safely be retracted to afford a proper view of its neck, (2) a broad base to the aneurysm.

Neck ligature

In 26 patients direct ligation of the neck of the aneurysm by a clip (2 cases), or silk or linen thread, was performed. In 13 cases a control puncture of the aneurysm's sac with a fine needle was advisable. Tables I, II and III show the immediate and late results in this series of cases. A postoperative angiogram was performed in 20 cases and revealed that the aneurysm was completely eliminated. Not one of these patients suffered from later recurrent hemorrhages.

Our experience lends support to the opinion that stalk ligature is at present the ideal method for intracranial saccular aneurysm because it reduces the risk of recurrent bleeding without eliminating the circulation through the anterior communicating artery.

When this technique was not possible, one of several alternative procedures was employed.

Muscle Wrapping

Wrapping of the aneurysm with muscle (1 case), or Eastman 910 and fascia temporalis (2 cases), was done in 3 patients. As seen in Table I, one patient (risk group A) expired. Two other patients are still living and well, three and four years respectively after the operation.

This method was used in the cases where neck ligature was considered dangerous and a trapping not advisable.

Trapping

This method was carried out by us in 16 cases when stalk ligature could not be accomplished.

In 13 patients we ligated the anterior communicating artery on both sides of the aneurysmal neck or the aneurysm stalk along with the anterior communicating artery. In four of these cases a partial occlusion of one of the anterior cerebral arteries was done. Tables I, II and III show the operative results and mortality and morbidity in this series of thirteen cases.

In three patients the neck of the aneurysm and one anterior cerebral artery were occluded. Two of these patients died (groups B and C).

Our experience leads us to the conclusion that ligature of the communicating anterior artery on both sides of the neck of the aneurysm, when this appears feasible, can be done safely if there are no abnormalities of the circle of Willis. Also a partial occlusion of one of the anterior cerebral arteries can be done without damage if the blood pressure is normal.

In cases of trapping, the use of hypothermia during and in the postoperative period is advisable.

Aneurysms of Carotid and Posterior Communicating Artery

ZDENĚK KUNC

Neurosurgical Clinic, Prague (Czechoslovakia)

Surgery of carotid saccular aneurysms is the oldest form of brain vascular surgery. Nevertheless, opinions are still different and sometimes contradictory on even some basic problems. The topic is extensive, and therefore only some important questions can be discussed here.

At the Neurosurgical Clinic in Prague, 159 patients with saccular aneurysms of different localizations, 69 (43.39%) of whom with carotid aneurysms, have been surgically treated till this time.

In 62 cases (89.85%), aneurysms arose at the intradural course of the carotid artery, most frequently, in 49 cases (71%), at or near the junction of the carotid artery with the posterior communicating artery. A particular type was junctional dilatation of the posterior communicating artery which, though it was not considered a real aneurysm, could bleed, as was the case in 2 patients. Other localizations were less frequent: 4 at the bifurcation of the carotid artery, 4 at the origin of the ophthalmic artery, 2 at the medial and 2 at the external carotid wall, and in 1 case there were 3 aneurysms on the same carotid artery. Extradural localizations were found in 7 cases.

In 2 cases, bilateral aneurysms were found. The incidence is actually higher, for total angiography was not routinely performed in the past, as it is done, on principle, at present.

The danger of rupture of carotid aneurysms is high. In our cases, bleeding occurred in 92.75%, and in 53.62% twice or many times. The size of the ruptured aneurysms in patients under 50 years was seldom larger then $\frac{1}{2}$ to 1 cm, in older patients it was larger. It would, however, be incorrect to assume that aneurysms start bleeding only when they have become large. According to the Institute of Legal Medicine in Prague, fatal hemorrhage was caused in 75.5% of cases by aneurysms of 1–5 mm, and in 55.6% of cases by 1–3 mm large aneurysms. The most common and first focal symptom was oculomotor palsy, in 46.37% of patients.

Visual fields defects (11.59%) were conditioned by aneurysms filling the whole parasellar space, or arising at the medial carotid wall or at the ophthalmic artery. Choked discs (15.94%), hemiparesis to hemiplegia, temporary (50%) or permanent (21.73%), and aphasia (10.13%) were more often manifestations of widespread vasospasms than of a blood clot, which was found only in 7.24%. In all these cases different psychological changes were present.

The results of surgical treatment depend on many factors. The most important is the

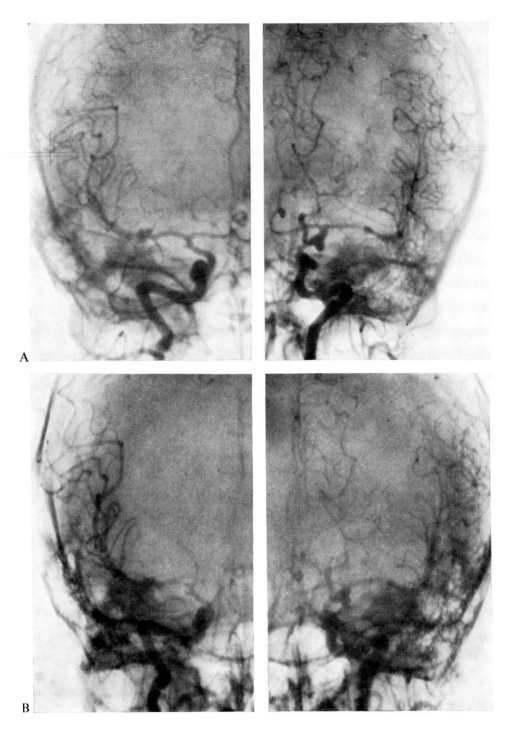

Fig. 1. A, bilateral angiogram after bleeding. B, widespread spasms 4 weeks later; angiography under hypothermia.

state of the patient following bleeding. In patients whose condition improves rapidly, good results can be achieved by acute as well as by delayed surgery. In 59 patients (85.5%) surgery was carried out 2–3 weeks or still later following bleeding. Earlier operation could become dangerous owing to peroperational rupture.

Coma or hemiplegia with psychological changes are a poor condition for any surgical procedure. The state is qualified by the degree of hemorrhage and the extent of vasospasm. To stop grave bleeding in time is difficult, as the carotid artery bleeds directly. If a poor state is caused by widespread vasospasm, the situation is not much better. All the methods used until now against vasospasm have been actually ineffective. Even the promising hypothermia brought disappointment, for rather than averting or suppressing cerebral vasospasms, it incites them. This maybe well demonstrated on the patient with 5 aneurysms, in whom a vasospasm fluctuated for a very long time (Fig. 1). Control angiogram 4 weeks after bleeding, performed under general anesthesia and hypothermia of 28° aggravated the vasospasm, which spread vehemently over both carotid systems. The patient became hemiplegic and disoriented. The same is our experience with hypotensive therapy.

Any surgical procedure will deteriorate the vasospasm, as the carotid artery is the most susceptible vessel to irritative impulses. Not only will neurological defects aggravate or become permanent, but the patient's life will be seriously threatened. Therefore, it is never advisable to operate a patient with carotid aneurysm while he is in a poor state. This is apparent from Tables I and II.

TABLE I

Working capacity	Invalidity	Mortality	Total
Cat. A* 2 = 20%	2 = 20%	6 = 60%	10
Cat. B** 43 = 72.88%	9 = 15.26%	7 = 11.86%	59

* Patients in coma or with major neurological disability.
** Patients in good condition.

The differences between the two groups are significant. In the first group the operation was carried out in 7 patients within the first days and 5 of them died, and in the second group 2–3 weeks or still later following bleeding.

TABLE II

CAUSES OF DEATH

Category A		Category B	
Hemorrhage	4	Brain infarction	2
Brain infarction	2	Postoperational rupture of aneurysm	1
		Arfonad circulatory stop	1
		Embolia	2
		Pneumonia	1
Total	6	Total	7

The survey of the causes of death merely emphasizes the difference between the two groups.

The influence of age on surgical results is shown in Table III.

TABLE III
AGE AND SURGICAL RESULTS
CATEGORY B

Age ys.	Working capacity	Invalidity	Mortality	Total
—50	26 = 89.65%	2 = 6.9%	1 = 3.45%	29
50+	17 = 56.7%	7 = 23.3%	6 = 20%	30
	Arterial hypertension		*Arteriosclerotic carotid artery*	
—50	37.9%		10%	
50+	43.33%		50%	

The difference between the results in the groups of patients under and over 50 years was very significant. Not alone age, but the extent of arteriosclerosis of the carotid artery makes conditions for surgical intervention unfavourable. It is necessary to obtain as much information as possible about arteriosclerotic changes. For the moment, the possibilities are unsatisfactory. Even proved arteriosclerosis, however, may merely suggest the adoption of cautious and rather conservative course in any type of surgery, but the likelihood of further bleeding must be decisive.

Should a carotid aneurysm revealed by chance be operated?

Some aneurysms have never bled. They may remain without symptoms. Some of them reach an extremely large size and ultimately manifest themselves as an intracranial tumor, mostly a pituitary adenoma. Little is known about the development and features of this type of aneurysms. A systematic study may be probably useful for a better selection of patients for conservative or surgical therapy respectively. The problem of preventive operation remains open. Surgery may be considered only if it is guaranteed to be safe. This is not so at present. The choice between extracranial and intracranial surgery is documented in Table IV.

TABLE IV

CATEGORY B

	Working capacity	Invalidity	Mortality	Total
Extracranial carotid occlusion	16 = 72.72%	4 = 18.18%	2 = 9.07%	22
Intracranial procedures	27 = 72.98%	5 = 13.51%	5 = 13.51%	37

Invalidity and working capacity are proportionately higher in the first group, but mortality, on the contrary, is lower. For closer estimation of the course of carotid occlusion, 18 cases have been followed up at intervals from 2 months to 9 years after operation, by carotid angiography of the non-operated side and by vertebral angiography. Only 6 aneurysms were found to be obliterated, 2 diminished, and 10 persisted unchanged, 3 bled again, 2 of whom died. Besides this, in 3, new contralateral aneurysms were revealed. They might have arisen due to developmental defects in media, under the influence of an increased bloodstream.

The aneurysms usually filled through the vertebral system, the bloodstream of which increased with the dilatation of the system and the enlarging of collaterals between the external carotid and vertebral artery (Fig. 2). This supports the prevailing opinion

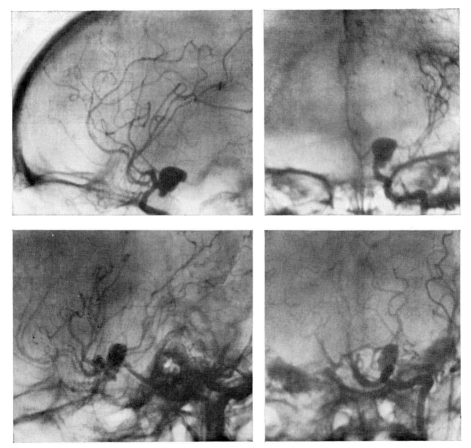

Fig. 2. Angiograms prior to operation and after common carotid occlusion. The aneurysm is filled through the vertebral system.

on the desirability of a direct surgical attack on the aneurysm. It is absurd to sacrifice the main brain vessel if there is no certainty that the aneurysm will be obliterated. Carotid occlusion is not without risk as neither the testing of collateral circulation, nor gradual occlusion can entirely prevent cerebral infarction. The procedure has no advantage for the treatment of arteriosclerotics either. A new aneurysm can arise on the contralateral side, furthermore the procedure constitutes a handicap for the event of arteriosclerotic insufficiency of the remaining carotid artery. There are few aneurysms completely inoperable by any direct method, so that carotid occlusion must be taken into account.

Direct operation on the aneurysm is, at the present time, considered feasible in the majority of cases. A small temporal craniotomy, urea, and dissection of the lower part of the Sylvian fissure provide sufficient approach. Aneurysms most frequently arise at the posterior carotid wall with their periphery hidden under the plica petro-clinoidea lateralis, often compressing the oculomotor nerve. Dissection should be limited to the neck of the aneurysm.

Temporary clamps are not free from irritative effects, and are not suitable for the arteriosclerotic carotid artery. If the space is filled by the aneurysm, they can impede rather than facilitate the operation.

The posterior communicating artery often fuses with the neck of the aneurysm, sometimes it is hypoplastic or absent, so that it is replaced by the aneurysm. The artery can usually be closed together with the aneurysm. The hypothalamic, subthalamic and thalamic nuclei are also supplied from the vertebral artery. Occlusion would be fatal only if the artery substituted the posterior cerebral artery, or if the anterior chorioidal artery was its branch.

Intracranial treatment was carried out in 45 cases; 33 clippings, 4 ligatures, 1 muscle wrapping, 4 cotton-wool wrappings, 1 Eastman coating, and 2 explorations.

In 8 of our cases, surgery was terminated with extracranial carotid occlusion, which became the definite therapy. It was carried out either for peroperational complications or for greater radicality.

Clipping was preferred, as it is less likely to incite a vasospasm than ligature; it does not reduce the diameter of the carotid artery when the aneurysmal neck is too large; besides it is simpler, but requires perfect forceps and clips. Arteriosclerotic changes or pouches arising close to the origin of the aneurysm should be carefully observed, as the neck can be easily ruptured. A tear spreading in the carotid wall may become extremely dangerous. In 2 cases, an unusual carotid injury developed in arteriosclerotic vessels. A tear at the entrance of the carotid artery into the intradural space, far from the site of the aneurysm, occurred during the clipping of a very large neck, probably due to traction. The breach gradually enlarged so that the vessel was completely broken. The only solution was to plug its lumen with a tampon and clip off the ophthalmic artery. Also a spontaneous rupture of a thin pouch, and so of the carotid artery itself, occurred during the exposure.

Such events should not be treated hastily by intracranial carotid occlusion, as the results are very bad. From 7 patients, 5 died and 2 became hemiplegic.

The treatment of aneurysms at the medial carotid wall and of ophthalmic aneurysms may be technically difficult. Their operability depends on the site and size of the aneurysm.

In aneurysms at the bifurcation, both branches may sometimes originate from the sac so that only its diminution by ligature is possible.

A difficult problem present giant aneurysms, not rare on the carotid artery. They are operable if they have a narrow and accessible neck (Fig. 3).

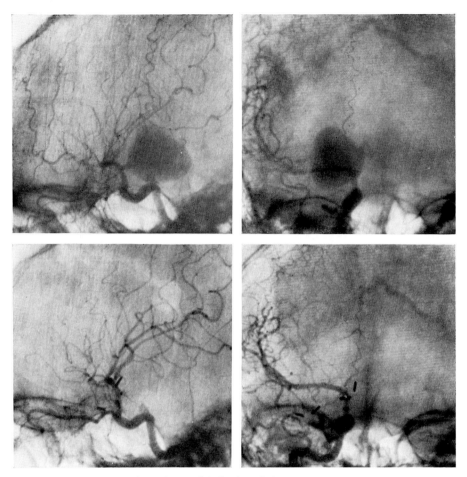

Fig. 3. Successful clipping of giant aneurysm.

A plastic coating of the vessel walls is a still a controversial technique, for its toxicity risk. Also it is seldom realizable in aneurysms inoperable because of their extent, as it is absolutely necessary to cover the whole surface of the aneurysm. Therefore, we obtained more experience in other localizations.

In some inoperable cases, thrombosis by pilojection or electrically induced clotting may be suitable, but we have no personal experience with these procedures.

Surgical Experience and Results on 159 Consecutive Cases of Intracranial Direct Attack to Saccular Aneurysms of the Internal Carotid and its Branches

PAOLO E. MASPES AND GIOVANNI MARINI

Neurosurgical Clinic of the University of Milano, Milano (Italy)

Purpose of this communication is to report the data concerning our most recent experience on direct intracranial attack to saccular aneurysms of the internal carotid and its branches. These data come from a series of cases which can be considered homogeneous from many aspects: all patients have been studied and treated in the same Neurosurgical Center, by the same surgical staff, within a relatively brief length of time, following the same criteria for surgical indication and using equal operative techniques such as direct attack to the aneurysmatic sac, moderate hypothermia and eventual intraoperative temporary interruption of blood flow to the lesion. We have also had the opportunity of getting a satisfactory follow-up control on our patients. We are thus able to present here together with the immediate surgical results, what is most important to the single patient, *i.e.* the capability to resume his usual life and activities, being cured from the distressful lesion.

263 Patients were admitted between April 1959 and June 1966 to the Neurosurgical Clinic of the University of Milano for subarachnoid hemorrhage from ruptured intracranial saccular arterial aneurysms. In every case the vascular malformation was proved angiographically. The few aneurysms belonging to the vertebro-basilar territory are not included in the number.

Table I shows sex and age of the patients and site of the aneurysms. It has to be noted that the great majority of cases belongs to the age group between 30 and 60 years and there is a predominance of young males and aged females, in accordance to the data published by the Report on the Cooperative Study of Intracranial Aneurysms and Subarachnoid Hemorrhage, 1966.

The saccular lesion is almost always localized to the anterior portion of the circle of Willis. Few cases belong to the intradural carotid siphon proximal to the posterior communicating artery; others are on the region of the main branching of the middle cerebral artery and very few on the distal branches of the carotid tree.

159 Patients underwent surgical operation with direct intracranial attack to the aneurysmatic sac. They represent 60% of the 263 cases with intracranial aneurysms proved by angiography.

References p. 321

TABLE I

INTRACRANIAL SACCULAR ANEURYSMS
(April 1959 - June 1966)
Total number: 263

Age	under 20	21–30	31–40	41–50	51–61	61–70	total
Males	6	16	35	46	38	5	146
Females	7	6	15	33	42	14	117
Total	13	22	50	79	80	19	263

Site

Intradural carotid
{ first segment: 15
posterior comm. artery region: 72
bifurcation: 21

Anterior communicating artery region: 93
Middle cerebral artery: 58
Others: 4
Multiple: 28

With the purpose of better evaluating the surgical results and as it has been done by the majority of the authors, we divided our cases according to their preoperative condition. We thus have two categories: favorable risk and poor risk patients. Following the criteria announced by Pool and Potts (1965), our "poor risk" patients include those in poor physical condition because of serious cardiovascular or systemic disease. They also include those whose neurological condition is considered precarious because of marked persisting confusion, stupor, coma and/or a major neurological disability such as hemiplegia. They are only 8.7% of our cases while the others who represent the great majority, have been considered as "favorable risk" being free from serious cardiovascular or systemic disease and in a reasonably good state of general health.

With respect to neurological condition, favorable risk patients include those who have recovered from a subarachnoid hemorrhage, who are alert or perhaps moderately or intermittently confused and drowsy but have no major neurological disability such as hemiplegia or aphasia. Patients with third or sixth cranial nerve signs or minimal neurological signs such as hemiparesis, have been included in our favorable risk group provided they were otherwise intact. Patients with multiple aneurysms, large aneurysms, or vascular hypertension have also been listed as favorable risk if their physical and neurological condition allowed this classification.

Table II shows operative mortality in relation to preoperative condition of our cases.

Operative mortality in favorable risk patients is only 12% while in unfavorable risk cases it is 70%.

The very high mortality of the latter group, generally operated in coma, shortly after the hemorrhage, is common to all series in the literature. For this reason and following what has been done by Pool and Potts (1965), we take here into consideration only the favorable risk patients, because of the accepted very high operative mortality

TABLE II

OPERATIVE MORTALITY IN RELATION TO PRE-OPERATIVE CONDITION

	No. of cases	Deaths	Percentage
favorable risk	145	18	12%
unfavorable risk	14	10	70%

of the unfavorable risk cases whose surgical indication has been considered only in particular cases.

Table III shows operative mortality according to age and blood pressure. As for blood pressure, the state of hypertension is referred only to the condition before the onset of subarachnoid hemorrhage, because there usually is a transitory phase of hypertension after the bleeding. It has to be noted that the rate between operative mortality above and under 50 years of age is two to one, while there is no great difference according to blood pressure.

TABLE III

OPERATIVE MORTALITY ACCORDING TO AGE AND BLOOD PRESSURE
(Favorable risk patients)

	No. of cases	Deaths	Percentage
under 50 years	102	10	9.5%
above 50 years	43	8	18.6%
normotensive	107	12	11%
hypertensive	38	6	15%

Table IV shows operative mortality according to the site of the aneurysmatic sac. Against what is generally reported in the literature, it has to be noted here the relative low mortality for the aneurysms of the region of the anterior communicating artery. This is probably due to the particular method of surgical treatment we have been using, consisting in bifrontal approach with intraoperative preventive temporary interruption of blood flow in both anterior cerebral arteries (Maspes and Marini, 1963).

Table V shows operative mortality according to interval between last hemorrhage and operation. In accordance with the largest reported series, mortality is higher during the first week, lower in the second and average afterwards.

Operative mortality according to surgical technique is reported in Table VI.

It has to be pointed out here that in 118 cases out of 145 (81% of the operated cases) we have performed radical treatment of the lesion with exclusion of the aneurysmatic sac from circulation, by clipping or ligature of the neck or local trapping. In the other 19% of the cases we have also made direct attack to the sac followed by wrapping of the malformation with various means, muscle, cotton, or more recently with plastics. Surgical mortality is 13% of the radically treated cases and 7% of the wrapped sacs.

References p. 321

TABLE IV

OPERATIVE MORTALITY ACCORDING TO LOCATION OF THE ANEURYSM
(favorable risk patients)

		No. of cases	Deaths	Percentage
intradural carotid	first segment	7	0	0%
	posterior comm. a. region	47	9	19%
	bifurcation	14	1	7%
anterior communicating artery region		51	6	11.7%
middle cerebral artery		26	2	7.6%

TABLE V

OPERATIVE MORTALITY ACCORDING TO TIMING
(Interval between last hemorrhage and operation – favorable risk patients)

	No. of cases	Deaths	Percentage
up to 7 days	6	2	33%
8–15 days	11	1	9%
15–30 days	32	5	15%
1 month–2 months	64	7	10%
over 2 months	32	3	9.3%

TABLE VI

OPERATIVE MORTALITY ACCORDING TO TECHNIQUE
(favorable risk patients)

	No. of cases	Deaths	Percentage
clip aneurysm or local trapping	118 (81%)	16	13%
wrapping	27 (19%)	2	7%

TABLE VII

RESULTS OF THE FOLLOW-UP CONTROL ON THE 145 OPERATED CASES
(from 7 years to 4 months - favorable risk patients)

	No. of cases	Percentage
no news	15	11%
operative mortality	18	12%
late mortality	8	5.5%
poor	9	5.5%
good or excellent	95	66%

TABLE VIII

LONG-TERM RESULTS ACCORDING TO THE CONDITION ON ADMISSION.
COMPARISON BETWEEN OPERATED AND NON-OPERATED CASES (Jan. 1964–June 1966)

	Cases	Good or Excellent	Poor	Deaths
Unfavorable Risk				
operated	13	5 (38%)	1 (8%)	7 (54%)
non-operated	33	5 (15%)	11 (33%)	17 (52%)
Favorable Risk				
operated	51	45 (86%)	3 (4%)	5 (10%)
non-operated	22	5 (22%)	1 (6%)	16 (72%)

We have then controlled the present condition of our patients, from seven years to four months after the intracranial operation. We were not able to obtain news from 15 cases.

Of the remaining 130 patients (89% of total number), 18 represent the operative mortality and 8 died over 6 months following surgery (5 for an event related to the aneurysm, one for gastric hemorrhage, one for heart failure and one for unknown cause). We have then divided the 104 patients living at the time of the follow-up control in two categories: "poor" are those patients presently inabilitated to work or social life, whose inability was caused in some way by the surgical operation; "good or excellent" are those patients who completely recovered and those who returned to their usual work or activity even though slightly handicapped by oculomotor paresis or weakness of a limb. 9 patients are reported as "poor" (5.5%); 95 (66%) of the total number of the operated cases are "good or excellent".

In order to compare the follow-up results between operated and non-operated cases, we finally made a study on *all* patients with intracranial saccular aneurysm hospitalized in a selected and relatively short period of time.

Between January 1964 and June 1966 we admitted to our Center 119 patients with cerebral aneurysms. All were documented angiographically.

The data, according to preoperative condition, are reported in Table VIII.

Table VIII gives us the opportunity of making two important remarks: in unfavorable risk patients, mortality is almost equal between operated and non-operated patients (54% *vs.* 52%), although the percentage of good or excellent results is more than double in the group of the operated patients (38% *vs.* 15%). The second remark is that in the favorable risk group, there is a great difference in the mortality rate between operated and non-operated patients (10% *vs.* 72%) and in the percentage of excellent or good results (86% *vs.* 22%).

REFERENCES

Maspes, P. E., and Marini, G., (1963); Aneurysms of the Anterior Communicating Artery. Results of Direct Surgical Treatment. *Acta Neurochir.*, **11**, 479–494.

Pool, J. L., and Potts, D. G., (1965); *Aneurysms and Arteriovenous Anomalies of the Brain.* New York. Hoeber Medical Division, Harper and Row.

Locksley, H. B., Sachs, H. L. and Sandler, R. (1966); Report on the Cooperative Study of Intracranial Aneurysms and Subarachnoid Hemorrhage. Section III. J. *Neurosurg.*, **24**, 1034–1056.

Arterial Vertebro-Basilar Aneurysms

E. LAINE

Chef de la Clinique Neuro-Chirurgicale, Lille (France)

DEFINITION OF THE SUBJECT

The subject to be discussed is contained within the anatomical limits described in the following (Fig. 1):

Inferior limit: vertebral artery penetrating into the subarachnoid space, near the first medullary segment.

Superior limit: cranial extremity of the basilar artery and origin of the posterior cerebral arteries up to their junction with the posterior communicating arteries: limit corresponding to the level of the third cranial nerve.

In this range, extensive studies of the aneurysms of the vertebro-basilar system are rare. The publications based upon a homogeneous series of observations including a valid therapeutic chapter may be counted on one's fingers. Moreover, the number of cases studied barely exceeds ten or twenty in each report.

Etiology — Relative frequency

Without ignoring the studies based upon one or two privileged observations, we may state that at the level of the vertebro-basilar network, arterial aneurysms are not as frequently encountered as in the territory of the internal carotid artery. This is differently interpreted by the various authors. Earlier anatomical studies (McDonald and Korb, 1939; Dandy, 1944; Richardson and Hyland, 1941) gave a proportion of 18 to 22% of intracranial aneurysms; in general, this ratio was most probably increased by including syphilitic aneurysms which are no longer seen at present.

It is, no doubt, more reasonable to adapt the figures of 6–6.5% advanced by Walton and Walsh, making allowance for the probability that the progress of vertebral angiography might slightly increase this proportion.

However, in agreement with Logue, we find that an estimation of 8 to 10% (figure equally adopted by Norlen) is sufficient to consider that vertebral angiography should form a part of the routine examination just like carotid angiography in cases of meningeal hemorrhage, except where such an intervention is absolutely contraindicated due to severe organic defects.

Anatomical pathology

From an anatomical point of view, we again find without surprise the different types of arterial aneurysms: *saccular, without pedicle,* and *fusiform.* This last variety — the volume of which sometimes becomes considerable — behaves like the true tumors of the posterior fossa. Examples have been noted by Alajouanine Castaigne, by Hamby and Krayenbühl and in isolated observations by several other authors. An important point is that these fusiform aneurysms practically never bleed. Within the limits of our study, we shall not deal with these forms, offering little possibility for the surgeon, and shall proceed to discussing saccular aneurysms.

In order to evaluate the relative incidence according to site on the vertebro-basilar system, we have combined the cases of Logue (12), of Drake (14), of Kenneth Jamieson (19-1), of Hook and Norlen (28-5) with our personal observations, making a total of 80 (Fig. 1).

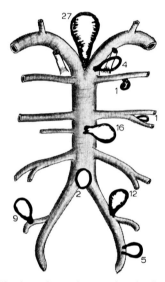

Fig. 1. Localization of saccular vertebro-basilar aneurysms.

Evidently, more or less extended *hematomas* or a *cerebellar infarction*, sometimes *an infarct of the brain stem*, indicate the gravity of the state of the patient (Logue and one of our own cases).

At the time of the rupture of the aneurysm, the hemorrhage generally diffuses into the subarachnoidal space. Sometimes a ruptured aneurysm causes the formation of thick layers of clots coating the cerebellum and the brain stem.

On the other hand, the fourth ventricle is in certain cases blocked by the presence of clots, in other cases it collapses due to pressure from a neighboring *subarachnoid hematoma*. This may account for the relative frequency of concomitant *hydrocephalus*, and the potential involvement of the cerebellar tonsils.

Accordingly, it is not exceptional that a hydrocephalus, most often of the communicating type, of subacute evolution develops even though an efficient intervention has suppressed the responsible aneurysm. This possibility constitutes an additional post-operative risk, due to which Jamieson lost 2 patients and Drake one.

The risks of *vertebral* or even *basilar thrombosis* are not negligible in aged patients with arteriosclerosis. This condition was fatal for one of our patients.

Before concluding this anatomical study, we must mention the proneness of the vertebral and basilar artery to spasms. Even a brief segmentary *spasm* may suffice to hinder the perfusion of the aneurysmal sac at the moment of the angiography. These spasms can spread over a broad area under the aneurysm; also, they may be extremely enduring to the point of having fatal consequences. Drake lost an operated patient due to a bilateral occipital infarction in the absence of thrombosis.

As far as the aneurysm itself is concerned, we note that its volume varies with the age of the aneurysm. Certain of them shrink or, in very fortunate cases, disappear due to the thrombosis; others steadily increase in volume. The example which Hook and Norlen permit us to report shows this well. Interestingly, at least in the case of the basilar aneurysms, this growth is realized at the expense not only of the wall of the sac but also of the collar whose fragility increases.

Finally, the vertebro-basilar aneurysm may well associate itself with another congenital malformation. The illustration presented associates a vestigial trigeminal artery with an aneurysm of the basilar artery located exactly at the mouth of the anomalous artery (Fig. 2).

Clinical study

The clinical aspect of the arterial aneurysms of the vertebro-basilar system is evidently very different depending upon whether it deals with a variety of pseudo-tumors with no subarachnoid hemorrhage or, instead, a ruptured aneurysm.

We shall not discuss here the rare pseudo-tumoral forms which are distinguished mainly by their irregular evolution marked by sudden aggravations, as a result of intra-parietal hemorrhages and the formation of an artificial sac arising from a dissecting aneurysm.

Ruptured aneurysms

Most of the vertebro-basilar aneurysms are discovered after rupture. The relative frequency of these hemorrhages is about 90%. They show a tendency to multiple and rapid relapses, which could be expected from the analogous behavior of aneurysms of the cerebral hemispheral region.

The accompanying *meningeal syndrome* does not much differ from that seen after a subtentorial cerebellar hemorrhage. One might, however, wonder whether its initial localization in the posterior fossa does not lend it certain special characteristics.

Lateralized and posterior cephalalgia — slightly retarded in relation to the neurological signs when they occur — rather discrete stiffness of the neck, fairly striking frequency of retinal hemorrhages are symptoms of a certain value which characterize

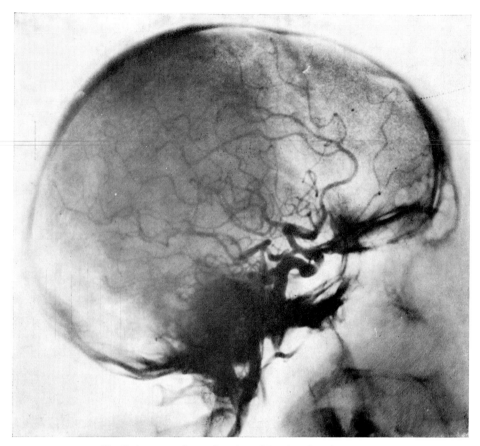

Fig. 2. Aneurysm located at the origin of a trigeminal artery.

the meningeal syndrome following rupture of an aneurysm in the posterior fossa. No definite diagnostic value should, however, be attached to these symptoms.

Is it possible to find, by analyzing the *pathological symptoms due to the brain stem*, more reliable symptoms for localizing the site of an aneurysm?

Dimsdale and Logue have undoubtedly given greatest attention to this problem.

The *pyramidal signs*, when they exist, can be very evocative. Hemiparesis, or total hemiplegia comparable to those after an injury of the region of the cerebral hemispheres are sometimes seen. Much less common are — during a meningeal hemorrhage — *bilateral perturbations*: *quadriplegia* reported by Dandy (1944), M. H. Cairns (1952) and Drake (1965) and especially *paraparesis* affecting the distal part of the lower limbs. Logue rightly attaches to them great importance. He encountered them in 5 patients out of 12 (observations 3, 4, 6, 7 and 12); Hook and Norlen reported a similar observation.

The onset of such paraparesis may be violent, and at times very su den. Important fact: it is often the *first sign of trouble*, heralding other clinical manifestations — mainly meningeal signs. The fact that in some cases the patient soon recuperates the use of his legs, *e.g.*, as soon as cephalalgia sets in, indicates that this course is merely the dissolution of the tonus. But in other cases genuine paraparesis can be present, which does not regress before a rather long time.

Just as striking can be the troubles of the bilateral *reflex function* and their localization in the lower limbs. A bilateral Babinski sign is generally found after meningeal hemorrhage of some importance. But hyporeflexia, even a bilateral patellar and milfoil areflexia such as we found, is a remarkable sign. We wish to compare the bilateral areflexia which we found in rather high proportion of the arterio-venous or cirsoid aneurysms of the same vertebro-basilar system.

One must also bear in mind the possibility of *sensory disturbances*, curiously *bilateral*, 'pins and needles' sensations in the legs noted by Logue (obs. 5) and by Norlen (obs. 13), pains beginning in the feet and progressing upward toward the root of the limbs and invading the trunk before reaching the neck.

Functions of the cerebellum

The observations of most authors are rather disappointing. Apart from an occasional case of ataxia, dysdiadochokinesia or hypermetria, no other signs were noted, but in reality these findings are relatively rare. Logue claims that cerebellar signs are almost totally absent. He recalls the tentative explanation of Elkington of the paradox: resistance of the cerebellum to anoxia, richness of its anastomotic network. We believe that the components of the cerebellar syndrome are not as rare as has been maintained. As Kremer remarked, some of the violent attacks of paraparesis of the lower limbs are actually crises of the dissolution of the tonus. Also, we feel that not enough attention is paid to the hypotonia of cerebellar nature, such as the tests of hand-waving or heel–buttocks can disclose even in uncooperative subjects. We found distinct cases of hypotonia in 4 out of 5 observations of aneurysm of the vertebral artery or of the posterior-inferior cerebellar artery in our series, without, however, including our 6 cases of basilar aneurysm.

The different *cranial nerves* are involved in different degrees. Among them, the oculomotor nerves — especially the IIIrd — are the most frequently concerned. Troubles of vertical or lateral eye movements are not rare. Rather than carrying out an analytical study of the cranial nerves we attempted to regroup the symptoms in order to reveal their connection with the different localizations.

Here, it should be stated that there is only *one syndrome* of almost *certain value*. It concerns the *vertebral artery and the inferior posterior cerebellar one*. This syndrome includes:

1. 'Drop attacks' and paresis of both legs, whether the posterior-inferior cerebellar (Logue, 3, 7 and 12; Norlen, 12) or the vertebral (Logue, 4, 6) arteries are involved.

2. The dysesthesias, the 'pins and needles' sensations of both legs (vertebral a., Logue 5; posterior-inferior cerebellar a., Norlen 13).

3. The association of dysarthria (Norlen 5 and 15; Jamieson 14; Laine 3), with, however, one exception, with basilar localisation (Norlen 4).

4. Trouble in oculomotor function in lateral sense (Laine 2 and 3).

References p. 345–346

5. Some signs of irritation of the Xth and XIth nerves, for example coughing in response to irritation of the Xth cranial nerve (Jamieson).

Other signs may be added. Cerebellar signs, among them hypotonia, do not have the same precise localizing value. Lesions of the VIIIth and IIIrd nerves may contribute to the symptoms listed above. However, this is not observed unless the vertebral artery and posterior-inferior cerebellar one are involved.

Is it possible to discern any other *circumscribed anatomo-clinical form*?

It appears that *trigeminal neuralgia* or, conversely, *trigeminal hyp-* or *anesthesia*, are not observed except if the superior cerebellar artery is involved; they are, however, rare.

Troubles of vision or of oculomotor function, including Parinaud's syndrome were also observed in cases of aneurysms localized on the lower arteries. Perhaps these troubles are slightly more frequent in cases of higher localization, as may be expected.

It is certain that the intense and sometimes prolonged *spasm* which is *produced by the rupture of the aneurysm* extends far above the splitting to the point of inducing serious *circulatory insufficiency* and, in consequence, very diffuse symptoms. Obser-

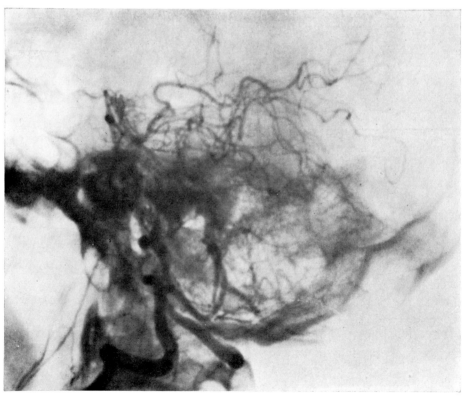

Fig. 3. Aneurysm of the left vertebral artery. Marked spasm of the basilar artery.

vation 6 of our series demonstrates such a case. In a 30-year-old male, a sudden subarachnoid hemorrhage was accompanied by left hemiparesis, right hypotonia and, especially, right ophthalmoplegia. In addition, he had difficulty in looking upward with the left eye. Vertebral angiography revealed an aneurysm of the left vertebral artery above which the basilar artery was intensely contracted to the extent of being only filiform (Fig. 3).

Because the circulatory disorders consequent to the rupture of the aneurysm diffuse over the entire subjacent area, only the vertebral and postero-inferior cerebellar varieties are accompanied by specific symptoms, while it is impossible to find any that should be typical of aneurysms in the superior regions.

To conclude the clinical study, it should be mentioned that the proportion of *vertebro-basilar aneurysms*, the rupture of which is accompanied only by a *meningeal syndrome*, is far from negligible. This is shown in 11 of the 28 cases of Hook and Norlen; Jamieson found it 9 times out of 19 cases.

Bearing in mind the frequent relapses in cases of meningeal hemorrhages due to vertebro-basilar aneurysms, and the gravity of the accidents which they may produce, one cannot but agree with all expert authors that a complete angiography is necessary, as soon as the patients' condition allows it.

Para-clinical examinations

Only by *angiography* an aneurysm responsible for an incident can be discovered and its site be ascertained. Other para-clinical examinations will not yield much information.

The *electroencephalogram* generally registers the sequence of slow bilateral synchronous waves, projecting to the frontal and occipital regions. It does, however, localize the origin of the meningeal hemorrhage in the posterior fossa. Its utility is especially of a prognostic nature. In particular, the finding of a sustained alpha rhythm in a patient in deep coma would support the existence of hemorrhagic lesions in the brain stem of such severity that it would be useless to intervene.

Although by *ventriculography* or *fractional pneumoencephalography* an aneurysm could exceptionally be spotted, *e.g.*, in a case of David; these techniques are unfit for systematic examination. They would not normally be applied in the pseudo-tumoral forms.

Vertebro-basilar angiography has not been applied until the past few years, except with much reticence, while bilateral carotid angiography has been used repeatedly for a long time.

These reservations may be explained partly by the cautious attitude towards surgical treatment. To what end — believed many authors, such as Walton (1956) and Walsh (1957) — force the patient to take the risk of a vertebral angiography only to discover an aneurysm very likely inaccessible to surgery?

This negative attitude has, fortunately, changed. In agreement with Logue, Norlen, Drake, the team of David and of Fischgold in 'La Pitié' we believe that *in each case of meningeal hemorrhage a complete angiogram should be made* and that, frequently, *vertebral angiography should be performed bilaterally, the same as carotid angiography.*

We have come to this conclusion at the expense of one of our patients:

Obs. 7: A 43-year-old female presented with subarachnoid hemorrhage accompanied by left transitory hemiplegia. The carotid angiogram revealed a large right sylvian aneurysm. It was ligated and removed without difficulty. Post-operative results were perfect. After a reassuring arteriographic control the patient left the department on the 12th day, without sequelae. She returned 8 days later with a much more serious hemorrhage, in a state of deep coma, complicated by grave vegetative disorders, especially of the respiratory function, to the point that immediate tracheotomy was performed. Marked left hemiplegia had reappeared, there was also hypotonia of the four limbs, the osteo-tendinous reflexes were absent in the legs. Due to a right axillary catheterization with Seldinger's sound, we performed simultaneously right carotidian arteriography showing that the sylvian artery was normal, and right vertebral angiography, which showed no abnormality either on this artery or on the basilar artery

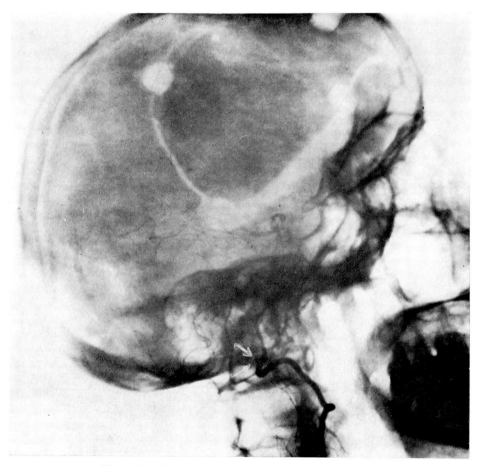

Fig. 4a. Small aneurysm of the left vertebral artery (arrow).

and its branches. Finally left vertebral angiography — carried out as a last resort — revealed the source of the vascular accidents in the form of a small aneurysm of the left vertebral artery pressing against the bulbo-medullary junction. Despite a fairly easy ligature, the patient died (Fig. 4a and b).

We think it necessary to submit the patient to a short preparatory perfusion of a 10% glucose solution in saline with papaverine hydrochloride added, of Solurutine and, in the case of important arterial hypertension, moderate doses of Hydergine.

One must, however, be aware that even under these ideal conditions *an aneurysm may* momentarily *be overlooked*. An example recently published by Weibel shows that angiography must be repeated in order to avoid failure of detecting the aneurysm.

One point deserves special attention (Fig. 5). Some *aneurysms of the basilar bifurcation* seem to directly prolong the artery without a discrete well-defined collar. Even

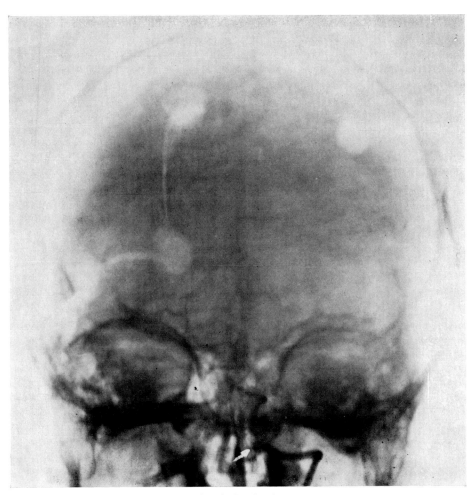

Fig. 4b. See fig. 4a.

more, *above the aneurysm the artery shows* relatively frequently *an ectasia* more or less large, from which posterior cerebral — sometimes even superior cerebellar — arteries stand out. This aspect is encountered in the superior network. As we have seen one of these aneurysms break close to the posterior cerebral, literally cutting off the basilar artery, we have learned to be wary of this aspect.

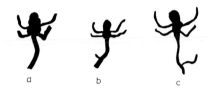

Fig. 5. Aneurysms of the basilar bifurcation.

Therapy

The indications of therapy and the possibilities of intervention remain to be considered.

The study of the spontaneous evolution of these dangerous vascular malformations and the operative risks and failures encountered by many authors should not be overlooked.

All publications agree that recurrence of the hemorrhage is extremely frequent — if not a constant feature — when it has a vertebro-basilar origin. They all agree on the extreme gravity of a relapse. 11 of the 16 patients of the statistics of Hook and Norlen, who had no small ruptures, and this was true for 10 of them died before the end of the 9th week. Out of the 10 patients of Dimsdale and Logue who were not operated, 5 died and only one has a valid survival. The 4 patients of our series who were not operated died.

The spontaneous fatal issue makes it necessary to attempt everything in order to remedy this situation.

Dimsdale and Logue (1959) were the first to protest against the general reluctance to operate. After them, Drake (1961), then Hook and Norlen (1963) and again Drake (1965) presented vigorous arguments in favor of the therapeutic intervention. Having operated on our first patients almost 15 years ago, we feel entitled to contribute our experience.

Dimsdale and Logue's theoretical considerations which make the vertebro-basilar aneurysms accessible to the surgeon are generally known. The situation, is however, not always simple; particularly when *aneurysms grafted on to the posterior wall of the basilar artery are pressed against the peduncle* or the protuberance, their dissection can be very dangerous. The *aneurysms* of the basilar bifurcation, especially when they *develop backward*, are in close relationship with the many meso-diencephalic perforating arteries (Fig. 6) which they contact. We agree with Drake that this is a very unfavorable anatomical disposition. The thrombosis, or the inclusion in the ligature of these arterioles has unavoidably catastrophic consequences.

We also must think of the troublesome *tendency of* the extremity of *the basilar artery to enlarge close to the site of the aneurysm*, thus impeding surgery. It is not

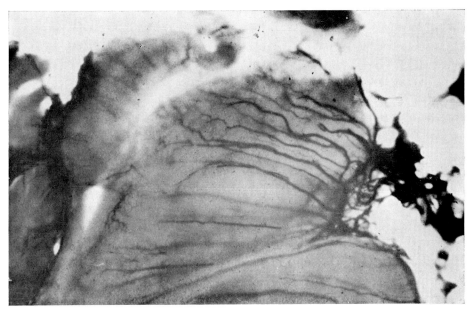

Fig. 6. Figure kindly loaned by Pr Lazorthes.

surprising therefore that Norlen felt obliged to admit that the problems posed by this variety of aneurysm are not fully resolved and that it is often difficult to foresee whether or not the aneurysm will be accessible to surgical intervention.

Anesthesia

The unpredictability of the result of an operation explains why the operator must take every possible safety measure and why anesthesia is most important.

It is certain that the benefit of perfusions of mannitol hypertonic solutions with or without urea is substantially enhanced by the evacuation of the CSF by lumbar drainage. In fact, the latter procedure is an indispensable adjuvant. Also, respiratory depression may be very useful, but risks of operating in contact with the brain stem must not be overlooked. Finally, hypothermia — moderate or deep — with cardiac arrest appreciably facilitates the work of the operator. We believe that age is a limiting factor, but Drake utilized with success deep hypothermia in a 63-year-old patient.

Surgical approach

The problem of the surgical approach need not be discussed at length in the case of the aneurysms of the vertebral artery or of the postero-inferior or antero-inferior cere-bellar arteries. The approach can only be *posterior* and the position of the patient — either sitting or lateral — can but facilitate access to the aneurysmal sac.

In the case of aneurysms of the basilar artery or of its bifurcation, the *sub-temporal approach* — after incision of the tentorium cerebelli — is the best one. Logue advised in 1959 a temporo-occipital approach, but found the group of the superficial Labbé veins and the Vth, VIIth and VIIIth cranial nerves in deeper layers embarrassing; also, he had trouble with a constant contra-lateral hemianopsia, which fortunately, regressed.

For our part, we prefer an anterior temporal approach completed, when the dissection of the aneurysm appears difficult, by the resection of the extreme point of the temporal lobe; this latter method leaves few sequelae, even on the dominant hemisphere. The IIIrd and the IVth nerves are certainly more exposed by this approach, but the space is large enough to permit avoiding them. Hook and Norlen appear also to favor such an approach, the possibilities of which are amply illustrated by Drake: a voluminous aneurysm implanted on the vertebro-basilar juncture is tied very correctly by the upper end.

Treatment of the aneurysmal sac

The techniques for the treatment of the aneurysmal sac are not different from those used in case of aneurysms of the carotid system, and need not be discussed in detail.

The ideal treatment consists in the ligature or the setting of a clip on the neck or the base of the aneurysm. It must be emphasized that certain varieties demand a careful dissection of the aneurysm and that it is desirable, whenever it is implanted on the neighboring artery by a large enough base, to fasten it rather than to clip it and not to pose the ligature until the sac has been deflated. In other words, the circulation must be very briefly interrupted so that in such cases moderate hypothermia is indicated. In the case of large aneurysms of the basilar bifurcation pointing up, or — especially — posteriorly, their close relationships with the meso-diencephalic perforating artery make the deflation of the sac even more imperative, right from the beginning of the dissection. That is why in these cases profound hypothermia becomes almost indispensable. Moreover, when the aneurysmal sac is voluminous and there is a chance of its flattening the contiguous vascular and nervous formations, its removal is, no doubt, advisable.

No other methods exist, except where ligature or clipping are impossible.

Time for intervention

Granting that the neurosurgeon operating late, after two or three weeks, has the advantage of appreciable operative comfort and security, it is none the less true that a fairly large number of patients will in the meantime have severe relapses. I consider surgery best on the 3rd or 4th day, whenever possible. There are many reports of a relapse where operation was delayed, to support this principle. Drake often intervened in the first 24 hours, which seems to us a bit too early.

The pre-operative condition and the site of the aneurysm are even more important for the final result than the time of the surgical intervention. If the gravity of the pre-operative state is a result of hemorrhage or of the infarction of the brain stem, nothing can be done, irrespective of the segment involved.

On the other hand, the discovery during the angiography of an extended and intense spasm deserves our attention. To operate without delay in these conditions is certainly not advisable unless, of course, there is a hematoma in the cerebellum or a thick subarachnoid basal effusion. The dissection of the contiguous arteries of the aneurysm can only prolong the duration of the spasm and aggravate circulatory insufficiency. In such cases we prefer to delay operation for a few days in the hope that vasodilators, notably papaverine and — if necessary — novocain infiltration of the inferior cervical ganglia should establish a better pre-operative state.

RESULTS OF THE SURGICAL TREATMENT (Tables I to V)

The analysis of the results of surgical therapy makes it necessary to distinguish between different localizations. Only the sufficiently important ones shall be discussed here.

Aneurysms of the cerebellar arteries (Table I) assure best post-operative results with the minimum of effort.

No mortality was noted among the patients of Dimsdale-Logue, of Hook-Norlen, or our own. The sequelae are minor. The return to an active life is often complete.

It is true that the patients were operated on under satisfactory conditions, in light coma (M) or in good condition (B). Besides, as it was to be foreseen, the results of the ligature of the collar are definitely superior to those of trapping.

Aneurysms of the vertebral artery (Table II) are almost equally easy to be treated. All patients who were in good pre-operative condition tolerated the intervention well and enjoyed a good functional state afterwards.

We lost one patient who was presented in a state of very deep coma, although the ligature of the aneurysm was easy. Due to a contralateral pyramidal deficit during a first relatively benign hemorrhage we suspected a sylvian aneurysm to be the cause, instead of a vertebral aneurysm (Fig. 4) which was actually responsible; we operated on the sylvian aneurysm which was completely inactive.

From a functional point of view, sequelae are apparently more serious than in the case of cerebellar aneurysms.

It is the collar ligatures which, once again, assure the best results. When they are not possible, the trapping or the ligature of the vertebral artery above the aneurysm is the acceptable procedure. In the case of a 58-year-old female patient, mother of 8 children, with arteriosclerosis, we preferred embedding the aneurysm in muscle — as we estimated that she could not support the ligature of the vertebral artery.

The aneurysms of the initial part of the posterior cerebral artery (Table III) have likewise a favorable localisation. Only one death has been reported (Jamieson) but the patient was originally in poor condition. Trapping, in this variety, does not necessarily cause hemianopsia, since the posterior communicating artery, where it is normally developed, provides a valid substitute.

In our experience, the ligature of the collar gave excellent functional restoration in spite of the basilar atheroma, the gravity of which was revealed by angiography. After 4 months of almost normal life, the patient had a fresh vascular accident in the form of a mortal mesenteric infarction. This deprived us of a following control, but death cannot be attributed to the intracranial intervention (Fig. 7).

TABLE I

POSTERIOR INFERIOR CEREBELLAR ANEURYSMS (5 operated / 9 cases)

Case	Sex/age	Duration of illness	Interval since hemorrhages	Number of hemorrhages	Condition at operation	Surgical procedures	Died	Post-operative course		
								Survivors		
								Interval	Activity	Residual defects
Hook Norlen 17	F 31		3 weeks	1	B	Trapping			Full time	slightly impaired vision
Hook Norlen 27	M 61		3 weeks	4	B	Trapping			Part time	?
Hook Norlen 1	F 50	2 months		0	B	Trapping excision		17 years	Part time	?
Dimsdale Logue 3	M 35	9 days	2 days	4	M	ligature on sac		2 years	Light work	Nystagmus difficulty in balancing on one leg
Laine 1	M 27	4 weeks	10 days	2	M cerebellar hematoma	ligature on neck		11 years	Full time	Right hypotonus
SUPERIOR CEREBELLAR ANEURYSM										
Dimsdale Logue 1	F 56	21 days	16 days	4	B	Trapping superior cerebellar		7 years	Full time	slight contracture facial Vth sens. loss

B: good   B+ : very good   M: drowsiness, confusion   C: coma   C+: coma carus   C++: coma + vegetative disorders

TABLE II

VERTEBRAL ANEURYSMS (10 operated/17 cases)

Case	Sex/Age	Duration of illness	Interval since hemorrhages	Number of hemorrhages	Condition at operation	Surgical procedures	Post-operative course			
							Died	Survivors		
								Interval	Activity	Residual defects
Dimsdale Logue 6	M 55	10 days	10 days	2	B+	vertebral clip proximal		2 years	light work	horizontal nystagmus, joint sense impaired in toes
Hook Norlen 22	F 57	7 weeks	7 weeks	1	B	Explor.			Part time	?
Hook Norlen 24	F 36	5 weeks	5 weeks	1	B	clip neck			Full time	?
Jamieson 17	F 31	15 days	15 days	1	B	Trapping		4 weeks	?	ataxia, hypoglossal paralysis
Jamieson 19	F 46		4 days		B	clip neck			Full time	0
Dimsdale Logue 5	F 47	10 days	10 days	2	M	vertebral clip proximal		18 months	impaired	ataxia, low visual acuity
Jamieson 15	F 42	1 day	1 day	1	M	Trapping	†			
Jamieson 16	F 42	4 days	1 day	2	M	vertebral clip proximal	†			
Jamieson 18	M 40	6 weeks	6 weeks	2	M	clip on neck ligature		?	impaired	low visual acuity
Laine 7	F 43	6 weeks	4 days	2	C++	on neck	†			
Laine 9	F 58	15 days	15 days	1	B	wrapping		9 months	Full time	:

B: good B+: very good M: drowsiness, confusion C: coma C+: coma carus C++: coma + vegetative disorders.

References p. 345–346

TABLE III

ANEURYSMS AT THE ORIGIN OF CEREBRAL POSTERIOR ARTERY (4 operated/4 cases)

Case	Sex/age	Duration of illness	Interval since hemorrhages	Number of hemorrhages	Condition at operation	Surgical procedures	Died	Post-operative course Survivors		
								Interval	Activity	Residual defects
Jamieson 1	M 21	1 month	1 month	1	B	Trapping cerebral posterior		10 years	Full Time	left hemiplegia, left hemianopsia, IIIrd palsy
Jamieson 3	F 34		7 weeks	1?	M	2 aneurysms left: clip on neck right: trapping		5 months	O	communicating hydrocephalus, impaired vision
Jamieson 4	F 29		6 days	1	M	Trapping	48 hours †			
Laine 11	M 43		5 days	1	M	ligature on neck		4 months	Part time	Right IIIrd palsy (4 months later mesentery infarct)

B: good   B+: very good   M: drowsiness, confusion   C: coma   C+: coma carus   C++: coma + vegetative disorders

TABLE IV

ANEURYSMS OF BASILAR ARTERY TRUNK (9 operated/18 cases)

Case	Sex/age	Duration of illness	Interval since hemorrhages	Number of hemorrhages	Condition at operation	Surgical procedures	Died	Post-operative course		
									Survivors	
								Interval	Activity	Residual defects
Jamieson 12	F 44	5 days	5 days	1	M	clip neck hematoma	†			
Jamieson 13	F 57	3 months		0	C	clip on left and right vertebral	†			
Jamieson 14	M 36	some months	1 day	2	C++	hematoma exploration		6 months	light work	hemianopsia
Drake 1	M 50	3 weeks	1 day?	3	M	clip on neck		1 year	Full time	O
Drake 6	M 23	10 days	6 days	2	C	clip on neck		1 year	Full time	O
Drake 8	M 66	20 days	6 days	2	M	clip on neck	†			
Drake 10	M 52	?	3 weeks	3	M	ligature sac		6 months	impaired communic. hydro-cephalus	impairment memory, initiative
Drake 12	F 54	5 years	10 weeks	3	B	clip part of sac		some weeks	well	IIIrd palsy
Drake 14	M 65		11 days	1		coat of plastic		3 weeks 3 weeks		Receptive dysphasia

B: good   B+: very good   M: drowsiness, confusion   C: coma   C+: coma carus   C++: coma + vegetative disorders.

References p. 345–346

TABLE V

ANEURYSMS OF BASILAR BIFURCATION—ANTERIOR VARIETY (6 operated/7 cases)

Case	Sex/age	Duration of illness	Interval since hemorrhages	Number of hemorrhages	Condition at operation	Surgical procedures	Post-operative course Died	Survivors Activity	Survivors Interval	Survivors Residual defects
Hook Norlen 9	F 43	4 months	8 weeks	3	B	clip on neck		13 years	Part time	?
Drake 2	F 45	6 weeks	20 hours	4	M	clip on neck		8 months	O	low visual acuity, central visual defect, Korsakoff-like state
Drake 3	F 45	14 years	1 day	3	C	clip on neck	3rd day			
Drake 5	M 48	8 days	1 day	2	M	clip on neck	3 months later without recovery			
Drake 7	M 63	2 days	2 days	1	M	deep hypothermia clip on neck		2½ months		recovered all his faculties except memory and speech
Drake 13	F 51	13 days		1	B	wrapping		6 weeks		O

B: good   B+: very good   M: drowsiness, confusion   C: coma   C+: coma carus   C++: coma + vegetative disorders

TABLE VI

ANEURYSMS OF BASILAR BIFURCATION — SUPERIOR VARIETY (7 operated/9 cases)

Case	Sex/age	Duration of illness	Interval since hemorrhages	Number of hemorrhages	Condition at operation	Surgical procedures	Post-operative-course			
							Died	Survivors		
								Interval	Activity	Residual defects
Hook Norlen 18	F 53		7 weeks	2	M	clip on neck	2 months later			
Jamieson 5	M 53	4 weeks	10 days	3	M	wrapping in muscle and gauze	5 days later			
Jamieson 6	F 42		4 days	1	B	clip on neck	2 days later			
Jamieson 7	F 43		5 days	1	B	clip on neck		?	Full time	Right IIIrd palsy. Transient left hemiplegia
Jamieson 9	M 36		16 days	1	B	clip on neck and origin of the left posterior cerebral	5 days later			
Laine 4	M 24	10 days	8 days	2	C++	Suture basilar bifurcation	1 day later			
Laine 8	M 20	6 days	6 days	1	M	ligature on neck		2 years	Full time	O post-operational arteriogram correct

B: good   B+: very good   M: drowsiness, confusion   C: coma   C+: coma carus   C++: coma + vegetative disorders

References p. 345–346

TABLE VII

ANEURYSMS OF BASILAR BIFURCATION — POSTERIOR VARIETY (9 operated/11 cases))

Case	Sex/age	Duration of illness	Interval since hemorrhages	Number of hemorrhages	Condition at operation	Surgical procedures	Post-operative course			
							Died	Survivors		
								Interval	Activity	Residual defects
Hook Norlen 6	M 45	10 years	5 weeks	2	M	exploration	5 months later			
Hook Norlen 12	M 42	4 years	2/8 weeks	4	M	failure of clipping	6 weeks later			
Drake 4	F 52	7 days	36 hours	2	B	clip on neck	few hours			
Drake 9	F 30	9 days		1	B	ligature on neck		6 months	O	4 limbs spastic, aphasia, IIIrd palsy
Drake 11	M 48	6 weeks	6 weeks	2	B	ligature on neck	7 months without improvement			
Jamieson 8	F 56	3 months	few days	2	B	clip on neck		3 months	O	severely handicap.
Jamieson 10	M 32	?	8 days	1	M	clip on neck	10th day			
Jamieson 11	F 52	11 days	7 days	2+	B	clip on neck	4th day			
Laine 5	M 16	30 days	30 days	1	B	ligature on neck		10 years	Full-time teacher	left sup. quadranopsia

B: good   B+: very good   M: drowsiness, confusion   C: coma   C+: coma carus   C++: coma + vegetative disorders

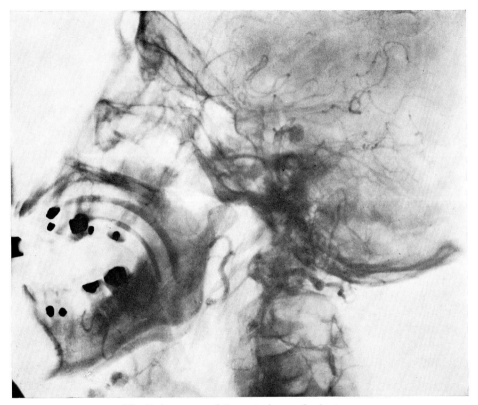

Fig. 7. Aneurysm of the posterior cerebral artery.

Aneurysms of the basilar artery (Table IV) remain apparently amenable to operation. Indeed, Jamieson, lost two patients out of three, but Drake reports on an imposing series of successful operations: five recoveries out of six; two perfect functional restorations, one patient in excellent condition but handicapped by paralysis of the IIIrd nerve; one patient retained serious memory difficulties, but his condition following the operation was complicated by communicating hydrocephalus, a sequeal of the meningeal hemorrhage. The last patient, aged 65, remained aphasic: he was submitted only to a minor intervention, the wrapping of the sac in a plastic film.

Aneurysms of the basilar bifurcation (Table V) give rise, no doubt, to most problems. In order to specify more effectively the operative indications, we divided them into three groups:

(a) the anterior varieties are the least dangerous of the three groups. Out of 6 cases, two patients died, in spite of the correct application of a clip on the collar of the aneurysm. They had been previously comatose, one in light, the other in deep coma. The four others are alive, but two of them or at least one, have memory troubles of the Korsakoff type.

(b) with *the superior varieties* the prognosis is different. Five out of seven patients operated on died. We have seen an aneurysm barely detached from the surrounding clots, tear at the base of the basilar artery, literally cutting it off, without having at-

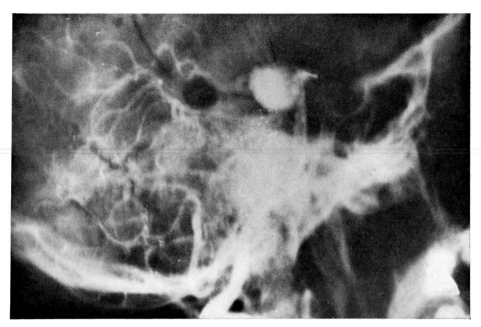

Fig. 8a. Aneurysm of the basilar bifurcation, posterior variety.

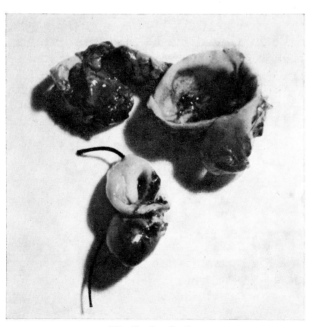

Fig. 8b. See fig. 8a.

tempted to mobilize the aneurysm. This drama occurred before techniques of artificial hypothermia existed. A suture, even though correctly done, of the distal end of the basilar artery could not save the patient because of an obviously too prolonged circulatory arrest.

We observed a tendency of the basilar artery to enlarge at its extremity. This is, perhaps, the reason why these varieties are so dangerous, even though easily accessible, so that clipping them was invariably successful.

Our second patient recovered, without sequelae.

(c) *the posterior varieties*, on the contrary, are not the most favorable ones. Six deaths out of nine represent a heavy balance. Out of the three survivals, two remained seriously handicapped. Only one good result is noted in this category: a young male (14 years) operated upon by us ten years ago for a very large aneurysm. He is a teacher, suffering only from a residual quadrantanopsia (Fig. 8).

We shall not review the reasons for the many failures sustained by the most brilliant surgeons. The difficulty of dissection in a milieu of many meso-diencephalic arterioles, as important as they are fragile, justifies the application of very important resources. Profound hypothermia finds here, without doubt, one of its best indications.

CONCLUSIONS

In the light of the surgical risks of the superior or posterior varieties of vertebro-basilar aneurysms, is there any point in discussing the operative indications? The fatal issues reported above, which almost unavoidably result from spontaneous evolution, relieve us from doing so.

A neurosurgeon worthy of this title should have the courage of assuming complete responsibility. Only the patients who obviously are irreparably lost, seen their catastrophic condition due to the aneurysmal rupture or the existence of organic defects beyond surgical help, should be left to their destiny. For all the others we must fight, and we must engage this battle as early as possible following the first meningeal hemorrhage.

Finally, it is from an early etiological diagnosis of a hemorrhage, by means of a correct and complete angiographic exploration that a better prognosis of the dreadful malformations can be expected; far more so than from the technical progress which neurosurgery and anesthetics may still accomplish.

REFERENCES

ALAJOUANINE, T., LEBEAU, J. AND HOUDART, R. (1948) La symptomatologie tumorale des volumineux anévrysmes des artères vertébrales et basilaires. *Rev. Neurol.*, **80**, 321–337.

DANDY, W. E. (1944) *Intracranial arterial aneurysms*. Comstock Publ. Co. — Inc. (Ithaca N.Y.), VIII, 47.

DAVID, M., ANGELERGUES, R. AND HECAEN, H. (1956) Un cas de migraine prosoplégique par anévrysme artériel de la fosse cérébrale postérieure. *R. Neurol. Par.*, **94**, 716–718.

DIMSDALE, H. AND LOGUE, V. (1959) Ruptures posterior fossa aneurysms and their surgical treatment. *J. Neurol. Neurosurg. Psych.*, **22**, 202–217.

DRAKE, C. G., (1961) Bleeding aneurysms of the basilar artery. Direct surgical management in four cases. *J. Neurosurg.*, **18**, 230–238.

DRAKE, C. G. (1965) Surgical treatment of ruptured aneurysms of the basilar artery — experience with 14 cases. *J. Neurosurg.*, **23**, 457–473.

HOOK, O., NORLEN, G. AND GUZMAN, J., (1963) Saccular aneurysms of the vertebral basilar arterial system. A report of 28 cases. *Acta Neurol. Scand.*, **39**, 271–304.

JAMIESON, K. G. (1964) Aneurysms of the vertebro-basilar system, surgical intervention in 19 cases. *J. Neurosurg.*, **21**, 781–797.

LAINE, E. AND GALIBERT, P. (1966) Aneurysmes artério-veineux et cirsoïdes de la fosse postérieure. A propos de quarante observations. *Rev. Neurol.*, **2**, 276–288.

LCGUE, V. (1964) Posterior fossa aneurysma. *Clin. Neurosurg.*, **II**, 183–219.

Remarks on the Direct Attack on Intracranial Aneurysms

G. MORELLO

Istituto Neurologico di Milano, Milan (Italy)

This contribution is about some aspects of operating policy in direct attack on intra cranial aneurysms. Direct attack now seems to afford the greatest guarantees of real efficacy, especially when the sack is excluded from the circulation, but it is a method which is taxing the surgeon. And so several expedients were devised to ease his task, mostly to facilitate exposure of the sack and prevent rupture of it during the exposure manoeuvers. For this purpose hypotension and local or total circulatory arrest came into use and, to protect the brain from the consequences of a decrease or interruption in the blood supply, hypothermia. These surgical expedients have been widely used and have certainly been of great help in direct attack, but it soon became clear that they are not without snags. Laboratory investigations into their effects showed that, like any other method inducing abnormal physiological conditions, they cannot be regarded as harmless. In any case, direct attack can now be facilitated by simpler means. And so the initial enthusiasm for these surgical adjuvants wore off a bit and I feel we should discuss whether they are indispensable in every case or not. Only experience of many cases and of many surgeons can supply an answer. It is with the intention of providing material for discussion that I shall now report on our experience at the Istituto Neurologico of Milan from 1949 to date.

During this period we operated on 245 intracranial aneurysms. Fourteen were sub-clinoid aneurysms and as they are unsuitable for direct attack, they are not relevant to our purpose. The remaining 231 were aneurysms of the supraclinoid carotid artery or of its intracranial branches. There have been three periods in our policy for treating such cases.

In the first (from 1949 to 1960) the operations were performed in normothermia and moderate hypotension (down to 70 mm Hg) induced by ganglion blockers. Eighty aneurysms fall into this group and there were 15 deaths (18.7%). Twenty-six were treated by wrapping with muscle or by ligation of the feeding vessel. Fifty-four, that is 67.5% of the total, were excluded from the circulation by clipping of the neck or by trapping; twelve patients died (22.2%).

In the second period (from 1961 to 1964) all patients were operated on in moderate hypothermia (28–30°C) and controlled respiration. Eighty-six aneurysms were operated on during this period and ten patients died (11.6%). Fifteen of these were treated by wrapping or by ligation of the feeding vessel. Seventy-one, that is 82.5% of the

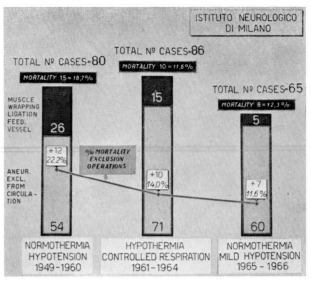

Fig. 1. Results in three periods of different treatment.

total, were excluded from the circulation and there were ten deaths (14% of the group). While we were still using hypothermia, my coworkers and I began to wonder whether it was really necessary; in the end we decided to give it up and to operate in normothermia and mild hypotension (about 100 mm Hg) induced by hyperventilation and fluothane narcosis.

In the third period (1965–1966) sixty-five aneurysms were operated on with 8 deaths (12.3%). All were exposed: five were wrapped and 60, that is 92.3% of the total, were excluded from the circulation, the number of deaths being 7 (11.6% of the group).

As the operation selection criteria did not change over the three periods, that is, operations were never performed on moribund or deeply comatose patients, the results of the three periods are comparable. They show that mortality from direct attack fell in the hypothermia period but fell again when hypothermia was abandoned. This suggests that the higher success rate was due to greater surgical skill resulting from greater experience and not to hypothermia. This tallies with other accounts that have appeared recently, one of which is based on a large series, showing that hypothermia does not improve the success rate of direct attack. I don't think one should infer that hypothermia is to be abandoned altogether, but I do think that it should be used only when it may be foreseen that deep hypotension or circulatory arrest is necessary. These two techniques are certainly very useful but they are not risk-free. Hence I feel that they should not be used systematically but should be confined to particular cases, i.e. for aneurysms which angiography has shown to be very large or unusually difficult to approach. Such cases are not frequent and most aneurysms, instead, can be exposed and treated satisfactorily without disturbing the cerebral circulation, a thing to be avoided unless indispensable. Thus, in the great majority of cases I believe hypothermia to be neither necessary nor useful.

There is another point of general operating technique which I think deserves discussion and that is: whether cerebral incisions or amputations are necessary or advantageous for the exposure of aneurysms. Even recently techniques have been described whereby supraclinoid carotid aneurysms are reached through an incision in the tip of the temporal lobe or aneurysms of the anterior communicating artery by resection of the frontal pole. Procedures of this kind were certainly often necessary in the past and may be so in special cases even today. But now that, with osmotics and hyperventilation, slack brains are a frequent occurrence, manoeuvers for exposing aneurysms are much easier and I think one can and should manage without sacrificing cerebral tissue, which does carry a risk. Many aneurysms can be exposed without injuring the brain in any way. A large number of anterior communicating aneurysms, for example, can safely be reached by subfrontal route. Since January 1966 at the Istituto Neurologico of Milan 17 of these have been clipped, with a single fatality, 14 of them being approached by subfrontal route.

Direct attack on aneurysms has made great strides in the past fifteen years. To overcome the initial difficulties several kinds of expedients and adjuvants were thought up. These have been of help and still are but, now that we have more experience and have gained greater confidence in ourselves, I think we should use them sparingly and conserve the anatomical and physiological integrity of the brain as far as possible, remembering that the simplest way is usually the best.

Some Remarks on the Question of the Saccular Aneurysms

L. ZOLTÁN

Budapest (Hungary)

The saccular aneurysm of the cerebral vessels became universally known since the routine use of angiography has gained ground. A large number of works have been published dealing with the etiology, pathology, and the clinical and therapeutical aspects of aneurysms.

Numerous studies have been conducted, based on vast material, yielding prognostic and katamnestic conclusions. Hardly any problems were left open, and the lectures presented gave account of an improvement of surgical therapy, as a result of extensive experience. In consequence, the official discussor has no easy task, for what more can be said about the subject, seeing the mass of publications by most distinguished investigators? To give a survey is also rather difficult, since besides the publications based on large material aiming to form general opinion, there are many casual publications, which may eventually modify wholly or partly, the opinions universally held. Nevertheless, I shall attempt to sum up our present knowledge of the question.

1. Though subarachnoidal bleeding can be due to a variety of causes, the most frequent one is the rupture of a cerebral aneurysm.

2. Single bleedings occur less frequently; much more frequent are recurrent bleedings.

3. The risk of a new bleeding diminishes with the time.

4. In a clinical state caused by bleeding, two factors are of paramount importance: age and the state of consciousness. The latter is determined, according to recent investigations, not only by the volume and the localization of the bleeding, but also by the hemodynamic state of the great vessels (Walter–Schütte).

5. The tools of the conservative therapy of a bleeding aneurysm are rather scanty, and recovery is actually left to the organism, namely to its balancing power. Therefore, surgical therapy: the complete exclusion of the aneurysm from the circulation and, thereby, the definitive elimination of a rupture of the sack, appears to be method of choice.

This optimistic view seems, however, to have been somewhat shaken in the past ten years by the katamnestic evaluation of numerous patients by McKissock and co-workers, Benson, and others. As opinions still differ on this subject, I should like to discuss it briefly.

It has been established from prolonged observation of operated and non-operated patients that no significant difference exists between the survival rate of the two categories, taken into consideration even the operative mortality. If we accepted this view, then a radical operation in these cases would not seem to be justified.

I think, this conclusion not altogether acceptable, especially if we consider recent splendid surgical results. Conservative therapy for "poor risk patients" should be seriously considered. Mortality rates (*e.g.* Pool 60%) compared with good recovery of the patients who overcame the acute state of the rupture with no new bleeding within 6 weeks, undoubtedly suggest the value of non-surgical treatment — says also Sencer. On the other hand, conservative therapy cannot be considered as the right one in cases of good risk, as the recent data of Richardson seem to confirm. Hamby, Pool, McKissock, Norlen, Krayenbühl, Laitinen and — we understand — Kunc and many others report besides very low mortality rates, also on very good postoperative recovery. This is due not only to the evolution of surgical techniques, but also to the surgeon's skill. Anesthesiology and other procedures connected with surgery show also rapid evolution, *e.g.* techniques of dehydration, hypotension and hypo-thermia. The latter is another question that requires further study. After early en-thusiastic response adverse opinion seems to gain ground concerning the favorable effect of hypothermia on mortality. Leaving apart the problems of deep and local hypothermia, about which neither literature data, nor my own experience are suf-ficient, I would like to point out one thing: the temporary elimination of the aneurysm from the circulation seems to diminish the risk of its rupture during surgery (see Maspes-Marini, Pool, etc.). It makes the isolation of the sac easier even in rather complicated cases, and the adjustment of clips, ligature, muscle or plastic substances to the aneurysm safer and more adequate. This procedure can be carried out some-times even in normothermia. For complete restoration of the cerebral function, and for prevention of postoperative edema, etc., it seems safer to carry out temporary occlusion under hypothermia. Neurosurgeons with vast experience could obtain excellent results without interrupting the regional circulation or without inducing hypothermia, respectively, especially in the group of benign cases. The impressive papers of Pool and others deserve our attention, and with more experience with this technique, it will be possible to consider a radical operation also for some of the less favorable cases.

Undoubtedly, for the surgery of saccular aneurysms the individual estimation of the case, the general neurological state of the patient and the technique of the surgeon are decisive. Yet, like in other fields of the medical sciences, generally the analysis of conclusions must be derived from growing experience. I have the impression that general opinion is gradually coming to approve of intracranial radical operation, where such intervention is indicated on the ground of age, the stage of consciousness, the neurological picture and the presence of the spasms of vessels at the time of the operation.

I believe that in the questions of the advantage of operative intervention and of the benefit of moderate hypothermia it will soon be possible to come to an agreement. The lectures delivered here will no doubt, contribute greatly towards such an agreement.

A Controlled Trial of Delayed Surgery for Intracranial Arterial Aneurysms. - First Results

G. af BJÖRKESTEN and H. TROUPP

Neurosurgical Clinic, Helsinki (Finland)

Since the early days of aneurysm surgery it has been more or less an axiom that once an intracranial arterial aneurysm has bled it should be operated on. This view has been based upon the fact that so many statistics comparing series of operatively and conservatively treated patients showed figures in favour of surgery. Most of these series were, in fact, not comparable, as they were not composed in the same way: the operatively treated series generally consisted of the most favourable cases, whereas the conservatively treated series included patients admitted in a hopeless state after haemorrhage, patients in bad general condition or with concomitant diseases preventing surgery, patients with technically inoperable aneurysms, and also patients who were scheduled for operation but died before surgery. It is quite clear that such a division affects the mortality and morbidity figures for the conservatively treated patients to such an extent that they can no longer be used as a real basis when judging the risks justifiable in connection with planned surgical treatment.

McKissock, Richardson and Walsh (1960, 1962, 1965) were the first to correct this inconsistency in the selection of patients. In controlled trials with entirely comparable series of operated and unoperated aneurysm patients they have shown that surgery does, in fact, benefit some groups of patients; for other groups they have not yet been able to show any difference.

The Atkinson Morley's Hospital group admit their patients and perform their operations very early after haemorrhage. Our aneurysm patients are admitted late; shortage of beds and distances of up to 600 miles do not allow us to admit subarachnoid haemorrhage patients in the acute stage. After having dealt with more than 1800 cases of subarachnoid haemorrhage during the '50s and up to the end of 1963, we realized that a controlled trial was necessary in the assessment of our results.

This trial was started on April 1st, 1964, and up to Sept. 30th 1966, 123 patients had been included. All patients reported on here have thus been followed up for periods varying between 6 months and $2\frac{1}{2}$ years.

54 patients had an aneurysm of the anterior communicating artery, 35 an aneurysm of the middle cerebral artery, and 34 had an aneurysm of the internal carotid artery. Only these three locations were included in the trial. In all instances this was the only aneurysm found; patients with two or more aneurysms and patients who in addition to an arterial aneurysm had an arteriovenous malformation were omitted. All patients

References p. 356

underwent bilateral carotid angiography and at least unilateral vertebral angiography as well.

At the stage at which our patients are admitted, generally 2–6 weeks after haemorrhage, the natural mortality is definitely much lower than during the acute stage (Pakarinen, 1967); consequently we were very careful in our selection of patients for the trial. In fact, only about one third of the aneurysm patients admitted to our department were included. When a patient was considered suitable for inclusion, *i.e.* his aneurysm had been considered operable and his general condition did not discount surgery, the time of a possible operation was fixed; the statistical decision, operative or conservative, was then made. If the patient suffered from a recurrent haemorrhage before the time fixed, he was excluded from the trial.

In the operatively treated group a direct intracranial attack on the aneurysm was performed and a ligature of the stalk of the aneurysm was aimed at in all cases; in a few cases, however, the attempt was unsuccessful, and a proximal clipping or a reinforcement of the aneurysmal wall had to be resorted to. Urea or Mannitol was used in most cases, but not hypothermia nor hypotension. The conservative treatment consisted of strict bedrest for at least 6 weeks.

There were no operative deaths. One patient died later from recurrent bleeding: a secondary rupture of an aneurysm reinforced with oxycel. Five conservatively treated patients died from a recurrent haemorrhage. All deaths occurred within six months after the first bleeding.

The results for the three different types of aneurysm are shown in Tables I to III. A good result means that the patient is able to work and has no symptoms or signs whatsoever. A fair result means a patient capable of working in spite of slight disorders, often of a subjective nature. A poor result means a markedly reduced working capacity, or total disability.

TABLE I

ANTERIOR COMMUNICATING ARTERY
(54 patients)

Treatment	Result			
	Good	Fair	Poor	Dead
Surgical	14	5	7	1
Conservative	14	6	4	3

TABLE II

MIDDLE CEREBRAL ARTERY
(35 patients)

Treatment	Result			
	Good	Fair	Poor	Dead
Surgical	5	7	6	–
Conservative	4	8	4	1

TABLE III

INTERNAL CAROTID ARTERY
(34 patients)

Treatment	Result			
	Good	Fair	Poor	Dead
Surgical	8	6	1	–
Conservative	5	7	6	1

TABLE IV

INTERNAL CAROTID ARTERY
(21 patients with aneurysms regarded as specially suitable for operation)

Treatment	Result	
	Good + Fair	Poor + Dead
Surgical	9	–
Conservative	6	6

The tables show that there are no overall differences between the operatively and the conservatively treated groups. A closer analysis shows that the difference in late mortality, 1 operated and 5 unoperated patients, is not significant. The only statistical difference between operated and unoperated aneurysms is found in the internal carotid group among aneurysms classified as specially suitable for operation. If good and fair results on one hand are compared to poor results and deaths on the other, the difference between operated and unoperated patients is statistically almost significant (Table IV).

Apart from this single example, and in spite of the fact that up to now there has been no operative mortality at all, we have not yet been able to prove convincingly that our delayed surgery for arterial intracranial aneurysms benefits the patients. To reach any definite conclusion, the trial must be continued. Recent electron microscopic investigations (Nyström, 1963) have shown that after a subarachnoid haemorrhage there are signs of a reparative process visible in the wall of the aneurysm at the site of the rupture; this may, perhaps, sometimes strengthen the wall to such an extent that no further bleedings occur. Nevertheless, the incidence of recurrent haemorrhages in the conservatively treated group may well increase during prolonged follow-up, thus making a difference in results statistically significant. In any case it seems evident that a possible difference in results between operative and conservative treatment in the later stage after a subarachnoid haemorrhage would definitely not be as great as was previously supposed. This fact must be given serious consideration when judging the operability of aneurysms.

References p. 356

REFERENCES

McKissock, W., Paine, K. W. E., and Walsh, L., (1960); An analysis of the results of treatment of ruptured intracranial aneurysms. Report of 772 consecutive cases. *J. Neurosurg.*, **17**, 762–766.

—, Richardson, A., and Walsh, L., (1960); "Posterior-communicating" aneurysms. A controlled trial of the conservative and surgical treatment of ruptured aneurysms of the internal carotid artery at or near the point of origin of the posterior communicating artery. *Lancet*, **ii**, 1203–1206.

—, —, and —, (1962); Middle-cerebral aneurysms. Further results in the controlled trial of conservative and surgical treatment of ruptured intracranial aneurysms. *Lancet*, **ii**, 417–421.

Nyström, S. H. M., (1963); Development of intracranial aneurysms as revealed by electron micrscopy. *J. Neurosurg.*, **20**, 329–337.

Pakarinen, S., (1967); Incidence, aetiology, and prognosis of primary subarachnoid haemorrhage. *Acta neurol. Scand.*, suppl. 29, 128 pp.

Richardson, A., McKissock, W., and Walsh, L., (1965); Anterior communicating aneurysms. In: *Intracranial Aneurysms and Subarachnoid Haemorrhage*. Fields, W. S., and Sahs, A.L. Thomas, Springfield, Ill.

Arterial Embolism as a Cause of Hemiplegia after Subarachnoid Hemorrhage from Aneurysm

J. N. TAPTAS AND P. A. KATSIOTIS

Departments of Neurosurgery and Radiology, Saint Savas Hospital, Athens (Greece)

Hemiplegia after subarachnoid bleeding is said to be due to an intracerebral hematoma or an arterial spasm. Angiography in these cases, a routine procedure, will generally demonstrate the cause of the hemorrhage as well as that of the neurological disorders.

Segmental narrowing of arterial lumen is evident in most aneurysmal subarachnoid haemorrhage and is attributed to arterial spasm. Such arterial images, single or multiple, are usually localised on the principal arterial trunks and are no more observed a few weeks after the bleeding. The aneurysm itself, as known, may not be injected during angiography.

Mechanism of arterial spasm is not clear: irritation of the arterial wall due to extravasated blood, meningeal reaction to subarachnoid hemorrhage or humoral modifications (serotonine secretion) have all been invoked but not proved.

Paretic neurological disorders after subarachnoid haemorrhage cannot often be attributed to an hematoma. Norlén and Barnum[3] found no hematoma in 7 out of 10 patients in whom the only evident abnormality on angiography was arterial spasm or absence of injection of a cerebral arterial branch. Whether arterial spasm alone is the cause of neurological disorders after subarachnoid hemorrhage from aneurysm is not clear. It is known[2] that patients over 55 do not generally present arterial spasm after subarachnoid bleeding and thus Taveras and Wood[4] consider that spasm alone cannot explain ischemic cerebral accidents.

In our opinion a possible cause of neurological accidents after subarachnoid bleeding is thromboembolisation originating from blood clot at the site of the aneurysm which has bled. The following case favors such a pathogenesis. In a patient who developed right hemiplegia with aphasia 15 days after a subarachnoid hemorrhage, left carotid arteriography three days after the appearance of hemiplegia showed a round filling defect in the carotid just above the origin of the posterior communicating artery (Fig. 1), multiple arterial spasm, a slowing-down of the circulation in the temporo-occipital region and delayed filling of the inferior branch of the angulary artery. The filling defect was evident on three planes. On a second series of angiographs, twenty days later, the defect and the arterial spasms had disappeared and the inferior branch of the angular artery was filled normally, while at the same time the hemiplegia and the aphasia had already started to regress. The aneurysm itself could not be filled until $2\frac{1}{2}$ months later a third series of angiographs showed, specially on oblique

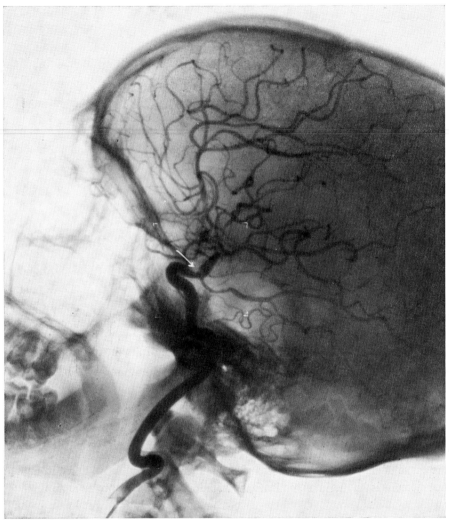

Fig. 1. Filling defect in the internal carotid artery.

projection, the neck of the aneurysm at the site of the endarterial filling defect (Fig. 2). The filling defect seen in three planes probably represented a clot obstructing the aneurysm and its neck, and we thought that the hemiplegia was thus due to arterial embolism.

Few works have been published about angiography in cerebral embolisation and generally concern extracranial causes of embolism. In such cases delayed injection of arterial branches was noted as a result of obstruction due to emboli. Slowing of cerebral circulation in case of arterial spasm is known. Recanalisation of an obstructed arterial branch has also been observed in patients having presented cerebral accidents after extracranial embolism[1].

The fact that spasm of cerebral arteries cannot be provoked experimentally except by direct mechanical irritation of the vessel, or by impact of a solid embolus in the

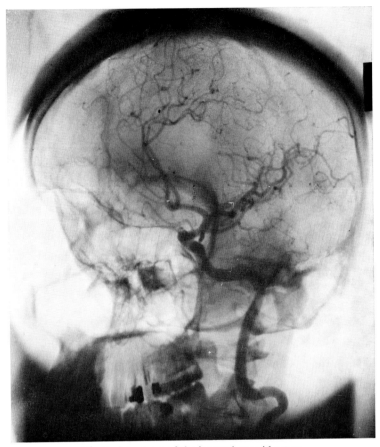

Fig. 2. Aneurysm of the internal carotid artery.

artery, permits to advance the hypothesis that the arterial narrowing observed after aneurysmal hemorrhage may be due to microembolism originating from blood clot formed in the burst aneurysm. This mechanism in case of controlateral spasm would only be possible with aneurysms below the circle of Willis, below or at the level of the bifurcation of the internal carotid. The failure of filling of a distal branch, such as the inferior branch of the angular artery in our case, is difficult to explain on the basis of spasm, such a hemodynamic phenomenon is better explicable by an embolic mechanism. The process of embolism would equally explain certain hemiplegias which sometimes supervene several days after successful operation for intracranial aneurysm. In cases without cerebral hematoma these postoperative neurological complications are also usually attributed to spasm.

In conclusion, it is felt that the angiographic study of the case presented, allows to attribute the onset of hemiplegia two weeks after subarachnoid haemorrhage to arterial embolism, and that embolism or microembolism could be the cause of neuro-logical complications after haemorrhage from an aneurysm, or after an operation for intracranial aneurysm in cases where no cerebral hematoma exists. As far as the

References p. 360

authors know, such a pathogenesis has not hitherto been considered. The segmental narrowing of arteries so often observed in angiograms after aneurysmal subarachnoid bleeding, and the failing of filling of a distal branch, could also be the arteriographic expression of microembolism originating from thrombus in the burst aneurysm.

REFERENCES

1. DALAL, P., SHAH, M. ET AIYAR, R. R. (1965) Les données de l'artériographie dans l'embolie cérébrale. *Lancet*, **1**, 358–361.
2. FLECHTER, T. M., TAVERAS, J. M., AND POOL, J.-L., (1959); Cerebral vaso-spasm in angiography for intracranial aneurysms. *Arch. Neur.*, **1**, 38–47.
3. NORLÉN, G. AND BARNUM, A. S. (1953) Surgical treatment of aneurysms of the anterior communicating artery. *J. Neurosurg.*, **10**, 634–650.
4. TAVERAS, J. M. AND WOOD, E. H. (1964) *Diagnostic neuroradiology*. Williams and Wilkins Co., Baltimore, pp. 1684–1691.

Reinforcement of Intracranial Aneurysms with Adherent Plastics: Selverstone Method

LUCJAN STEPIEN

Warsaw (Poland)

Some cases of the intracranial aneurysms cannot be treated classically by ligation or clipping of the neck of the sac. In many aneurysms of the anterior communicating and middle cerebral arteries one is faced with the necessity of ligating the parent vessel or wrapping it in a bit of muscle or gauze, hoping that a fibrous perivascular capsule would occur. However, it is well known that recurrent hemorrhage is most often to occur within two or three weeks after the first. Therefore many investigations have been undertaken in order to devise a reliable method for immediate protection of the aneurysm without impairment of the blood supply of the brain.

The reinforcement of the walls of intracranial aneurysms with adherent plastics was first suggested by Selverstone, and the technique developed and presented at the meeting of the American College of Surgeons in 1957 (Selverstone and Ronis, 1958). Since that time, the Selverstone method has been used with great success in the treatment of intracranial aneurysms (Selverstone, 1961; 1962), in experimental arterial surgery (Selverstone *et al.*, 1962) and for reinforcement in the course of the great vessels (Collow *et al.*, 1962).

Synthetic materials to be applied to the arterial wall must fulfill certain criteria.

1. The materials should adhere intimately to the moist surface leaving no dead space between the material and the adventitia of the aneurysm.

2. The materials should be nontoxic systemically and should not provoke undue tissue reaction nor induce intravascular thrombosis.

3. Reinforcement of the aneurysm should be produced directly by the materials, and should not depend upon a delayed fibrotic tissue reaction.

4. To minimize danger of erosion of the vessel wall the materials should be flexible and permit retention of the elasticity of the underlying vessel.

After testing a large number of synthetic materials Selverstone and Ronis (1958) selected an artificial latex of *polyvinyl-polyvinylidene chloride copolymer* (PVC) and an *epoxy-polyamide, 2-component resin* (EP). The PVC is dispersed in water in the form of spherules, 0.2 micron in diameter. Upon evaporation of the water, polymerization takes place, to form a dry, transparent, waterproof film. This film adheres so intimately to the aneurysm, that it cannot be removed without taking the adventitia with it. PVC alone does not provide an adequate protection against rupture of the aneurysm. Therefore, the thin coat of PVC is reinforced by the second layer of the EP resin.

The polymerization of the second coat proceeds in 45 minutes and the resulting coat is nontoxic, insoluble, dimensionally stable, flexible and does not rupture by the pressure even higher than 1,000 mm Hg.

We are especially grateful to Professor Bertram Selverstone who kindly operated with us the first two patients and who is sending us generously the necessary plastic materials.

TECHNIQUE

The aneurysm is explored in routine fashion without preliminary exposure of the internal carotid artery in the neck. Intravenous urea, hyperventilation and lumbar drainage of cerebro-spinal fluid is usually used. The aneurysm as well as portions of the vessel leading to and from the aneurysmal sac are exposed completely. We believe that exposure of the aneurysm by removal of the adjacent, usually softened and hemorrhagic brain tissue and preservation of the arachnoid overlying the vessel and the aneurysmal sac is an important aspect of this technique and constitutes a good protection against the bleeding. In fact, extreme care is taken not to retract the aneurysm nor to manipulate vessels leading into the area so that rupture of the aneurysm very seldom occurs and a minimum of vascular spasm is produced.

Using an artist's hairbrush the aneurysm and adjacent vessels are then coated with the artificial latex PVC. This first coat should be as thin as possible, in order to insure its uniform adherence to the aneurysm and vessels. After one or two minutes the first coat is reinforced with the EP resin. Reasonable firmness is attained within 45 minutes although several hours are required for full polymerization. As soon as the aneurysm has been coated, one may close the incision in routine fashion while the polymerization proceeds.

RESULTS

From September 1965 until the date of this presentation, the technique described above has been employed in 35 cases, as shown in Fig. 1.

ANEURYSMS TREATED BY COATING WITH ADHERENT PLASTICS

Internal carotid	11
Anterior commun.	1
Anterior cerebral	1
Middle cerebral	9
Total	35
Males	21
Females	14

Fig. 1.

There were 11 cases of internal carotid, 14 of anterior communicating, 1 of anterior cerebral and 9 of middle cerebral aneurysms. There were 21 males and 14 females.

The age of our patients varied from 11 to 62 years.

TABLE I

NEUROLOGICAL CHANGES

	No changes	Meningeal signs	Papill-edema	Paralysis III n.	Hemiparesis	Hemi-anesthesia	Aphasia	Uncon-sciousness	Total
Internal carotid	2	4	1		4			1	11
Anterior communic.	1	9	3	4	4		2	1	14
Anterior cerebral			1						1
Middle cerebral	2	4	1	3	4	3			9
Total	5	17	6	7	12	3	2	2	35

References p. 365

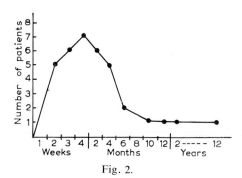

Fig. 2.

TABLE II

RESULTS

Vessel	Excellent	Good	Death	Total
Internal carotid	5	4	2	11
Anterior communic.	13	—	1	14
Anterior cerebral	1	—	—	1
Middel cerebral	7	2	—	9
Total	26	6	3	35

The interval between the first bleeding and operation varied from 2 weeks to 12 years, the majority being between 2 weeks and 4 months. In 21 cases there was only one and in 14 patients two and more bleedings before operation.

Table I summarizes the chief neurological symptoms which were found before operation. In 5 patients no neurological changes were found and in 17 other only meningeal signs were present. More or less pronounced hemiparesis was revealed in 12 cases, oculomotor paralysis in 7, papilledema in 6, hemianesthesia in 3, aphasia in 2 and unconsciousness in 2 patients.

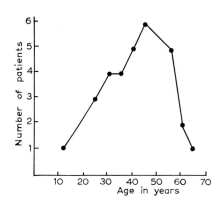

Fig. 3.

The operative results (Table II) after coating the aneurysms with adherent plastics are excellent in 26 patients — all of them were neurologically intact after operation. In 6 patients with pronounced neurological deficit before operation quick improvement was observed after coating of the aneurysms. The results may be classified as good.

There were 3 postoperative deaths in our series. One patient died three days after coating internal carotid aneurysm because of rupture of the second aneurysm on the middle cerebral artery. The second patient with the aneurysm on the internal carotid artery and with general arteriosclerosis died 4 days after operation because of cerebral edema. The third patient with the aneurysm on the anterior communicating artery died 3 weeks after operation because of severe bronchopneumonia.

In concluding we would like to say that reinforcement of intracranial aneurysms with adherent plastics modo Selverstone enlarged the field of intracranial vascular surgery and permits us to approach certain aneurysms that heretofore have been rejected. This technique is especially useful in the treatment of anterior communicating and middle cerebral artery aneurysms.

REFERENCES

SELVERSTONE, B., (1961); Treatment of intracranial aneurysms with adherent plastics. *Clinical Neurosurgery*, **9**, (Proc., Congr. Neurol. Surg., New York), Williams and Wilkins, Baltimore.

—, (1962); Aneurysms at middle cerebral "trifurcation": treatment with adherent plastics. *J. Neurosurg.*, **19**, 884–888.

SELVERSTONE, B., AND RONIS, N., (1958); Coating and reinforcement of intracranial aneurysms with synthetic resins. *Bull. Tufts-New Engl. med. Cent.*, **4**, 8–12.

—, DEHGHAN, R., RONIS, N., DETERLING, R. A., Jr., AND CALLOW, A. D., (1962); Adherent synthetic resins in experimental arterial surgery. *Arch. Surg. (Chic.)*, **84**, 80–84.

Methods of Circulatory Arrest

F. JOHN GILLINGHAM

University of Edinburgh (Scotland)

The operative ablation of a ruptured intracranial aneurysm must be carried out during the first seven days after the haemorrhage if recurrence with increased mortality and morbidity is to be prevented. A few patients will bleed again before the seventh day but most aneurysms rupture again between the seventh and twenty-first day of the first episode. Unfortunately successful operative treatment is not easy to achieve in this relatively acute stage and the complexity of management as regards the type and timing of operation and selection of patients is well borne out by the mass of literature accumulating on this subject.

In my own experience over the period 1950 to 1965 about half the patients with ruptured intracranial aneurysms who are admitted following a major intracranial haemorrhage have had a clear-cut minor episode with the onset of sudden severe nuchal pain or headache, usually without loss of consciousness, a few days or weeks before. It is also quite clear that operative treatment within a few days of this minor episode whilst the patient is alert, without significant intellectual or neurological deficit and only suffering from meningism, is associated with a low mortality and morbidity in spite of being within the relatively acute stage. Yet operative treatment in the drowsy or stuporose patient is associated with a high mortality and morbidity (Gillingham, 1958; Tables I, II and III).

There are unfortunately other factors which influence the success of operative treatment. The size of the sac, its site and anatomical relationships, the physiological age of the patient and the state of his cardio-vascular system and of his cerebral blood vessels, the tendency to cerebral arterial spasm and the presence of atheroma, and finally the experience of the surgeon and his team and that of the neuro-radiologist who has brought to the surgeon all the information he requires without risk to the

TABLE I

ASSESSMENT OF OPERATIVE RISK
(Botterell)

Grade One	Conscious with/without meningism
Grade Two	Drowsy, without neurological deficit
Grade Three	Drowsy, with neurological deficit
Grade Four	Major deficit, with deterioration
Grade Five	Near moribund patient

References p. 376

TABLE II

POLICY OF SURGICAL MANAGEMENT OF RUPTURED INTRACRANIAL ANEURYSMS
1950–65

1950–1952 Morbidity and mortality very low. (Gillingham, 1958)	Definitive surgery of aneurysmal sac or carotid ligation in the neck more than three weeks after haemorrhage. Grade One. No hypothermia.
1952–1954 Early morbidity and mortality very high.	Immediate angiography and operation in all patients. Grade One to Grade Five. No hypothermia.
1954–1965 Morbidity and early mortality low.	Immediate angiography and operation within a few hours if patient alert and without neurological deficit (Grade One). Definitive surgical treatment of sac otherwise delayed until patient alert and with minimal deficit taking the calculated risk of a recurrent haemorrhage. Angiography used early only if spasm less likely and clot suspected (*e.g.* hemiparesis, field defect, pineal shift, lateral shift on echo encephalogram). Evacuation of clot and ventricular drainage of hydrocephalus to speed up recovery if indicated. No hypothermia.

TABLE III

(a) SURGICAL MANAGEMENT OF ANTERIOR COMMUNICATING ANEURYSMS 1950–65
TOTAL = 64 (7 CASES OF MULTIPLE ANEURYSMS EXCLUDED)
Correlation of operative results with operation risk (Botterell)

Grade	No.	Result				
					Deaths	
		Early return to full activity	Modified activity	Major deficit Invalid	Early (months)	Late (years)
One	33	26	3	0	4	2
Two	19	8	1	3	7	1
Three	9	4	1	1	3	2
Four/Five	3	0	0	0	3	0

TOTAL OPERATIVE MORTALITY 17/64

patient. With all these factors influencing decision it is difficult to carry out statistically sound controlled studies and relate the results of the method of treatment compared with another or those of one group of surgeons with another. Much will depend upon interpretation of results after analysis in depth and in those patients who die it is essential to perform careful autopsy studies to help to determine the exact cause of failure of the method.

With this background we have approached the appraisal of the various ancillary methods which theoretically at any rate might improve the surgical treatment of ruptured aneurysm, in particular circulatory arrest or elective profound hypotension. One of the main problems of operative technique is the definition of the aneurysmal neck without rupture of the sac, particularly in the early days after rupture. Sudden

(b) SURGICAL MANAGEMENT OF MIDDLE CEREBRAL ANEURYSMS 1950–65
TOTAL = 56 (4 CASES OF MULTIPLE ANEURYSMS EXCLUDED)
Correlation of operative results with operation risk (Botterell)

Grade	No.	Result			Deaths	
		Early return to full activity	Modified activity	Major deficit Invalid	Early	Late
One	27	23	1	(←2) 3	0	4
Two	6	5	1	0	0	1
Three	19	5	10	1	3	1
Four/Five	4	0	(←1) 1	(←1) 1	2	0

(←) Improving on a long-term basis.

(c) SURGICAL MANAGEMENT OF ANEURYSMS OF THE INTERNAL CAROTID ARTERY
1950–65
(POSTERIOR COMMUNICATING AND ANTERIOR CHOROIDAL)
Total = 58.

Grade	No.	Haematoma	Spasm	Result			Deaths	
				Early return to full activity	Modified Activity	Major deficit Invalid	Early	Late
One	30	–	2	26 ←———(1) (1)———→		1	2	1
Two	13	1	1	10	–	1	2	2
Three	14	2	4	7 (1)———→	1	3	3	2
Four/Five	1	1	1	–	–	1	0	0

(d) COMPARISON OF DIRECT APPROACH AND COMMON CAROTID LIGATION
(INTERNAL CAROTID AND POSTERIOR COMMUNICATING OR
ANTERIOR CHOROIDAL JUNCTION ANEURYSMS)
CRANIOTOMY – DIRECT APPROACH

Grade	No.	Early return to full activities	Return to modified activities	Disabled	Early Deaths	Late Deaths
One	3	1	1	–	1	–
Two	3	2	–	–	1	2
Three	4	2	–	1	1	–

COMMON CAROTID LIGATION

Grade	No.	Early return to full activities	Return to modified activities	Disabled	Early Deaths	Late Deaths
One	27	25	–	1	1	1
Two	10	8	–	1	1	–
Three	10	5	1	2	2	2

major bleeding which follows obscures the field and tempts the surgeon to be inaccurate and rough. Because of continuing bleeding there is a rapid ischaemia of the territory of supply of the artery involved. Traction of the striate vessels or accidental occlusion of them or of major vessels add to this ischaemia resulting in morbidity or mortality. Moderate hypotension by reducing the blood pressure to 60 or 80 mm Hg either with or without moderate hypothermia employing arteriotomy (Gardiner, 1946; Gillingham, 1953) or Arfonad, or Halothane, has been used in most neurosurgical departments during the past fifteen years. Providing it is used during the approach to the sac in a fit patient who is alert before operation and there is no undue retraction it is usually safe and helpful. It is however somewhat uncontrollable and the restoration of the normal pressure sometimes slow. Moderate hypothermia is of less proven value and profound hypothermia carries a high mortality. Small and Stephenson (1964) and Obrador (1965) reported the combination of moderate hypothermia with occlusion of the venae cavae and aorta through a thoracotomy with total interruption of the circulation for eight to ten minutes. The results were encouraging and although attractive in some ways the addition of major chest surgery raised doubts about its broad application. More recently Small et al. (1966) replaced this method by one using the cardiac pacemaker for producing profound and easily reversible hypotension. Because the circulation is virtually arrested during cardiac pacing to between 200 and 250 pulses per minute, only four to six minutes of profound hypotension to 20 to 30 mmHg could be regarded as reasonably safe in a normal individual and about half that time in a patient suffering from recent ischaemia of the diencephalon following ruptured aneurysm. This now appeared to be a considerable step forward and from July 1965 we began a study of the method in selected patients in whom the operative risk was increased because of a large sac or one with particularly difficult anatomical relationships.

The team consisted of three surgeons who carried out the operative procedures, two anaesthetists, two cardio-physiologists and a biochemist.

The technique used is as follows:

Premedication is with Chlorpromazine 25 mg. Following induction and intubation with thiopentone and succinyl choline, anaesthesia is maintained with nitrous oxide and oxygen supplemented by phenoperidine and curare. Ventilation is controlled throughout using intermittent positive negative pressure ventilation. 550 ml of 25% mannitol is employed as an osmotic diuretic to reduce intracranial bulk.

Intra-arterial and venous pressure lines are inserted into the femoral artery and vein and connected to their recorders, and the electrocardiogram connected. A cardiac pace-maker electrode is inserted into the antecubital vein in the right arm and directed under fluoroscopy into the apex of the right ventricle and wedged there. The electrode is connected to the pace-maker and its action tested. Meantime cooling has begun using heat exchanger blankets. The patient is now transferred to the operating theatre. The craniotomy and exposure of the aneurysm are begun. During the final approach to the aneurysm the surgeon will decide whether hypotension will be needed or not, and the cardiologist and anaesthetist informed. A maximum of four minutes profound hypotension is considered reasonable, and six minutes the maximum permitted time. Thus the surgeon has a very limited time during which he must complete the critical part of the operation.

Hypotension can be produced immediately to aid the final approach to the neck of the sac and its safe dissection or a full definition of the sac if it is necessary. It is unwise as will be seen from the analysis of the results to wait until the sac has ruptured before hypotension is induced (Table III, a, b, c). Yet the temptation is to wait for as long as possible in view of the short period of hypotension available. Good timing allows rapid fall in the tension of the sac, easier dissection, much less risk of rupture and the opportunity to clip or ligate the neck of the sac with less risk of tearing it. If necessary the blood pressure can be restored within seconds if time is running out and lowered again after a few minutes, although the safe interval has not yet been determined.

In fourteen patients pacing was carried out for periods of up to four minutes using a unipolar electrode catheter under moderate hypothermia of an average temperature of 31°F. Pulses of 2–6 V and 2 msec duration were used. Electro-cardiogram, arterial and venous pressures were monitored and blood samples were taken for pH, pCO_2 and oxygen saturation. The ease with which pressure may be lowered is variable and probably depends on such factors as depth of anaesthesia, hypothermia and the state of electrolyte balance. At rates varying from 240 to 400 beats per minute ventricular fibrillation may be produced resulting in circulatory arrest and requiring external massage and defibrillation. This occurred in four patients. With avoidance of acidosis and of excessive hypothermia however, arterial blood pressure may be lowered to 30–35 mmHg for several minutes without producing ventricular fibrillation: at that pressure mixed venous oxygen saturation remained as high as 60–65 per cent, indicating overall adequate body perfusion.

In two patients atrial fibrillation occurred followed pacemaking; one of these reverted spontaneously to sinus rhythm while the other was converted to sinus rhythm by synchronised defibrillation. No other adverse cardiac sequelae were encountered.

Cardiac pacing was not employed in four patients because it was felt during the final exposure of the aneurysm that hypotension would not be required. In the remaining fourteen it was used on ten occasions to control haemorrhage and on the other four as a precautionary measure during the final dissection and definition of the aneurysm and to facilitate its clipping and/or wrapping.

The first six patients in the series were ventilated mechanically but no attempt was made to keep the PaCO$_2$ within normal limits. A level of 23 to 27 mm Hg was accepted as satisfactory. The arterial pH at body temperature was kept in the range of 7.38 to 7.52 by the addition of bicarbonate to the intravenous infusion. The volume required varied between 150 and 300 mequiv. One patient did not have cardiac pacing employed and no arrhythmia occurred. Of these six, one and of the remaining eight who were paced, three developed ventricular fibrillation after two to four minutes ventricular stimulation. Closed cardiac massage was used to maintain the circulation. All reverted to normal rhythm by the use of the external cardiac defibrillator.

In the remaining patients the $PaCO_2$ was adjusted to fall in the range of 35 to 40 mmHg at body temperature by the addition of the appropriate quantity of carbon dioxide to the inspired gas mixture. CO_2 was estimated by respiratory end tidal sampling and simultaneously in the laboratory by arterial sampling. There was close agreement between both methods of estimation. Arterial pH was corrected as required by the injection of sodium bicarbonate. When the pCO_2 was kept within the normal range the quantity of bicarbonate required was from 50 to 100 mequiv. Only one patient has had ventricular fibrillation since CO_2 levels have been controlled.

The addition of carbon dioxide to the inspired gas mixture controlled as indicated above has no significant effect on the intracranial pressure or on brain volume, or on its apparent vascularity. It does prevent peripheral vasoconstriction at low temperature so that cooling and rewarming are facilitated. Pooling of cold blood in the extremities is avoided and with it the development of metabolic acidosis from this cause.

The results of operative treatment of ruptured intracranial aneurysms during the period July 1st 1965 to July 31st 1966 are shown in Table IV, a, b, c. Only those aneurysms treated intracranially were included. The numbers are too small and the variables too great to be of significance in determining whether elective profound hypotension is of value, particularly when one bears in mind the relatively encouraging results shown in Table III, a, b, c, d.

TABLE IV

(a) ANTERIOR COMMUNICATING ANEURYSMS
ELECTIVE HYPOTENSION USING PACEMAKER, WITH OR WITHOUT VENTRICULAR FIBRILLATION
Total = 6

Operation Risk:			Result of Operation:			
Good	Fair	Poor	Return to normal activities	Slightly reduced activities, improving	Disabled	Dead
4	2	0	2	2	1	1

Good Risk = Botterell Grade One. No evidence of cerebral or cardio-vascular disease. Under age 60. Aneurysmal sac of size less than 8 × 6 × 6 mm. No evidence of multiple aneurysms.
Fair Risk = Botterell, Grade Two. Minimal cerebral or cardio-vascular disease. Under 60. Aneurysmal sac of size less than 10 × 6 × 6 mm. No evidence of multiple aneurysms.
Poor Risk = Botterell Grades Three to Five. Definite cerebral or cardio-vascular disease. Over 60. Aneurysmal sac of size more than 10 × 8 × 8 mm. Multiple Aneurysms.

Standard Operating Conditions (Pacemaker in situ in 2 but not used).
Total = 6

Operation Risk:			Result of Operation:			
Good	Fair	Poor	Return to normal activities	Slightly reduced activities, improving	Disabled	Dead
4	1	1	3	0	0	3

(b)
MIDDLE CEREBRAL ANEURYSMS
Elective Hypotension using Pacemaker with or without Ventricular Fibrillation.
Total = 6

Operation Risk:			Result of Operation:			
Good	Fair	Poor	Return to normal activities	Slightly reduced activities, improving	Disabled	Dead
1	4	1	1	2	2	2

Standard Operating Conditions (Pacemaker not inserted).
Total = 1

Operation Risk:			Result of Operation:			
Good	Fair	Poor	Return to normal activities	Slightly reduced activities, improving	Disabled	Dead
1	0	0	1	0	0	0

(c)
CAROTID { POSTERIOR COMMUNICATING / ANTERIOR CHOROIDAL } ANEURYSMS
Elective Hypotension using Pacemaker with or without Ventricular Fibrillation.
Total = 2

Operation Risk:			Result of Operation:			
Good	Fair	Poor	Return to normal activities	Slightly reduced activities, improving	Disabled	Dead
1	1	0	1	1	0	0

Standard Operating Conditions (Pacemaker in situ in 2 but not used).
Total = 4

Operation Risk:			Result of Operation:			
Good	Fair	Poor	Return to normal activities	Slightly reduced activities, improving	Disabled	Dead
1	2	1	0	2	1	1

References p. 376

However, two main features are apparent in the three groups of aneurysms studied. Firstly, that poor risk patients are better treated expectantly, no matter what ancillary aids are available. Secondly, that the whole group of middle cerebral aneurysms managed under hypotension fared badly and this is quite inconsistent with previous experience for they have proved to be the most amenable. It would suggest that other factors are playing a part in determining morbidity and mortality in this end-artery aneurysm when profound hypotension is employed. For example, disturbance of the autoregulating mechanisms by manipulation of the main trunk and branches of the middle cerebral artery with resulting spasm of the distal small branches (Haggendal, 1965). Under conditions of hypotension a contralateral facio-brachial monoparesis or monoplegia and associated sensory deficit with less obvious involvement of the lower limb would be expected and this is the pattern we have seen as a temporary or more permanent deficit. It was more evident in the poor and fair than in the good risk patient. For the same reason temporary clips on the major vessels would seem to be an unwise step. On the other hand, the anterior and posterior communicating aneurysms, lying as they do within the Circle of Willis and with better collateral supply, fare better and there is sufficient evidence that this method of profound hypotension should be given a more extensive trial in these lesions, especially if it is used during the final approach to the sac and its definition rather than after it has ruptured. Even so the time limit would seem to be ten minutes, possibly five, provided the patient is a good or fair risk for operation. As will be seen from Table V ventricular fibrillation should be avoided at all cost.

If ventricular fibrillation occurs, the venous pressure tends to rise and venous bleeding can be troublesome at a critical time during the operative procedure. Also when sinus rhythm is restored the blood pressure can rise suddenly to a high level and again obscure the field at a critical stage of the operation, with rupture of the aneurysm at the site of clip occlusion or ligation of the sac.

Of the two patients who died, one with a large middle cerebral aneurysm, and one with an anterior communicating aneurysm, both were subjected to prolonged hypotension for more than fifteen minutes, and required defibrillation and closed cardiac massage. The patient with the middle cerebral aneurysm was severly disabled and died

TABLE V

ELECTIVE HYPOTENSION WITH VENTRICULAR FIBRILLATION
3 Anterior Communicating and 1 Middle Cerebral Aneurysm
Total = 4

Operation Risk:			Result of Operation:			
Good	Fair	Poor	Return to normal activities	Slightly reduced activities, improving	Disabled	Dead
3 (Ant. Comm.)	1 (Mid. Cerebr.)	0	1 (Ant. Comm.)	1 (Ant. Comm.)	0	2

in one month of a recurrent haemorrhage (sac incompletely wrapped with cotton gauze) and the patient with the anterior communicating aneurysm died in a few days of widespread and severe cerebral ischaemia. Autopsy was performed in both instances.

Appraisal of the value of profound hypotension is also difficult because present techniques and instruments for dealing with aneurysmal sacs are still not perfected and their long-term value is only now being assessed. For example, almost every known clip has at some time opened up or been pushed off the sac by its pulsation and tension, some at operation and some after years and with recurrent bleeding. Ligation of the neck of the sac is a better technique but it involves more manipulation, takes longer and sometimes because of a broad neck or the presence of an atheromatous plaque at the neck, the major vessel is compromised by kinking or thrombosis. The long-term value of common carotid ligation in the neck is only now being fully assessed for aneurysms of the carotid artery and those anterior communicating aneurysms which fill from one side. Provided the operation is carried out carefully and after detailed assessment of the collateral circulation the long-term results are very reassuring (Table III,d).

SUMMARY

1. Ruptured intracranial aneurysm is best managed surgically as soon as possible after the first episode of bleeding to prevent recurrent haemorrhage, provided the patient is alert and without significant deficits. Under these conditions and without special ancillary techniques such as hypothermia and hypotension results are good except in those cases when the sac is large or has special difficulties of access.

2. Elective controlled hypotension employing the cardiac pacemaker is of value in certain instances.

ADVANTAGES OF TECHNIQUE

1. Provides a rapid controllable fall of blood pressure which can be reversed rapidly and which can be of value in certain types of aneurysms difficult to approach such as anterior or posterior communicating or basilar aneurysms.

2. The changes in blood pressure can be short and rapid and easily controlled.

DISADVANTAGES

1. Time-consuming, requiring a large team of skilled personnel who may not always be available.

2. The hypothermia and increased length of anaesthesia time may not be of benefit to the patient.

3. High ventricular rates and prolonged lowering of the blood pressure to 25 mmHg may produce ventricular fibrillation.

4. The safe working time for the surgeon to secure the aneurysm is very short,

and in the region of three to four minutes, but may be longer in the patient who is fully alert before operation.

5. A sudden drop in the cerebral blood flow which occurs in sudden hypotension may give rise to the 'watershed lesion' described by Meyer and by Zulch and Behrend, due to failure of vasodilatation and opening up of anastomotic channels.

6. The technique is inadvisable in the presence of ischaemic heart disease.

ACKNOWLEDGEMENTS

I would like to thank our anaesthetic colleagues in the Department of Surgical Neurology (Doctors Allan Brown and Jean Horton), Doctors Arthur H. Kitchin and J. Bath of the Department of Cardiology of the Western General Hospital who have been largely responsible for this study and have contributed sections of this paper. Dr. Christine G. Thomson of the Teaching and Research Unit of the Western General Hospital has been responsible for the biochemical studies. The surgical team consisted of the author, Mr. Phillip Harris and Mr. John Shaw, and I am grateful to them for their considerable contributions.

REFERENCES

GARDINER, W. J. (1946) *J. Amer. Med. Ass.*, **132**, 572–574.

GILLINGHAM, F. J. (1953) *Edin. Post. Grad. Lect. Med.*, **6**, 496–506.

GILLINGHAM, F. J. (1958) *Annals of Roy. Coll Surgeons Eng.*, **23**, 89–117.

L. HAGGENDAL, E. (1965) *Acta Neurologica Scandinavica*, Suppl. 14, 104–109.

MEYER, A. (1963) In: *Greenfield's Neuropathology*, 2nd ed., edited by R. M. Norman, ch. 4. London: Arnold.

OBRADOR, S. (1965) *Revista Clinica Espanola*, **97**, 1–4.

SMALL, J. M. AND STEPHENSON, S. C. F. (1966) *Lancet*, **1**, 570.

SMALL, J. M., STEPHENSON, S. C. F., CAMPKIN, T. V., DAVISON, P. H., AND McILVEEN, D. J. S., (1966) *Lancet*, **1**, 571.

ZULCH, K. J. AND BEHREND, R. C. H. (1961) In: *Cerebral Anoxia and the Electroencephalogram*, edited by J. F. Meyer and H. Gastaut, ch. 14. Illinois: Thomas.

Methods of Circulatory Arrest

KRISTIAN KRISTIANSEN

Oslo (Norway)

OFFICIAL DISCUSSION

Complications and catastrophies occurring during or after operations for saccular aneurysms, arteriovenous malformations and highly vascularized brain tumors are permanent neurosurgical problems. Preventive measures include controlled hypotension, partial or complete circulatory arrest and hypothermia techniques in different combinations. In spite of all experimental and laboratory work and of widespread clinical efforts there is still disagreement with regard to principal questions, the main reason being our limited knowledge of the reactions of the intracranial vessels to pathological conditions and stimuli. The amazing ability of the cerebral arteries to stop the hemorrhage from a ruptured aneurysm is unexplained, but it must depend upon reduction of local flow due to constriction of the wall of the feeding vessel, a reaction which is just what we need during a craniotomy. Socalled "arterial spasms" may on the other hand result in alarming consequences and seem to occur in a haphazard and uncontrolled fashion. Because we are not able to make use of the mechanisms guiding the behavior of the intracranial arteries, neurosurgeons have resorted to rather complicated and perhaps dangerous methods of circulatory arrest.

Since I have the honor of being the official discussor of the present subject I feel a sense of duty to draw attention to the negative aspects of the auxiliary procedures and raise the question of the justification of our methods of circulatory arrest. It is a moral obligation for those of us who have recommended or perhaps introduced debatable means to attain a goal, to reconsider the inherent difficulties and risks.

The complete arrest of brain circulation in combination with deep hypothermia requires as a rule major thoracic surgery and a prolonged systemic use of anticoagulants. The initial enthusiasm for this procedure seems to have diminished, although some reports from Japan give evidence of continued interest. Yonezawa (1964) stated that deep hypothermia can be achieved simply and safely without the use of extracorporeal circulation, but I have not been able to find details about his methods. Handa's paper (1964) on hemodilution and wash-out perfusion of the brain vessels and a bloodless operative field for $4\frac{3}{4}$ hours at a brain temperature of 15–25 degrees C is remarkable.

The selective profound brain cooling through carotid-carotid or femoral-carotid shunts (Kristiansen, 1964) is still an object for experimental research of which a recent

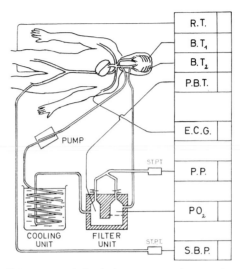

Fig. 1. Extracorporeal circulation system and types of recording.

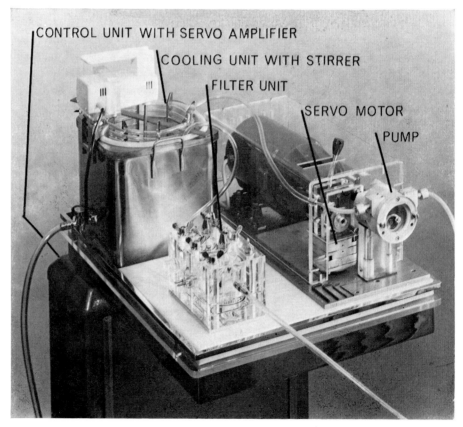

Fig. 2. Equipment for local brain cooling.

publication by Verdura *et al.* (1966) bears witness. This procedure demands cannulation of important arteries, extracorporeal circulation equipment and the use of heparin. If complete circulatory arrest is desirable a dissection of all the large vessels in the neck is necessary. Otha *et al.* (1966) have recommended another method of differential cooling of the brain to provide controlled profound hypotension but without complete arrest of brain circulation. Experiments have been reported where the exposed carotid arteries have been cooled with liquid nitrogen to obtain a selective brain hypothermia without cannulation of the arteries.

Our own method of selective brain cooling may be illustrated by a diagram (Fig. 1) showing the application of the extracorporeal circuit and the recordings.

The equipment necessary for the extracorporeal circulation is assembled on a movable stand (Fig. 2).

A considerable reduction in blood flow may, if required, be obtained by stopping the pump during the dissection of an aneurysmal sac. The duration of this incomplete circulatory arrest can be extended to 20–30 min or even more depending on the brain temperature level (Fig. 3).

Gött (1965) has reported his experience with a similar procedure. Marshall *et al.* (1964) and Dickinson *et al.* (1964) have recommended the use of this extracorporeal shunt as an aid in the surgical treatment of internal carotid stenosis by endarterectomy.

However, the added risks of the extracorporeal circulation have lately influenced our attitude. Since 1963 we have used selective cooling in only 6 patients whereas the method was applied in 27 cases before 1963.

During 1966, 40 patients were operated on for saccular aneurysms by direct intracranial approach without a single case of selective deep cooling. We used this method only in one patient with a large arteriovenous malformation.

I am somewhat afraid of temporary clamping of the intracranial arteries and prefer a slow dissection of the sac and, in case of rupture, direct suction on the sac to obtain

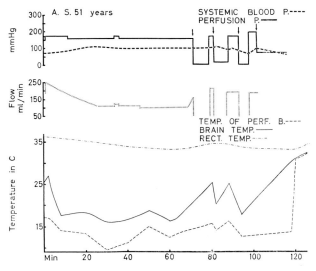

Fig. 3. Recordings from a patient. Arrows: Temporary arrest of extracorporeal circulation.

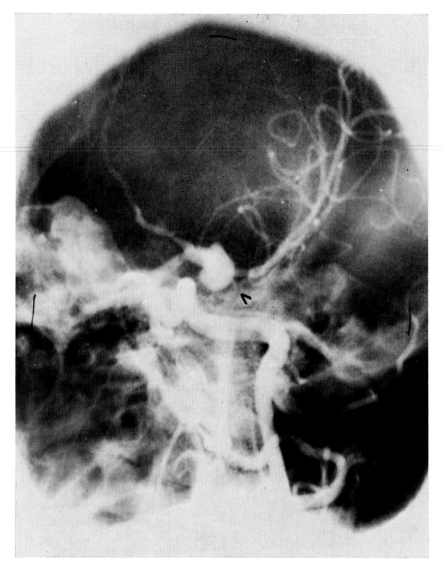

Fig. 4. Aneurysm of the most medial portion of the left middle cerebral artery.

a bloodless field. A complication due to the application of a temporary clamp occurred in a 49 year old woman who was admitted with a severe subarachnoid hemorrhage and a rightsided hemiparesis. The angiography showed a middle cerebral artery
aneurysm with a relatively rare location (Fig. 4). At operation the intracranial portion
of the carotid artery was found atherosclerotic. A Mayfield clip was placed temporarily
on the carotid artery and the neck of the aneurysm was occluded with a silver clip.
The postoperative angiogram showed a severe spasm in the middle cerebral artery
branches, and in addition a dissecting or false aneurysm on the carotid artery at the
site of the temporary clip (Fig. 5).

Le Beau *et al.* (1964) stated that a provisional clip may be the cause of postoperative

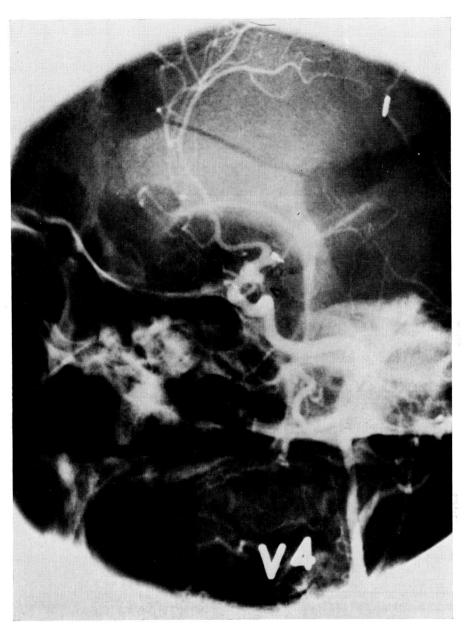

Fig. 5. Postoperative angiogram. False aneurysm at the site of temporary clamp.

infarction and in my opinion this possible complication must also be taken seriously into consideration.

The use of moderate hypothermia combined with an intraventricular cardiac pacemaker to induce a profound hypotension has been suggested by Small *et al.* (1966). Gillingham deserves credit for having taken up this method for further evaluation. To obtain a completely bloodless field ventricular fibrillation is required.

With modern synchronized equipment it may be possible to initiate and to discontinue this condition as required, but the time limitation of the circulatory arrest at moderate hypothermia is unavoidable. I have discussed this method with our cardiologists who are afraid of "pacing an old heart". The average age of our 40 operated patients in 1966 was 46 years and 15 of them were more than 50 years of age. In my opinion this method of circulatory arrest may be too hazardous in just the group of patients where auxiliary methods may be most desirable.

A completely different approach to the problem is the research on circulatory arrest under hyperbaric condition. Fasano and his collaborators have made an important experimental contribution which may give a fresh stimulus to further clinical investigations as indicated by Ingvar and Lassen in 1965. The combination of hyperbaric oxygen with a reduced cerebral blood flow or an incomplete circulatory arrest may be the next step in our attempt to improve the results of treatment of intracranial aneurysms, a problem that according to a leading article in The Lancet (1966) "remains to be solved again and again — and again".

I would like to finish with a slide showing the picture of an arteriovenous malformation hanging in my office. It is an original drawing by Miss Codding for Cushing and Bailey's book on tumors arising from the blood vessels of the brain from 1928. The picture carries an inscription from one of Cushing's successors Donald Matson: "Before hypothermia" — as a memento to apply sound surgical judgement with regard to ancillary methods. A meticulous approach, gentle handling of the intracranial structures, personal skill and experience reduce the number of cases which have to be submitted to the inevitable hazards of temporary circulatory arrest.

REFERENCES

CUSHING, H., AND BAILEY, P., (1928) *Tumors arising from the blood vessels of the brain. Angiomatous malformations and hemangioblastomas*. Baillière, Tindall and Cox, London.

DICKINSON, P. H., HANKINSON, J. AND MARSHALL, M. (1964) Internal carotid artery stenosis. *Brit. J. Surg.*, **51**, 703–709.

GÖTT U. (1965); Methodik und Erfahrungen mit der selektiven extrakorporalen Hirnkühlung für neurochirurgische Operationen. *Forts. Med.*, **83**, 943–945.

HANDA, H. (1964) Discussion. *Neurol. Med.-Chir.*, **6**, 200.

— (1966); Intracranial aneurysms. (Leading article.) *Lancet*, **I**, 581–582.

INGVAR, D. H. AND LASSEN, N. A. (1965) Treatment of focal cerebral ischemia with hyperbaric oxygen. *Acta Neurol. Scand.*, **41**, 92–93.

KRISTIANSEN, K. (1964) Physiopathology, Methods and clinical results of selective brain cooling. *Acta Neurochir.*, *Suppl. XIII*, 139–158.

LEBEAU, J., FONCIN, J. F. AND HANAU, J. (1965) Ramollissement et "oedème ischémique" du cerveau dans les ruptures des anévrismes intracraniens. *Ann. Chir.*, 1030–1049.

MARSHALL, M., HANKINSON, J. AND LESLIE, W. G. (1964) An extracorporeal circuit for unilateral brain perfusion and cooling. *Brit. J. Surg.*, **51**, 701–703.

OTHA, T., SAGARMINAGA, J. AND BALDWIN, M. (1966) Profound hypotension with differential cooling of the brain in dogs. *J. Neurosurg.*, **24**, 993–1001.

SMALL, J. M., STEPHENSON, S. C., CAMPKIN, T. V., DAVISON, P. H. AND MCILVEEN, D. J. S. (1966) Elective Circulatory Arrest by Artificial Pacemaker. *Lancet*, **I**, 570–572.

VERDURA, J., WHITE, R. J., AND ALBIN, M. S. (1966) Profound selective hypothermia and arrest of arterial circulation to the dog brain. *J. Neurosurg.*, **24**, 1002–1006.

YONEZAWA, T. (1964) Studies on deep hypothermia and permissible time of cerebral circulatory suspension. *Neurologia Medico-Chirurg.*, **6**, 199.

Arteriovenous Aneurysms of the Posterior Fossa

H. VERBIEST

Utrecht (The Netherlands)

Anatomically the posterior fossa is the intracranial space below the tentorium with its hiatus and above the level of the foramen magnum. Since estimating the localisation in patients is based on the roentgenological anatomy the greatest difficulty is experienced in cases of A.V.A. closely related to the tentorium, because the latter slopes downward laterally. Reuter *et al.* (1966) stress the importance of information obtained by analysing the position of the lesion relative to the venous sinuses. When on a lateral view it lies below a line drawn along the superior petrosal and transverse sinuses, it must be within the posterior fossa. Lesions which in the lateral view lie between this line and the straight sinus may be either supra- or infratentorial. In such cases an analysis of arterial supply, pneumography, and comparative studies of A.P. and lateral views may be helpful in establishing the exact localisation of the lesion. Transition forms of supra- and infratentorial A.V.A.'s may be presented by A.V.A.'s of the brainstem, the great vein of Galen, and some dural A.V.A.'s.

CLASSIFICATION OF POSTERIOR FOSSA A.V.A.'S

1. Intraparenchymatous A.V.A.
   - (a) cerebellar,
   - (b) pontine and/or bulbar,
   - (c) mixed forms.
2. Subarachnoid A.V.A.
   - (a) A.V.A. in cerebello-pontine cistern,
   - (b) some A.V.A.'s of the region of the vein of Galen. These are always transition forms, since the vein of Galen is localised supratentorially.
3. A.V.A. in the walls of the posterior fossa
   - (a) purely intradural A.V.A.,
   - (b) A.V.A. occupying all the layers of the wall of the posterior fossa.

CONCOMITANT ANOMALIES

These may be:
1. Persistance of fetal bloodvessels, or saccular aneurysms;
2. A.V.A. of the retina (Bonnet *et al.*, 1937, 1938; Olivecrona and Riives, 1948;

Wyburn, 1943) most frequently encountered in cases of A.V.A. of the brainstem, but also found in A.V.A.'s of cerebral or cerebellar hemispheres.

3. Association of retinal and brainstem A.V.A. with a facial naevus flammeus, bordering on the group of the phacomatoses.

Other accompanying lesions reported are: neurocutaneous syndromes, the so-called dysraphic disturbances and intracranial tumors, such as angiomas or gliomas. Extensive reference to this subject is given in Ley's monograph (1957).

In our personal series of 15 posterior fossa A.V.A.'s 4 patients had concomitant anomalies. One presented a bilateral cerebellar A.V.A., a round cell sarcoma in the occipital lobe, an occipital angioma, frontal meningeal sarcomatosis, thoracic kyphoscoliosis, a "monk cap" naevus and a cutaneous angioma in the area of the right scapula (Verbiest, 1961). Two other patients presenting a bulbopontine A.V.A. and an A.V.A. in the cerebellopontine cisterns resp. had an Arnold Chiari malformation.

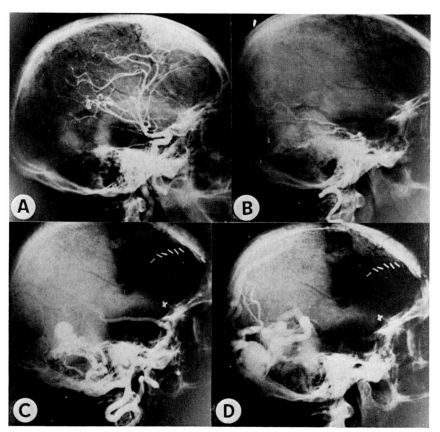

Fig. 1. A. Olfactory groove meningioma. Left internal carotid angiogram shows compression of carotid siphon and backward displacement of anterior cerebral artery. No filling of dural A.V.A. B. Same case. Left vertebral angiogram, no A.V.A. visualised. Note dilated groove of posterior meningeal artery. C. Same case. Left external carotid angiogram made 3 months after operative removal of olfactory groove meningioma shows A.V.A. supplied by posterior branch of middle meningeal and occipital arteries. D. Same case. Later phase of left external carotid angiogram.

In the 4th patient an intradural A.V.A. of the posterior fossa was associated with a meningioma of the olfactory groove (Fig. 1).

TYPES, SITES AND SYMPTOMATOLOGY OF POSTERIOR FOSSA A.V.A.

Besides the classification according to their localization in cerebellum, brainstem, or both, it is useful to define them on the basis of arterial supply and venous drainage. Laine *et al.* (1966) distinguish between proximal and distal cerebellar A.V.A.'s. The proximal forms are supplied by branches of the vertebro-basilar artery, whereas the distal lesions originate from ramifications of these branches. This distinction was

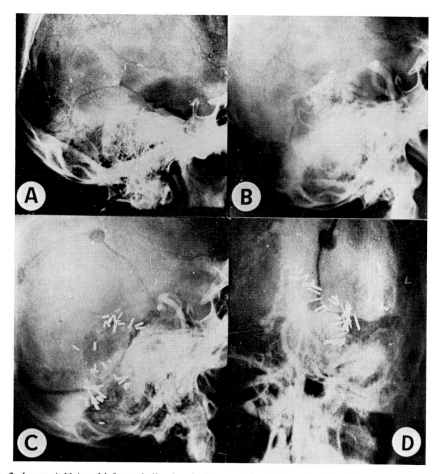

Fig. 2. Large A.V.A. of left cerebellar hemisphere and tentorium. A. Dilated groove of posterior meningeal artery. B. Vertebral angiogram demonstrating cerebellar A.V.A. The tentorial A.V.A. could not be visualized in the carotid and vertebral angiograms. C. Lateral view after excision of cerebellar A.V.A. by means of a combined suboccipital and transtentorial approach. D. A.P. view shows a residual abnormal vascular pattern in the midline area.

made because of certain particularities in their clinical picture and surgical accessibility. Draining vessels involved in posterior fossa A.V.A.'s may be: the galenic
draining group, the petrosal sinuses, the torcular, the straight and lateral sinuses.

Incidence

The first surgical treatment of a cerebellar A.V.A. was performed by Dandy (1928) in
1925. It consisted of posterior fossa decompression because of hydrocephalus and
ligation of the vertebral artery in a second stage, which resulted in some improvement.
The first excision of a cerebellar A.V.A. was performed by Olivecrona in 1932.
Because of a more systematic use of vertebral angiography an increasing number of
papers on preoperatively diagnosed A.V.A. of the posterior fossa, have appeared in
the past 15 years (for extensive references of literature see Krayenbühl and Yasargil,
1965; Pool and Potts, 1965; Verbiest, 1962).

The comparative frequency of posterior fossa and supratentorial A.V.A.'s is still
debatable. Krayenbühl and Yasargil (1958) collected from literature a number of
800 A.V.A.'s, supplied by either the carotid or vertebral arteries or by both. They
found that 6.2% was localized in the posterior fossa. In Laine's (1966) case material
it was 20%. Our personal case material consists of 61 supratentorial and 15 infratentorial A.V.A.'s, dural forms included, so that the infratentorial A.V.A.'s also
represent 20% of the material.

CLINICAL EVOLUTION

1. Intraparenchymatous posterior fossa A.V.A.

These lesions may present an acute or chronic clinical picture, an acute episode may
interrupt a chronic evolution. The acute manifestations are caused either by subarachnoid, cerebellar or brainstem hemorrhage. The development of a non-traumatic
acute subdural hematoma of the posterior fossa, as observed in one of our personal
cases of bilateral cerebellar A.V.A., is rare. Ciembroniewicz (1965) found only 6 cases
of non-traumatic subdural hematoma of the posterior fossa in literature but in all of
them the source of bleeding was obscure. Wright *et al.* (1965) reported one personal
case and one from literature where this hematoma was due to a ruptured posterior
fossa aneurysm. A clinical differentiation between cerebellar and pontine hemorrhage
is in many cases hardly possible. Their clinical pictures vary greatly and cerebellar
hemorrhages may be accompanied by symptoms of brainstem involvement. For this
reason it is important to apply all possible methods of examination, especially arteriography, to ensure the localization, since cases of cerebellar hemorrhage may sometimes
benefit from surgical treatment. In exceptional cases even surgical evacuation of a
pontine hemorrhage may be followed by good results, as was observed in one of our
patients, a girl of 11, who suddenly developed diplopia, followed in the next few days,
by disturbances of gait and left facial paralysis. She frequently vomited and after 1
week all eye movements were paralysed. Consciousness was normal. The pneumo-

encephalogram gave a picture of a pontine tumor with invasion of the 4th ventricle. Operation revealed a pontine hematoma bulging in the midline of the fossa rhomboidea over the whole length of the pons. The intrapontine clots were evacuated. The greatest lateral intrapontine extension was below the eminentia medialis. The wall of the hematoma showed hemangiomatous tissue, but no definite diagnosis could be made. Six months after operation there was only residual paresis of the left 6th and 7th cranial nerves.

A.V.A. with chronic clinical picture: Part of the patients have chronic complaints of headaches, migraine syndromes and trigeminal neuralgia without other apparent disturbances. They may be the prodromal symptoms preceding hemorrhage. Other cerebellar and brainstem A.V.A.'s give rise to slow, continuous or fluctuating, progressive neurological deficit. In addition these lesions may produce acute or chronic hydrocephalus.

The neurological picture of brainstem A.V.A.'s varies greatly, including involvement of cranial nerves, long tracts and cerebellar symptoms. Disturbance of ocular movement, nystagmus and Parinaud's syndrome are frequently present as well as mental disturbances.

Some, even large-sized, cerebellar A.V.A.'s produce few neurological symptoms. Others display signs and symptoms which cannot be attributed to their localization alone, such as bilateral cerebellar symptoms in unilateral cerebellar A.V.A., or pyramidal signs, hemihypesthesia, and cranial nerve deficit, the latter giving an impression of a bulbo-pontine process.

It is important to know that these entities exist, since as Laine and his collaborators (1966) rightly stress, the clinical picture not encouraging surgical intervention, some of such lesions can yet be removed with good results. The steadily progressive forms may give the clinical picture of a tumor. The intermittent or remittent forms must be differentiated from certain types of multiple sclerosis or vertebro-basilar insufficiency. In such cases the differential diagnosis should rely not only on details of semeiology but also on arteriography and, if necessary, on other neuroradiological procedures.

An objective or subjective bruit over the mastoid or occipital area is a valuable symptom. In literature it has been more frequently reported in the brainstem and Galenic than in the cerebellar A.V.A.'s.

2. Subarachnoid posterior fossa A.V.A.

(a) A.V.A. of the great vein of Galen

An excellent report on these lesions has recently been given by Gold *et al.* (1964), who collected 33 cases from literature and added 8 personal cases. They classified the patients in three age groups because of their characteristic differences in symptomatology. The symptomatic neonate presents signs of cardiomegaly and cardiac decompensation and, occasionally, of hydrocephalus. All but one of the cases reported died from cardiac failure and the remaining patient from meningitis. The infants invariably presented hydrocephalus and/or convulsions. Ten out of 19 children had an

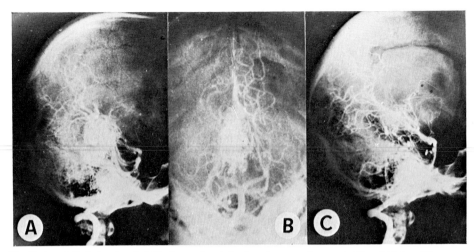

Fig. 3. A and B. Lateral and A.P. views of vertebral angiograms demonstrating A.V.A. of the upper vermis. C. Lateral vertebral angiogram following excision of A.V.A. by means of transtentorial approach.

intracranial bruit, and varying other symptoms such as i.a. cardiomegaly, psycho-motor retardation, pyramidal tract involvement. Of the older children and adults ten had a subarachnoid hemorrhage; they frequently complained of headaches and developed signs of long tracts and cranial nerves, ocular symptoms being present in 8 patients. The A.V.A. of the vein of Galen is a transitional, supra- and infratentorial, form. Although the shunt itself is located above the tentorium the supplying arteries and draining veins belong to either the supra- or infratentorial compartments or to both. Of the 41 patients collected by Gold *et al.* (1964) the vascular supply was un-

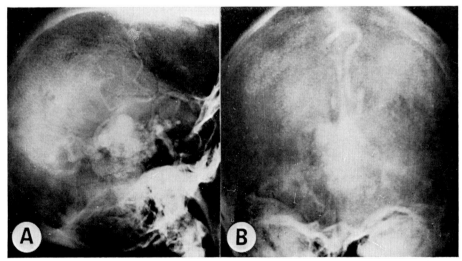

Fig. 4. A and B. Lateral and A.P. vertebral angiograms demonstrating A.V.A. of great vein of Galen, supplied by superior cerebellar arteries.

known in 4, pertained to the supratentorial compartment in 29, to both supra- and infratentorial space in 7 and in one only the supply came from the superior cerebellar artery alone. Additional cases and literature were reported by Gomez *et al.* (1963) and Lehman *et al.* (1966).

The only adult with mixed supra- and infratentorial arterial supply described in the literature was a patient of our personal series (Fig. 4). She was a 42 year old woman, who had been treated elsewhere under the diagnosis of multiple sclerosis because of temporal pallor of optic discs, diminished visual acuity, horizontal nystagmus to both sides, spastic atactic gait and increased tendon reflexes. Following a subarachnoid hemorrhage 3 months prior to admission she developed a paralysis of upward gaze, anisocoria and right-sided spastic hemiparesis. Arteriography revealed an A.V.A. of the vein of Galen supplied by the left posterior cerebral and both superior cerebellar arteries. In the patient's history there probably was another subarachnoid hemorrhage 19 years previously but this condition had not been recognized (Verbiest, 1961).

The occurrence of hydrocephalus in the A.V.A. of the vein of Galen may be due to mechanical obstruction of the aqueduct of Sylvius or increased intracranial venous pressure. The latter mechanism will be discussed under the paragraph on intradural A.V.A.

(b) A.V.A. in the cerebello-pontine cistern

It is generally accepted that the cerebello-pontine angle is a space bounded by the pons, the uppermost portion of the medulla oblongata, the anterior inferior surface of the cerebellum with the flocculus and brachium pontis, and the temporal bone. Only in cases where operation or autopsy has established that the A.V.A. is entirely or principally situated in the ponto-cerebellar cistern it should be classified as an A.V.A. of the cerebellopontine angle. In literature, however, this classification has also been applied to A.V.A.'s producing a pontine angle symptomatology unaccompanied by an exact description of their localization and even to cerebellar A.V.A.'s in which vascular loops cause traction upon the nerve roots in the pontine angle. So, for instance, Weersma's (1958) and Paterson's (1956) cases of cerebellar A.V.A. were classified by Dereux *et al.* (1960) as pontine angle A.V.A.'s. To our knowledge only 4 A.V.A.'s of the pontine angle have been described, which more or less answer to the criteria mentioned previously.

1. Bunts' case (1949): female of 36, subarachnoid hemorrhage, then right sided hemiparesis, hemihypalgesia, dysarthria, left sided paralysis of 6th and 7th cranial nerves and left Horner syndrome. Normal angiograms (!). Operation revealed A.V.A. in left pontine angle draining into superior petrous sinus.

2. Eisenbrey and Hegarty (1956): female of 30, trigeminal neuralgia for 20 years, then subarachnoid hemorrhage, deficit of 5th and 8th cranial nerves, diminished tendon reflexes of right arm and cerebellar symptoms. No further details concerning the location and draining of the A.V.A. were given. Vertebral angiography was performed after operation, and the picture reproduced in the author's paper leaves

some doubt whether the localization of the A.V.A. was restricted to the ponto-cerebellar angle.

3. Dereux *et al.* (1960): male of 45 with a 24 years history, starting with left sided dysesthesia and disturbance of equilibrium. Preoperative symptoms: left sided cerebellar symptoms, left hemihypalgesia, exaggerated left tendon reflexes, deficit of left 5th, 7th and 8th cranial nerves, disturbances of gait. No arteriography. Operative exploration reveals cystic arachnitis and tortuous vessels in left cerebello-pontine angle in area of 7th and 8th cranial nerves. Venous drainage not mentioned.

4. Verbiest (1962): female of 39, history of 1.5 years. Bifrontal headaches. Deficit of left 5th, 6th, 8th, 9th and 12th cranial nerves. Increased right tendon reflexes. Unsteady gait. Decalcification of left petrosal apex. No arteriography. Operative exploration revealed polycystic arachnitis in left cerebello-pontine angle and A.V.A. below 7th and 8th nerve roots, draining into abnormal dural venous sinuses. In this case the A.V.A. was complicated by an Arnold Chiari malformation.

In all 4 cases the diagnosis of A.V.A. was only made at operation. Occlusion of abnormal vessels resulted in worsening of the patient's condition in Bunts' case and considerable improvement in the cases of Dereux and Verbiest. The condition was not treated in Eisenbrey's patient, her neurological symptoms did not change during the one month follow-up, but she developed psychiatric disturbances.

3. A.V.A. in the wall of the posterior fossa

These lesions can be divided into:
(a) Pure dural A.V.A.; (b) Combined dural and cerebellar or pontine A.V.A.; (c) A.V.A. in more than one layer of the wall of the posterior fossa.

The angiographic finding of a posterior fossa A.V.A. exclusively filling from the external carotid artery is no proof of the lesion being localized in its wall. So, for instance, Ciminello and Sachs (1962) described an A.V.A. of the posterior fossa which was only supplied by the posterior meningeal and occipital arteries but the malformation was localized in the cerebellum.

(a) Pure dural A.V.A. of the posterior fossa
This group of anomalies in which the lesion is supplied by dural arteries and drained by dural veins and sinuses is very rare. The first descriptions of these lesions were published in 1951 by Fincher and by Verbiest. Fincher's case was a supratentorial, and ours a combined supra- and infratentorial dural A.V.A. From the scarce literature the distinction between the following 3 clinical forms can be made.

Dural A.V.A. producing hydrocephalus and an intracranial bruit. Our personal case (Verbiest, 1951) was a male of 54. Numerous arteries in the tentorium, occipital and suboccipital dura drained into the transverse sinus. The symptoms were pulsating bruit, vertigo, clonic jerks in homolateral foot, contralateral vestibular inexcitability and diminished hearing, which developed in the 4th month after a head injury. Besides, there was a hypertensive communicating hydrocephalus. The A.V.A. was not visualized in the carotid and vertebral angiograms. A similar case was described by Van der Werf (1964) in a child of 3. Symptoms: audible bruit and hypertensive hydrocephalus. The dural arteries drained into both transverse sinuses and the torcular. The A.V.A. was not visualized in the vertebral angiogram. The carotid angiogram showed supply by meningeal and transmastoid branches of the external carotid and a tentorial branch of the internal carotid. The operative report mentions only exposure of the supratentorial dura, the aspect of the dura is not described. The hypertensive hydrocephalus in both cases may be due to massive drainage of the dural arteries into the lateral sinuses with resulting increased venous pressure. A similar mechanism may be active in hydrocephalus accompanying an A.V.A. of the great vein of Galen.

Dural A.V.A. manifesting itself with repeated subarachnoid hemorrhages. Laine (1963) described a case in whom the only other symptom was a 3rd nerve paralysis. Pecker's (1965) patient, who had a mixed form, supplied by the occipital artery and meningeal branches of the vertebral artery, presented papilledema and bilateral 6th nerve paralysis. In Laine's case the subarachnoid hemorrhage probably arose in the subarachnoid portion of branches of the carotid and cerebellar arteries, which participated in the tentorial A.V.A. In Pecker's patient the hemorrhage might be due to rupture of a draining vein, crossing the cisterna magna and ending in venous convolutions on the posterior aspect of the medulla oblongata.

Dural A.V.A. presenting neurological deficit. This form was described by Laine (1963). The patient had repeated hemiplegias, the first two following a trauma, the third being spontaneous.

Other cases of dural posterior fossa A.V.A. have been published but the diagnoses were made on the arteriogram, no operations being performed (Obrador and Urquiza, 1952; Pool and Potts, 1965), or no descriptions of the operation given (Dilenge *et al.*, 1964).

A history of trauma preceding the onset of symptoms in a dural A.V.A. was reported in some of the cases (Fincher, 1951; Laine, 1963; Pakarinen, 1965; Verbiest, 1951).

Fontaine *et al.* (1957) believe that the trauma causes an enlargment of congenital arterio-venous shunts, so-called Sucquet's ducts, of the skull and dura mater.

(b) Combined intradural and cerebellar A.V.A.
Such a malformation was encountered in one of our patients (1961). A large left cerebellar A.V.A. was associated with a tentorial A.V.A. No direct vascular connections between both malformations were found (Fig. 2).

(c) A.V.A. in more than one layer of the wall of the posterior fossa
An impressive malformation involving the extracranial soft tissues, the petrosal bone and the dura was described by Tönnis (1936). During its radical removal it appeared that the malformation was supplied by the middle meningeal and occipital arteries. Röttgen (1937) described a case with similar vascular supply. A special group is formed by the communications between the occipital artery and the transverse sinus (Fontaine *et al.*, 1957; Newton and Greitz, 1966; Pecker *et al.*, 1966; Takehawa

and Holman, 1965; Verbiest, 1962; Van Wijngaarden and Vinken, 1966) (Fig. 5A). In most patients the only symptoms consisted of pulsating tinnitus and/or an audible bruit of sudden onset. In a few cases there were other symptoms such as attacks of vertigo, loss of hearing, fainting or transient symptoms pertaining to the ipsilateral

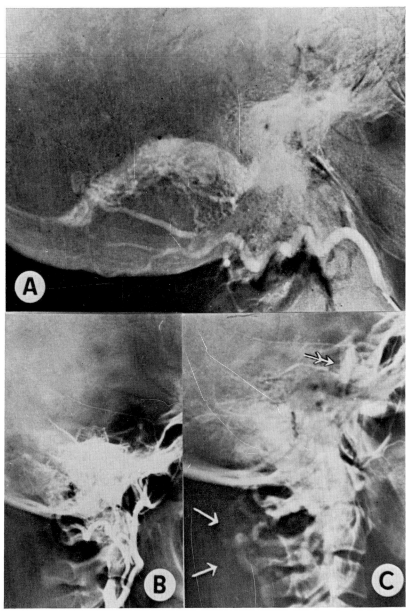

Fig. 5. A. Subtraction of angiogram of left occipital artery shows A.V.A. between occipital artery and transverse sinus. B and C. Other case. Phases of external carotid angiogram showing A.V.A. in posterior cervical muscles (→) and A.V. shunt to venous plexus of the clivus (→→). C is a subtraction picture.

hemisphere. Takehawa and Holman (1965) think that these communications result from connections between branches of the external carotid artery and the basal emissary veins. Very rare are connections between the external carotid artery and other venous sinuses of the posterior fossa, such as a communication between the occipital artery and the clivus plexus of veins described by Pool (1965). We had a similar case, which in addition presented an A.V.A. in the deep cervical muscles, supplied by the occipital artery (Fig. 5B and C) (Verbiest, in press).

RADIOLOGICAL DIAGNOSIS

Plain films of the skull may show alterations of vascular grooves, widened foramina, enlargement and/or erosion of the sella turcica, signs of hydrocephalus in infants and calcification in some cases of A.V.A. of the vein of Galen. Several cases reported had air studies because of a diagnosis of tumor. Pathological features in the pneumograms were communicating or obstructive hydrocephalus and filling defects in the 3rd and 4th ventricles or the basal cisterns caused by a mass or loops of abnormal vessels.

Arteriography is the most adequate diagnostic aid. For a surgical diagnosis selective angiography of the external and internal arteries and of both vertebral arteries is essential. Cerebellar A.V.A.'s may receive their supply from both carotid and vertebral arteries. Ciminello and Sachs (1962) described an A.V.A. of the vermis and right cerebellar hemisphere, which filled exclusively from the left external carotid circulation. In the supply of a dural A.V.A. may be participated by the internal carotid, posterior cerebral, vertebral and external carotid arteries.

The photographic subtraction technique of Ziedses des Plantes (1935) is a most valuable aid providing more detail information in the angiographic examination of posterior fossa A.V.A. A new development is the electronic subtraction (Holman and Bullard, 1963) using closed-circuit television. Its greatest advantages are: rapid technique, easy magnification of images and great possibilities for altering the over-all density or contrast features of the films. The videorecorder is another useful diagnostic aid.

OTHER DIAGNOSTIC TESTS

The experience with radioisotopic scanning in posterior fossa A.V.A.'s is very limited. In a personal case of A.V.A. between the occipital artery and the transverse sinus, where [^{197}Hg]Neohydrine was applied, no reliable information was obtained. The use of the phonocardiograph may be helpful in detecting and localizing bruits. In cases where the presence of an A.V.A. is suspected but angiography fails to demonstrate such a lesion, measurements of oxygen saturation of venous outflow may be helpful (Verbiest, 1951). There is no need to insist on the value of other diagnostic procedures, such as spinal fluid tap, cardiological examination, etc.

SURGICAL TREATMENT

Patients, in whom the A.V.A. is accidentally discovered during arteriography for another lesion (Fig. 1) should, if the lesion does not produce symptoms, have a regular check-up. Operation should be considered in case of hemorrhage, progressive neurological deficit, hypertensive hydrocephalus, trigeminal neuralgia, or, especially in infants, cardiological disturbances, but all depends upon the localization and extension of the lesion.

A pulsating bruit as an unique symptom, is a relative indication because frequently ligation of supplying arteries does not produce complete relief, while the symptom is not serious enough to justify a major operation, unless the bruit disturbs the psychic equilibrium. But even then this should be done in agreement with the psychiatrist.

SURGICAL PROCEDURES

Clipping of supplying arteries has been performed in A.V.A. of the brainstem or of the vein of Galen. Ligation of the vertebral artery in brainstem A.V.A. is a hazardous procedure. Laine (1966) criticizes ligation of other nutrient vessels in this type of malformation as well, because they may also supply neighboring nervous tissue, while on the other hand the distinction between normal and pathological vessels may be impossible. Only in those rare cases of brainstem A.V.A. producing a sub-arachnoid hemorrhage this author is of opinion that staged interruption of supplying arteries is justified.

In cases of trigeminal neuralgia root section or tractotomy has been performed (Dereux et al., 1959; Olivecrona and Riives, 1948). In one of our patients (Verbiest, 1961) interruption of the causative vascular loops relieved the patient, with the advantage of preserved sensibility. Before interrupting such loops it should be ascertained that they are not formed by elongated basilar or vertebral arteries.

In hypertensive hydrocephalus it is recommended to perform posterior fossa decompression and exploration of the malformation. If no relief is obtained a ventriculo-atrial shunting operation should be applied.

It is difficult to evaluate the benefit of surgical evacuation of a cerebellar hematoma. Good results have been reported but the mortality is high because of failure to recognize the condition early. As mentioned above surgical evacuation of an intra-pontine hematoma may result in considerable improvement in an exceptional case.

Complete excision of a cerebellar A.V.A. is the ideal treatment, but may be impossible in cases of a very large A.V.A., occupying both cerebellar hemispheres or involving the brainstem as well. The latter complication may not demonstrate in the angiogram. This was the case in one of our patients (l.c.), presenting a large cerebellar A.V.A. During excision we found that a large draining vein entered the brachium pontis. It ruptured during ligation. Although hemostasis was obtained the patient developed a postoperative hemorrhage from which he died.

Since ligation or clipping of supplying arteries may facilitate excision of the A.V.A. the surgical approach should be based not only upon the localization of the A.V.A. but also upon the accessibility of the supplying arteries.

The transtentorial approach is the operation of choice for A.V.A.'s of the upper vermis (Fig. 3) or the anterior superior portion of the cerebellar hemisphere. The suboccipital craniotomy allows removal of A.V.A.'s of the lower vermis or the inferior posterior portion of the cerebellum.

In large cerebellar A.V.A.'s a combined transtentorial and suboccipital approach is advisable (Fig. 2). This approach should also be considered in some A.V.A.'s of the pontine angle.

We will not enter into detail concerning the value of moderate hypothermia and temporary occlusion of the main arteries in the neck, but wish to stress the danger of using "cold" blood when large transfusions are required, especially in infants. Ventricular fibrillation and cardiac arrest is its imminent danger. This danger is greatest if the operation is performed under moderate hypothermia.

More experience is needed to evaluate the application of the ingenious freezing (Cooper and Stellar, 1963) or artificial embolization (Luessenhop et al., 1965) techniques to the parenchymatous posterior fossa A.V.A.'s. Surgery of pure dural A.V.A.'s may imply great hazard in extensive lesions or those involving the basal dura of the posterior fossa, requiring staged operations. The risks of the operations should not exceed those of the lesions for which they are applied. In A.V.A.'s between occipital artery and transverse sinus surgical occlusion of the occipital artery may result in diminishing pulsating tinnitus but in many cases it does not disappear completely.

REFERENCES

BONNET, P., DECHAUME, J., AND BLANC, E. J., (1937); *Méd. Lyon*, **18**, 165.
—, —, AND —, (1938); *Bul. Soc. Franc. Ophth.*, **51**, 521.
BUNTS, A. T., (1949); *Rev. Neurol.*, **81**, 442.
CIEMBRONIEWICZ, J. E., (1965); *J. Neurosurg.*, **22**, 465.
CIMINELLO, V. J., AND SACHS, E., (1962); *J. Neurosurg.*, **19**, 602.
COOPER, I. S., AND STELLAR, S., (1963); *J. Neurosurg.*, **20**, 921.
DANDY, W. E. (1928); *Arch Surg.*, **17**, 190.
DEREUX, J., AND DEBERDT, R., (1960); *Sem. Hôp.*, Paris, **36**, 1849.
—, NAYRAC, P., LAINE, E., GALIBERT, P., AND DELANDTSHEER, J. M., (1959); *Neurochirurgie*, **5**, 257.
DILENGE, D., DAVID, M., SIMON, J., AND MORICE, J., (1964); *Neurochirurgie*, **10**, 265.
EISENBREY, A. B., AND HEGARTY, W. M., (1956); *J. Neurosurg.*, **13**, 647.
FINCHER, E. F., (1951); *Ann. Surg.*, **133**, 886.
FONTAINE, R., DANY, A., AND BRIOT, B., (1957); *Neurochirurgie*, **30**, 30.
GOLD, A. P., RANSOHOFF, J., AND CARTER, S., (1964); Vein of Galen Malformation, *Acta Neurol. Scand., Suppl. 11*, **40**.
GOMEZ, M. R., WHITTEN, Ch. F., NOLKE, A., BERNSTEIN, J., AND MEYER, J. S., (1963); *Pediatrics*, **31**, 400.
HOLMAN, C. B., AND BULLARD, F. E., (1963); *Proc. Mayo Clin.*, **38**, 67.
KRAYENBÜHL, H., AND YASARGIL, M., G., (1958); *Das Hirnaneurysma*, Series chirurg., Geigy, Basel.
—, AND —, (1965); *Die zerebrale Angiographie*, Thieme, Stuttgart,
LAINE, E., AND GALIBERT, P., (1966); *Rev. Neurol.*, **115**, 276.
—, GALIBERT, P., LOPEZ, J., DELAHOUSSE, J. M., DELANDTSHEER, J. M., AND CHRISTIAENS, J. L., (1963); *Neurochirurgie*, **9**, 147.
LEHMAN, J. St., CHYNN, K., HAGSTROM, J. W. C., AND STEINBERG, I., (1966); *Am. J. Roentgenol., Rad. Therapy and Nuclear Med.*, **98**, 653.
LEY, A., (1957); *Aneurismas arteriovenosos congenitos intracranealis*, Acad. de Herederos de Serra y Russell, Barcelona.
LUESSENHOP, A. J., KACHMANN, R., SHEVLIN, W., AND FERRERO, A. A., (1965); *J. Neurosurg.*, **23**, 400.
NEWTON, Th. H., AND GREITZ, T., (1966); *Radiology*, **87**, 824.
OBRADOR, S., AND URQUIZA, P., (1952); *Folia psychiat. neerl.*, **55**, 385.

OLIVECRONA, H., Reported by Tönnis, 1936.

—, AND RIIVES, J., (1948); *Arch. Neurol. Psych. (Chic.)*, **59**, 567.

PAKARINEN, S., (1965); *J. Neurosurg.*, **23**, 438.

PATERSON, J. H., AND MC KISSOCK, W., (1956); *Brain*, **79**, 233.

PECKER, J., BONNAL, J., AND JAVALET, A., (1965); *Neurochirurgie*, **11**, 327.

POOL, J. L., AND POTTS, D. G., (1965); *Aneurysms and Arteriovenous Anomalies of the Brain*, Hoeber, New York.

REUTER, S., NEWTON, Th. H., AND GREITZ, T., (1966); *Radiology*, **87**, 1080.

RÖTTGEN, P., (1937); *Zentralbl. f. Neurochir.*, **2**, 18.

SORGO, W., (1938); *Zentralbl. f. Neurochir.*, **3**, 64.

TAKEHAWA, S. D., AND HOLMAN, C. B., (1965); *Am. J. Roentgen., Rad. Therapy and Nuclear Med.*, **95**, 822.

TÖNNIS, W., (1936). In: BERGSTRAND, H., OLIVECRONA, H., AND TÖNNIS, W., *Gefässmissbildungen und Gefässgeschwülste des Gehirns*, Thieme, Leipzig.

VERBIEST, H., (1951); *Rev. Neurol.*, **85**, 189.

—, (1961); *Acta Neurochir.*, **9**, 171.

—, (1962); *Psychiat. Neurol. Neurochir.*, **65**, 329.

—, (1967); In press.

WEERSMA, M., (1958); *Folia Psychiat. neerl.*, **61**, 315.

VAN DER WERF, M. A. J. M., (1964); *Neurochirurgie*, **10**, 140.

VAN WIJNGAARDEN, G. K., AND VINKEN, P. J., (1966); *Neurology*, **16**, 754.

WRIGHT, J. R., SLAVIN, R. E., AND WAGKER, J. A., (1965); *J. Neurosurg.*, **22**, 86.

WYBURN MASON, R., (1943); *Brain*, **66**, 163.

ZIEDSES DES PLANTES, B. G., (1935); *Fortschr. Geb. Röntgenstrahlen*, **52**, 69.

To the Discussion of Arterio-venous Anomalies

ADAM KUNICKI

Professor of Neurosurgery, Neurosurgical Clinic, Academy of Medicine, Cracow (Poland)

At the first Neurosurgical Congress 1957, Krayenbühl drew attention to intracerebral haemorrhages which are due to the tiny angiomas known as microangiomas of the brain. Eight years later the same author in collaboration with Siebmann published a series of 24 cases of that kind. In 15 cases the cause which induced the haemorrhage was revealed by means of angiography, operative treatment or post-mortem examination. In 9 cases the reason for the haemorrhage has not been ascertained beyond doubt. I should like now, on the basis of ten observations of my own, to call again

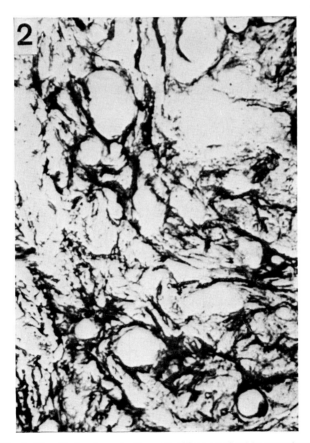

Fig. 1. Case 2. Angioma in the wall of intracerebral haemorrhage.

TABLE I

HAEMORRHAGIC CYSTIC ANGIOMAS

Case No.	Sex age	Obser. years	Onset	Location	Epilepsy before/post operation		Haemorrhage before/post operation		Intracranial hypertension before/post operation		Local function deficits before/post operation		Follow up
1	M 41	?	Acute	Temporal L.	—	?	—	?	+	?	+	?	No data
2	M 30	13	Chronic	Sens. Mot. R.	+	+	—	—	+	—	+	—	Full recovery
3	M 28	0	Acute	Temporal L.	—	—	+	—	—	—	+	—	Death 8 days after oper.
4	M 29	6	Acute	Parietal R.	—	+	+	—	—	—	+	—	Full recovery
5	F 27	5	Acute	Temporal L.	—	—	+	—	—	—	+	—	Full recovery
6	M 57	4	Acute	Frontal L.	+	+	—	—	—	—	+	—	Full recovery
7	M 22	4	Acute	Temporal L.	+	+	+	—	+	—	+	—	Full recovery
8	M 20	3	Acute	Parietal R.	—	+	+	—	+	—	+	+	Partial recovery
9	M 46	2	Sub-acute	Frontal L.	—	—	+	—	+	—	+	—	Full recovery
10	F 32	2	Sub-acute	Temporal R.	—	—	—	—	+	—	+	—	Full recovery
				Total	3	5	6	0	7	0	10	1	

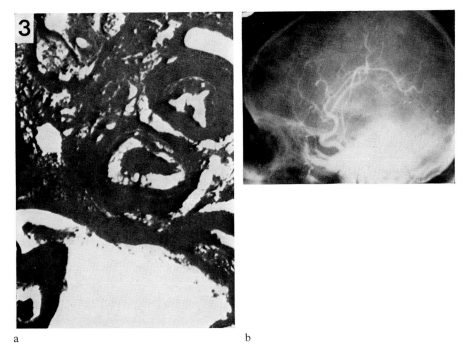

a   b

Fig. 2. Case 3. (a) Angioma in the wall of intracerebral haemorrhage, (b) Preoperative arteriogram.

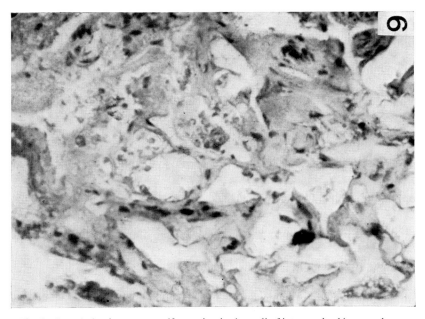

Fig. 3. Case 6. Angiomatous malformation in the wall of intracerebral haemorrhage.

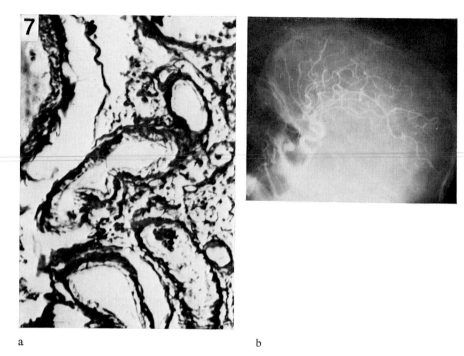

a b

Fig. 4. (a) Angioma in the wall of intracerebral haemorrhage, (b) Preoperative arteriogram.

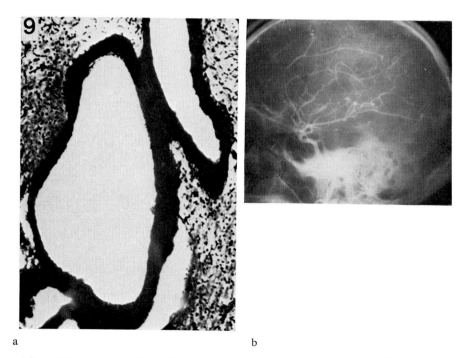

a b

Fig. 5. (a) Angioma in the wall of intracerebral haemorrhage, (b) Preoperative arteriogram.

the attention to these cases which, although not too frequent, still deserve interest in view of the good results attained by surgical treatment. Of 8 cases where angiograhpy was applied, in 4 the presence of angioma has been detected, while in the other 4 only a tumour of the brain has been recognized. In the remaining 2 cases the tumour was revealed by pneumoencephalography. In 7 cases papilloedema was found. All essential clinical data have been presented in Table I. In 7 cases the histological examination of tissue taken from the wall of the haemorrhage cavity has revealed the presence of pathological vessels forming the picture of racemous or cavernous angioma (Figs. 1, 2, 3, 4, 5, 6, 7). The numbers in the left corner of the pictures are in accordance with the numbers of the Table no. I. In three cases no tissue for histological examination was obtained. In 7 cases during postoperative observation which lasted respectively 13, 6, 4, 4, 2 years and 1 year, haemorrhagic symptoms did not occur. The patients have all resumed their previous jobs. One patient observed for three years is partly selfdependent. There are no data available about one of the patients and one died on the eighth day after surgery. The operation failed to relieve of epilepsy any of the three patients who had suffered from that disease prior to the operation, whereas in two patients the first epileptic attacks occurred after the surgical treatment.

To the Discussion of Surgical Treatment of the Encephalic Supratentorial Arteriovenous Aneurysms

ADAM KUNICKI

Professor of Neurosurgery, Neurosurgical Clinic, Academy of Medicine, Cracow (Poland)

Opinions differ as regards operative indications in the cases of angioma localized in the senso-motor area. There are numerous neurosurgeons who fear that the operative treatment would affect the functional state of limbs impaired by the angioma. On the other hand, however, there is a steadily increasing number of reports from which it appears that the removal of angioma from that area not necessarily must induce an intensification of the paralysis and that even an improvement of motion and sensitivity has been observed (Kunc, Norlén).

To illustrate that statement I would like to present two cases of patients where the angioma of that region had been removed without aggravating the pre-operative paresis (Plates I and II). Both patients can walk and move without aid, while their vital activity is restricted by the paresis of the upper extremity, which however had

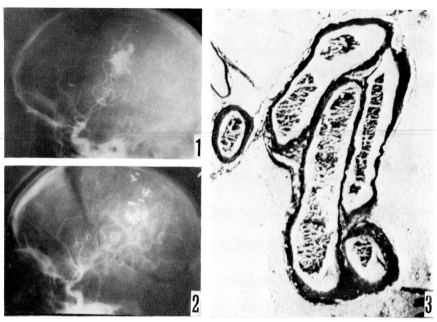

Plate I. 1 Angiography before operation. 2 Postoperative angiography. 3 Histopathology Perdrau stain.

existed still before the surgical treatment. In one of these cases the patient suffered also, apart from hemiparesis, from speech disturbances, which in the course of post-operative process have entirely disappeared.

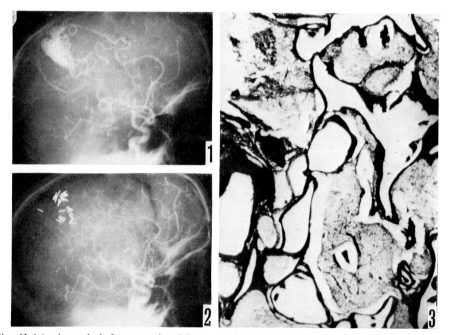

Plate II. 1 Angiography before operation. 2 Postoperative angiography. 3 Histopathology Perdrau stain.

Some Remarks to the Operability of the Centrally Located Arteriovenous Angiomas

L. ZOLTÁN

Budapest (Hungary)

The diagnostic and therapeutic problems of cerebral arterio-venous angiomas have almost entirely been solved. In consequence of epileptic fits, intracranial bleedings or, eventually, neurological symptoms, patients are generally admitted in special hospitals, where the existence of the angioma can be easily verified, and its localization with all hemodynamic details can be ascertained. In respect to the indication of an operation, a uniform view prevails. It is no longer doubtful that the adequate therapy of angiomas is surgery, and the best results can be achieved by radical removal, with an acceptably low mortality rate. The operation of angiomas seated in the central region, *i.e.*, in the territory supplying the midcerebral artery is, however, a disputed matter. Many authors, *e.g.* Svien and McRae, abstain from the operation of angiomas localized in this region, not so much because of the operative risk, as of the neurological deficit to be expected.

Since arterio-venous angiomas are congenital anomalies, the conjecture has been entertained for a long time that the parenchyma including the angioma is a worthless territory for the cerebral function, and its operative traumatization has no particular noxious consequences. On the ground of such considerations, the successful removal of large, central, eventually deep seated angiomas has been reported.

I wish to add here some positive data from our own experience. In our Institute we operated 74 out of 95 angiomas. Of these, 38 were either large ones, or near the motor cortex or the speech centers, or in the supplying territory of the mid-cerebral artery, respectively. From this group of patients (38) 4 died immediately after the operation, 1 after some months, in consequence of a new bleeding. The others recovered, and only two showed mild neurological symptoms. The good result was attributed to the fact that cerebral hemodynamics, which had been insufficient in consequence of the malformation, were normalized after the radical extirpation of the angiomas.

In our material no pathologic neurological symptoms could be observed in 8 cases from 27 malformations operated in the vicinity of the motor cortex, light palsy which improved in 12 cases, and moderate permanent palsy in 2 cases. Of the 5 operated patients with severe hemiplegia caused by an acute hematoma due to rupture of a malformation seated near the motor cortex, 3 improved. The radical removal of the 10

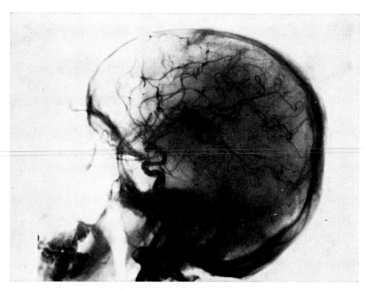

Fig. 1. On this angiogram the malformation is located among the arteries of the Sylvian group.

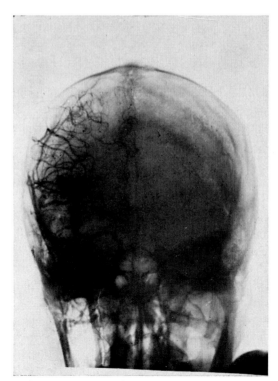

Fig. 2. The same malformation on the AP picture.

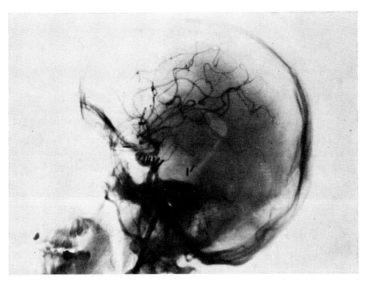

Fig. 3. On the postoperative angiogram it can be seen that the malformation could be radically removed without sacrifying even one important branch of the mid-cerebral artery.

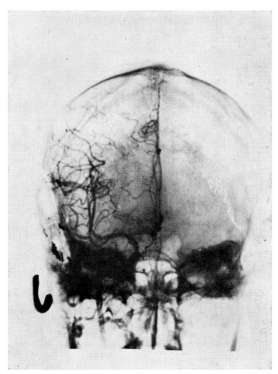

Fig. 4. The same fact is more clearly demonstrable on the post-operative AP angiogram.

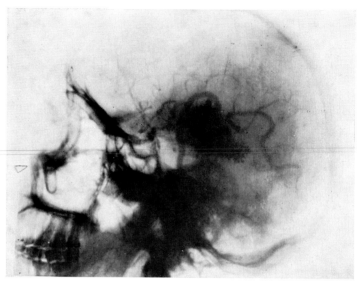

Fig. 5. Malformation located on the left side corresponding to the speech center of Wernicke.

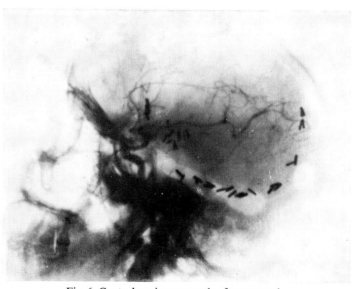

Fig. 6. Control angiogram made after removal.

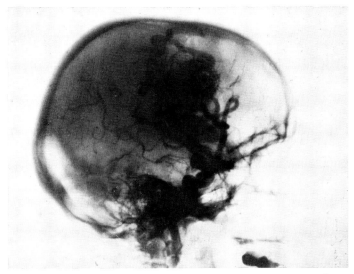

Fig. 7. Another angioma, situated corresponding to the sensory speech area.

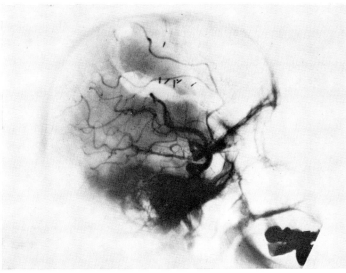

Fig. 8. Control angiogram after complete removal.

angiomas seated in the neighborhood of the speech centers never caused permanent lesion of the speech. Some figures are presented to illustrate this.

Thus we may establish that the radical removal of the malformations does not cause permanent severe symptoms, even in the vicinity of "indispensable" cortical or speech areas. This is partly, because the vessels forming the malformation do not participate in the cerebral blood supply, and partly, because the parenchyma in the vicinity of the anomaly is functionally ineffectual. The pathologic neurological symptoms are caused not so much by the cessation of the blood supply of the intact cerebral territories, as by the cortical excision that was done unintentionally in the course of the operation.

We found that after removal of the malformations causing severe impairment of the cerebral circulation, the latter was restored to normal in the vicinity of the pathologic change, and was improved also in distant cerebral areas, since on the post-operative angiograms there appeared arteries that could hardly have participated in the cerebral circulation before.

We believe that the radical removal of cerebral arterio-venous malformations is the most effective therapeutic method and we confirm the recommendation of Norlén, Pool, Kunz and other authors, not to restrict the intervention to the polarly seated angiomas only.

Since the anomalies often cause epilepsy that is refractory to medicamentous treatment, and since a malformation seated anywhere in the brain constitutes a permanent danger of bleeding, the view supporting preventive removal can also be supported.

Some Observations on the Surgery of Cerebrovascular Diseases

S. KOSTIĆ

Neurosurgical University Clinic, Belgrade (Yugoslavia)

During the past few years cerebrovascular diseases have been entering more and more into the domain of surgical treatment. This is largely due to new knowledge of these diseases, their pathogenesis, timely diagnosis, better pre-operative treatment and certain novelties and facilities in operative techniques. This success is reflected in the definite results and decreasing operative mortality. It is especially marked in radical intervention in the case of aneurysms and arterio-venous malformations.

However, notwithstanding the latest experiences, arachnoidal hemorrhage caused by vascular malformations, aneurysms and other diseases of unknown etiology is frequently still a source of considerable difficulty in making a timely and precise diagnosis, determination of surgical intervention and selection of operative methods.

Furthermore the steadily increasing incidence of these diseases, their vague and acute development, serious sequelae and high mortality rate, obstruct clinical study and diagnosis. Similarly, recurrent and severe, often fatal, hemorrhage, not infrequently prohibits any kind of treatment.

In order to gain better knowledge of these so-called negative characteristics of cerebrovascular diseases and of the difficulties arising in their treatment, we made an analysis of our own cases observed and treated at the Neurosurgical Clinic in Belgrade from 1961 to 1965. I must mention, however, that during this period we were unabe to admit to the Clinic all the cases of subarachnoidal hemorrhage. Although the actual number is far greater, we had during this period 94 cases admitted for acute subarachnoidal hemorrhage, most of them subcomatous or in a coma. During the same period we had 9,683 neurosurgical patients, among them 1232 operated for brain tumor or some other expansive intracranial process, and of this latter group the 94 cases of spontaneous hemorrhage constitute 7.63%. During the past few years, this percentage of cerebrovascular diseases has been steadily and markedly growing at our Clinic.

Our series of 94 cases included only aneurysms and vascular malformations of the brain with acute hemorrhage. Hemangiomas and angioblastomas, which were more frequent, as well as cases of subarachnoidal hemorrhage of uncertain etiology have not been included.

In this series we determined the cause of spontaneous hemorrhage to be solitary or multiple aneurysms of various localization in 2/3rds of the total cases, while the remaining cases revealed various forms of vascular malformations.

In selecting the cases suitable for surgery we took into consideration the general condition of the patient, age, the time elapsed since the first symptoms of hemorrhage, angiographic findings, various malformations and, in individual cases of aneurysms, localization and number, and finally the degree of the patient's consciousness on admission. According to these criteria, only 14 cases were found suitable for operation in this series during the period reviewed. They were 5 cases with aneurysms of various location, and 9 with vascular malformations suitable for extirpation. Of the 14 radically operated patients, 2 died after a few days, one of acute cerebral edema, and the other of thrombosis. In the remaining patients of this series, we performed palliative operations of various kinds or applied only conservative medical treatment.

In conclusion of the analysis of 94 patients suffering from vascular malformations and cerebral aneurysms with acute subarachnoidal hemorrhage, observed and treated at our Clinic between 1961 and 1965 we can state the following:

1. Serial cerebral angiography yields important data and facilitates the establishment of a correct and timely diagnosis.

2. Subsequent and unexpected hemorrhage is frequent in the period of clinical observation, the outcome usually being fatal.

3. In spite of meticulous pre-operative treatment and more favorable conditions for surgery, the number of cases suitable for radical intervention is still restricted.

4. Cerebrovascular surgery is undoubtedly producing better and better results, however such cases require above all accurate and timely diagnosis, comprehensive pre-operative treatment and, given certain surgical indications, prompt surgical intervention and a carefully chosen operative method according to each individual case.

Diagnosis and Therapy of Arteriovenous Malformations shown by Vertebral Angiography

J. WAPPENSCHMIDT, W. GROTE and K. H. HOLBACH

Neurosurgical University Hospital, Bonn (Germany)

(Director: Prof. Dr. P. RÖTTGEN)

Cerebrovascular malformations of the vertebral circulation system are much rarer than those of the carotid circulation system. This becomes even more evident considering aneurysms and arteriovenous malformations (AVM) of the posterior fossa which only can be demonstrated by the vertebral angiography. The vertebral angiography also shows in cases of supratentorial cerebrovascular malformations, that branches of the posterior cerebral artery (p.c.a.) can take part in supplying AVM mainly belonging to the carotid circulation system. In some cases these branches of the p.c.a. even are the only nutrient vessels of the supratentorial AVM. In such situations therapy offers especial problems and possibilities. Following we shall report on our experience in treating such AVM.

TABLE I

SPONTANEOUS INTRACRANIAL HEMORRHAGES
(Total of our patients with spontaneous intracranial hemorrhages)

Aneurysms	318	501	
Arteriovenous Malformations	183		534
Intracerebral Hemorrhages	33		
Subarachnoidal Hemorrhages of unknown origin	184		
	718		

As Table I demonstrates we were able to diagnose 318 aneurysms and 183 AVM causing intracranial hemorrhage or other symptoms. Only during the last years we regularly perform the vertebral besides the carotid angiography in the 718 cases of subarachnoidal or/and intracerebral hemorrhage. Therefore we think that the etiology in some of the 184 cases with hemorrhage of unknown origin could probably have been found by additional vertebral angiography.

Table II shows the number and the location of cerebrovascular malformations visualized by the vertebral angiography. In 12 cases of aneurysms 3 belonged to the

TABLE II

ARTERIOVENOUS MALFORMATIONS
(Cerebrovascular malformations shown by vertebral angiography)

Location	Group		Cases	Total
A. Supratentorial	1		8	
	2		4	
		a	3	19
	3	b	2	
		c	2	
B. Infratentorial	1		7	
	2		2	9
C. Extra- and Intracranial			4	4
				32

A1 paramedial (lateral ventricles and basal ganglia)
A2 medial (splenium of corpus callosum, midbrain)
A3 cortical-subcortical   a   lateral part of hemisphere
                b   medial ,,   ,,   ,,
                c   only cortical (not subcortical)
B1 Cerebellum and caudal brain stem
B2 Cerebellopontile angle

ANEURYSMS

	Vertebral artery	bas. artery	post. c.a.	Total
berry	3	3	4	10
fusiform	–	2	–	2
				12

vertebral artery, 5 to the basilar artery and 4 to the p.c.a. From 32 AVM 4 were located extracranially, 9 infratentorially, and 19 supratentorially.

Since we mainly are interested in the 19 supratentorially sited AVM we subdivided them again (Table II).

The group A1 consists of 8 paramedial AVM which are located in the region of the lateral ventricles and the basal ganglia. In the group A2 there are 4 cases of medial AVM located in the area of the splenium of corpus callosum and of the midbrain. 7 AVM of the group A3 were found in either the medial or lateral cortical-sub-cortical or only in the cortical region of the brain.

The group B1 (infratentorial AVM) consists of AVM located in the region of the cerebellum and of the caudal brain stem, the group B2 of those in the cerebellopontile angle. Comparing 21 infratentorial cases of cerebrovascular malformations with 480 supratentorial ones indicates that those of the posterior fossa are much rarer among our patients (4,4%).

The group C (combined extra- and intracranial AVM) consists of malformations which were located in the soft tissue of the occiput and of the temporal region expanding into the posterior fossa. They are mainly supplied by the external carotid artery. In such cases the vertebral angiography is necessary to visualize the intra-cranial portion of the malformation, which can be located in the dura mater — nutri-ent vessel ramus meningicus posterior — or in the tissue of the cerebellum.

As said above our main interest concentrates in the supratentorial AVM of group A. By comparing the total amount of 170 supratentorial AVM with the 19 cases of those being partly supplied by the vertebral circulation system we can suppose the latter being rather rare.

A few years ago we finished the diagnostical procedures after having demonstrated the AVM by carotid angiography. In the last years we perform regularly the vertebralis angiography, too.

In order to find the etiology of a subarachnoidal hemorrhage we usually first per-form the countercurrent angiography by injection into the right brachial artery per-mitting a simultaneous visualization of the infratentorial and supratentorial cerebral vessels. The rate of 19 : 170 which was mentioned before therefore does not reflect the real frequency.

In the main group A1 (Fig. 1) there are only subcortically and centrally sited AVM. These paramedially located AVM are mostly found in the posterior portion of the basal ganglia and only a few in their anterior parts. They touch the lateral ventricles or even extend into them. They also can be located within the lateral ventricles or in the region of the Island of Reil. In many cases it is impossible to demonstrate angio-graphically all these particulars. They can be visualized by the vertebral angio-graphy apart from carotid angiography because the basal ganglia and the chorioid plexus of the lateral ventricles are supplied by the posterior chorioid artery. The branches of the anterior chorioid artery, the central arteries rising from the medial cerebral artery and the branches of the posterior communicating artery are shown by the carotid angiography. If the p.c.a. is not connected to the carotid circulation system some nutrient arteries and also some portions of the AVM often cannot be demonstrated. In some cases the p.c.a. can even be the only nutrient vessel of the AVM.

The group A2 (Fig. 2) consists of AVM located in the midline behind the splenium of corpus callosum and in the region of the midbrain. There we found aneurysmal dilatations of the vein of Galen (we diagnosed 4 cases) and AVM. These malformations are supplied by central branches of the carotid artery and of the vertebral artery. Therefore they can be visualized by both the carotid and the vertebral angiography. Superficially located AVM can also be demonstrated by the vertebral angiography if their nutrient cortical vessels are connected to the p.c.a. In this group there are AVM of the occipital lobe which can only be shown by vertebral angiography. The vertebral angiography is also useful if an AVM of the occipital lobe wedge-shaped extends from the surface into the subcortical brain tissue; for the subcortical portion of these occipital malformations is partly supplied by the posterior chorioid artery.

This knowledge finally leads to the following discussion of some therapeutical problems. The paramedial AVM cannot be extirpated totally. The optimal treatment, the extirpation of the AVM, is only possible if it is located within the lateral ventricle. Therefore we examined whether the ligation of the main nutrient vessels (Figs. 1 and

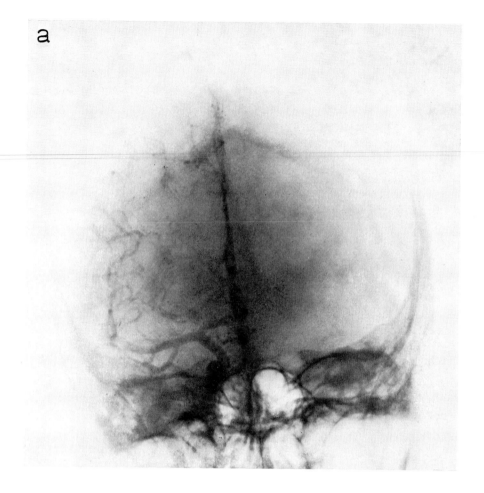

3) would reduce the danger of an hemorrhage and would improve the cerebral blood circulation.

The following case of group A1 represents an example of such a treatment. The AVM of a 16-year old patient having the size of a tomato is only supplied by the right p.c.a. This nutrient vessel was ligated just before splitting into its main cortical branches, as the postoperative angiograms show. The p.c.a. is still filled by collateral vessels distal from the ligation opacifying the clearly reduced AVM during the later phase of the angiography. In contrast to the preoperative arteriograms the branches of the carotid artery are earlier opacified than those of the p.c.a. and show a much better blood circulation of their peripheral region. Neurological deficits did not appear postoperatively. 4 patients of this group were operated on. In 3 cases the p.c.a. was ligated and in one case total extirpation of the AVM located in the lateral ventricle was possible. In 2 from 4 patients of group A2 (AVM of the midline) the nutrient vessels coming from different areas of the cerebral circulation system were ligated. Both patients died. A surgical treatment of these AVM and of the aneurysmal dilatations of the vein of Galen seems not to be possible at present.

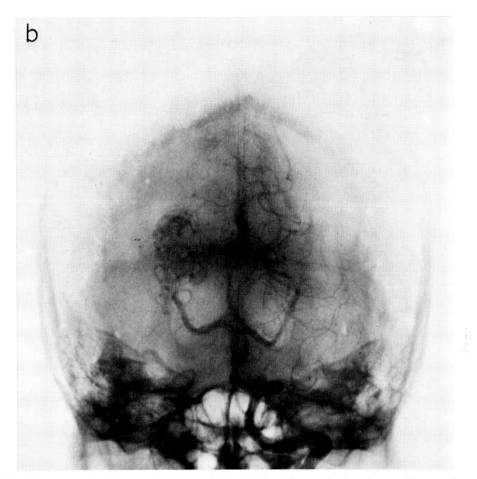

Fig. 1. Comparing the right carotid angiogram (a) with the right vertebral angiogram (b) we notice that the visualization of the AVM is better and that the AVM is more enlarged.

5 patients of the group A3 (superficially located AVM extending into the subcortical brain tissue) were operated on. 1 case of a left occipital AVM (Fig. 3) being supplied only by the p.c.a. was very impressive. After the ligation of the p.c.a. this AVM disappeared completely as the postoperative angiogram showed (Fig. 3). Postoperative deficits did not appear.

We also operated for combined AVM whose cortical portions were supplied by the p.c.a. and whose medial parts were supplied by the anterior chorioid artery. After the ligation of the p.c.a. only the part of the AVM supplied by the anterior chorioid artery could be visualized. The ligation of the anterior chorioid artery will be performed by a second operation.

The treatment of the 5 patients of this group was the following: twice the p.c.a. was ligated, twice the AVM was totally extirpated and in one case with an enlarged and expanded AVM being supplied by vessels of all 3 main cerebral arteries we just ligated an aneurysm of the pericallose artery. Futhermore we noticed in this case,

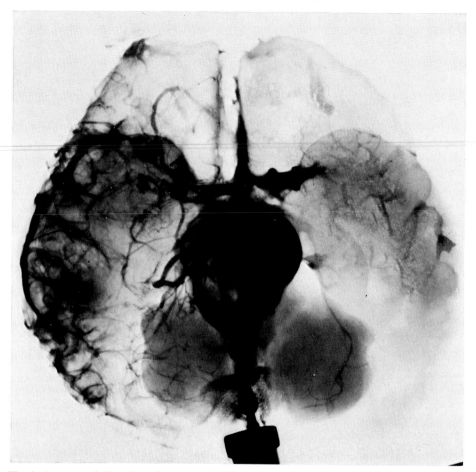

Fig. 2. Aneurysmal dilatation of the vein of Galen. The main nutrient vessel is the post. cerebral
artery (Preparation was made by injection).

that both anterior cerebral arteries rose from a common proximal trunk being only
connected to the left carotid artery.

There exist similar problems in treating infratentorial AVM. These malformations
usually cannot be totally extirpated because of their enlargement and location. Only
in 2 cases we completely extirpated an AVM of the cerebellopontile angle with success.
In 3 from 7 cases with AVM of the cerebellum we only were able to improve the
circulation of the cerebrospinal fluid and in 4 cases nutrient vessels were ligated.
Only 2 cases showed a satisfactory result.

SUMMARY

The significance of demonstrating the circulation system of the vertebral artery is
discussed regarding a representative number of cases consisting of 318 berry and
fusiform aneurysms, 183 arteriovenous malformations (AVM), 33 spontaneous intra-

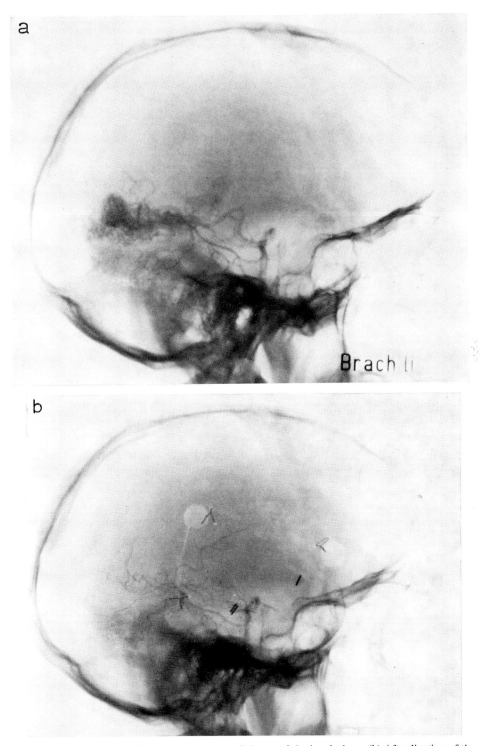

Fig. 3. (a) Left occipital AVM located in the medial part of the hemisphere. (b) After ligation of the homolateral post. cerebral artery the AVM cannot be demonstrated.

cerebral hemorrhages, and 184 subarachnoidal hemorrhages of unknown origin. The number of subtentorial AVM and aneurysms only demonstrated by vertebral angiography is small compared to the amount of supratentorial AVM diagnosed by the carotid arteriography. The main interest of this publication is given to the angiographic findings seen in cases of supratentorial AVM. The application of the vertebral angiography shows in such cases that AVM of a certain localization are supplied by the branches of the vertebral arteries. It is important to demonstrate the vertebral circulation system because the posterior chorioid artery very often mainly supplies the central and paramedial angiomas of the basal ganglia and of the lateral ventricle, and the subcortical part of the combined cortical and subcortical AVM. Since the posterior cerebral artery is not connected to the carotid circulation system in some patients we see an uncomplete or even no representation of the AVM in such cases by performing the carotid arteriography only.

According to the angiographic findings we can divide the AVM into three groups differing in localization and expansion of the AVM:

I. group: paramedial (ventricle and basal ganglia)

II. group: medial (splenium of corpus callosum and the area of the midbrain)

III. group: combined cortical and subcortical AVM.

The therapy of the AVM of each group is discussed. The paramedial and medial AVM form a special group, since their total extirpation, their optimal treatment, is only possible, if they are located in the lateral ventricle. Therefore we examined whether the danger of a hemorrhage could be reduced and whether the general blood circulation of the brain could be improved by ligating the main supplying arteries of the AVM. The results of the operated AVM indicate the following: the ligation of the posterior cerebral artery and of the anterior chorioid artery is of use in the paramedial AVM, for their expansion is reduced and the cerebral blood circulation is improved. The ligation of the posterior cerebral artery leads to a complete recovery in combined cortical and subcortical AVM of the occipital region if the AVM is only supplied by the posterior cerebral artery. An improvement can only be expected by ligating the supplying branches of the subtentorial AVM, if their blood is supplied by accessible arteries (like the arteria cerebelli superior or inferior posterior).

The Relative Importance of Atheroma in the Clinical Course of Arteriovenous Angioma of the Brain

J. E. PAILLAS, M. BERARD, R. SEDAN, M. TOGA AND B. ALLIEZ

The Neuro-Surgical Clinic and the Chair of Pathological Anatomy**, Faculty of Medicine,
Marseille (France)*

It has been stated that the presence of atheroma is a factor in the mechanism of rupture complicating the clinical course of arterial or arterio-venous intracranial aneurysms. In the case of arterial aneurysms this would seem true inasmuch as the hardened wall of the vessel will transmit the systolic pressure more intensely within the aneurysmal sac, which is rendered more fragile by the lipoid deposit at its neck. The first manifestation of this congenital malformation may therefore be its rupturing in old age. The role of atheroma in arterio-venous aneurysms is not so obvious, however.

To elucidate this problem we undertook a pathological study of excised arterio-venous angiomas and compared and contrasted the histological findings with the observed clinical ones. More than 100 specimens were examined, but useful anatomo-clinical correlations were possible in only 77 cases and it is these which we propose to discuss.

PATHOLOGICAL STUDIES

Macroscopic features of the malformations were described *in vivo* from angiographic studies and appearances at operation. For the purposes of our study the sites of malformation and the origins of the afferent limbs are unimportant. On the other hand we adhered to the classification by size[5], namely: small angiomas (under 2 cm in diameter), 32 cases; medium size angiomas (2–4 cm in diameter), 16 cases; and large angiomas (over 4 cm in diameter), 24 cases. Five specimens remained unclassified because of thrombosis or extensive hemorrhage.

The vessels inspected at operation and in fresh specimens after removal never showed the characteristic plaques of atheroma. They were only turgescent, abnormally tortuous and occasionally thickened, regardless of caliber.

Serial sections mounted in paraffin and prepared by the usual techniques, some being stained with Masson's Trichrome based on aniline blue, others variously impregnated (in particular by Weigert's method), permitted us to examine individual segments of the malformation and its elastic fibers. We usually[3] classify histological

---

* Head: Prof. Paillas.
** Head: Prof. Gastaut.

appearances by analogy with the stages of vascular embryogenesis as described by Streeter:

Stage 1 — represented by proliferation of undifferentiated vascular tissue often remaining in the blastema phase — 6 cases.

Stage 2 — represented by a mass of incompletely differentiated malformed vessels in which arterial, venous and capillary tissues were hardly distinguishable. The majority of the specimens (52) belonged to this group.

Stage 3 — is made up of differentiated malformations (19 cases); this differentiation is usually unidirectional, *i.e.*, either arterial (14 cases), capillary (2 cases) or venous (3 cases).

In our studies we ignored the interstitial tissue and concentrated on the cells of the coats of large numbers of malformed vessels. We were thus able to bring to light three main types of lesions, namely:

1. Sclerosis — in various forms:

simple sclerosis characterized by a variable degree of thickening of the parietal collagen fibers.

Fibro-hyalinosis associated with sclerotic thickenings in the wall, with the appearance of hyaline degeneration.

In other cases, sclerosis is associated with intramural fibrinoid deposits.

Generally speaking, sclerosis leads to thickening of the walls of the vessels and formation of a thick matrix with considerable reduction in the lumen almost to the point of complete disappearance.

The endothelium is either lifted and projects into the lumen or is affected by fibrosis. The endothelial cells often show a tendency towards either 'palisade' formation or desquamation. This parietal hypertrophy determines the formation of endo-luminal pads described by Conti and is also responsible for the frequently noted phenomena of stasis.

The elastic laminae are always grossly altered. Occasionally hyperplastic, they may be shown by special techniques to be doubled or even stratified. Most commonly, however, they are destroyed. The internal one is easier to define, but the external one may indeed be entirely lacking, even in normal cerebral vessels.

The tunica media shows important alterations if the sclerosis is particularly massive and may be associated with deposits of iron-containing pigment.

The tunica adventitia is most often congested and hemorrhagic and may contain abnormal deposits resulting from disintegration of the adjacent altered nervous parenchyma.

These sclerotic lesions are almost constant but involve neither the whole extent of the vascular wall nor the whole bulk of the abnormal vessels. In a single transverse section either all or a proportion of the elements of the wall will be involved. The lesions predominate in bigger vessels, but spare neither fine ones nor capillaries.

2. Histiocytic conglomerates consist of clear cells with irregular cytoplasm. After being imbedded in paraffin the cells are not foamy but optically empty, showing an excentric nucleus. They lie in groups, either under the intima or, more rarely, in the media. They are most often found underlying Conti's pads. They seem to be packed with cholesterol.

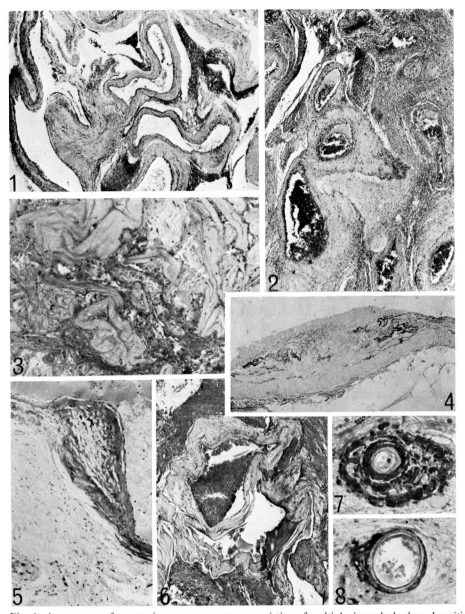

Fig. 1. Appearance of an arterio-venous aneurysm consisting of multiple, irregularly shaped cavities with walls thickened by Conti's pads.

Fig. 2. Severe sclerosis of the walls.

Fig. 3. Hyalinosis and obstruction of the lumen.

Fig. 4. Destruction of the elastic laminae in a fibrotic wall.

Fig. 5. An excess of foamy histiocytes in a thickened wall.

Fig. 6. Severe calcification of the intima and media of a malformed vessel.

Figs. 7 and 8. Annular calcium deposits (angioliths) and intra- and extra-parietal hemosiderotic deposits.

References p. 425

3. Calcium deposits are found in contact with sclerotic lesions or in their middle in particularly badly affected vessels. Isolated calcium deposits intimately associated with neither sclerotic lesions nor with intra- or extracellular deposits can, however, be found round apparently intact or only slightly affected capillaries. They form angioliths.

In conclusion, it must be pointed out that while sclerotic lesions were present in all the specimens examined, histiocytic conglomerates and calcium deposits were demonstrated only in 10 and 6 cases respectively. We found no crystals of fatty acids nor atheromatous porridge-like masses in the usual sense of the word, and no evidence of intra-parietal inflammation. Five specimens showed large iron deposits outside the sites of recent ruptures.

A careful study of the specimens shows an essential discrepancy between the prominence of the sclerotic lesions, whether associated or not with hyaline degeneration or fibrinoid deposits, and the slight evidence of fatty excess which is the principal manifestation of atheroma.

It is therefore impossible in the material in question to envisage the initial development of atheroma followed by atherosclerosis, which is the usual sequence of events in general pathology. The sclerosis is constant. The processes of formation of fat and calcium deposits are separate and rather rare, judging by their incidence in our material.

Fig. 3 clearly shows the distribution and incidence of the lesions in relation to the stage of differentiation of the walls of the malformed vessel. The most advanced and most characteristic lesions are confined to stage 2, which corresponds to the majority of angiomas or arterio-venous aneurysms of the brain.

The slowly evolving sclerotic lesions therefore do not appear in immature vascular tissue (stage 1). They selectively affect more bulky malformed vessels or more differentiated ones (stage 2). They seem to avoid fully differentiated tissue (stage 3). It must be admitted, however, that the vessels of the last group, once they become affected, may undergo regressive changes with loss of differentiated wall structure and become morphologically similar to malformations stage 2.

The possibility was conceived that the size of the angioma might influence the development of histiocytic conglomerates, endothelial proliferation, calcium deposits and iron deposits in 9 small, 4 medium and 2 big angiomas. However, histiocytic conglomerates with endothelial proliferation are almost all confined to small angiomas (7 cases) which represent instances of arterio-venous fistulae even better than large cirsoid aneurysms. It would seem therefore that the changes in the wall ('jet lesions') may be due to turbulence resulting from the local hemodynamic disturbances.

CLINICAL CORRELATIONS

1. With systemic atherosclerosis

As the parietal sclerosis is constant in cerebral angiomas it cannot be linked to generalized arteriosclerosis even if this also happens to be present in an aged subject. As it happens, our 9 cases with histiocytic conglomerates, which are nearest to atheroma, despite the absence of fatty acid deposits, were not atheromatous subjects. The possibility of coincidence could be also invoked if the operations for arterio-venous aneurysms were usually carried out at an advanced age, but in fact 89 of our 100 patients were under 50, and the oldest was 66.

Other reasons for the lesions superimposed on sclerosis must be thus found, and their possible consequences examined.

2. The role of age

The average age of our subjects was 33 years (30 in Houdart's series), and that of the 16 cases forming the group with histiocytic masses or calcium deposits was 32 years. The age distribution curve by decades in the latter group deviates slightly to the right compared with the general curve. The difference is not significant however, and that fact also made us presume the absence of any influence of systemic arterio-sclerosis.

3. Influence of duration of disease

The real duration is unknown, but let us consider the time interval between the onset of symptoms (headaches, epileptic fit, hemorrhage) and the date of operation, excluding those cases in which onset was marked by acute hemorrhage necessitating immediate operation. The interval was 1 to 5 years in 19 cases, 5 to 10 years in 8 cases and over 10 years in 9 cases. Of the 17 cases with angiomas showing the above-mentioned special histological features, 9 had a clinical history of less than 1 year, 6 between 1 and 5 years, 1 between 5 and 10 years, and 1 over 10 years.

It would therefore seem that the special histological changes either facilitate the development of the clinical manifestations of the lesion or else point to hemodynamic disorders, the intensity of which is such that clinical signs appear sooner rather than later.

Lesions including calcium deposits (5 patients, aged 29 to 40 years) seem to be correlated with the slow progress of the disease and play a role in the production of the clinical picture, in that this group consisted of 1 subject with migraine and 4 epileptics.

4. The role of chronic accidents in the pathogenesis of the symptoms

Two types of symptoms occurring in repeated attacks mark the progress of the disease: attacks of migraine and epileptic fits.

Migraine — by which one does not, of course, mean the headaches commonly occurring in many people, but true migraine — occurred in 9 of our patients (11.6%) and in 75 cases in the various series collected by Houdart[2] (11%). Corresponding figures for the groups of patients with special histological lesions and with histiocytic conglomerates were 4 out of 17 (25%) and 3 out of 9 (33%). These subjects thus seem to have a tendency towards attacks of migraine and the lesions might be a result of arterial spasms, whatever their ultimate cause.

Epileptic fits often mark the clinical progress of cerebral angioma. Apart from the known cases of hemorrhagic accidents, we found 13 cases of epilepsy in the group of 17 patients with special parietal lesions (84%) and only 24 cases among the remaining

60 patients (40%). The overall incidence of epilepsy in cerebral angioma is given as 30% by Houdart[2] and as 28% by Perret and Nishoika[6] (545 cases).

Of 5 patients with calcifications 3 were epileptics, and in the group of 5 patients with iron deposits (including one with calcifications) all were epileptic. It thus seems quite certain that the occurrence of epilepsy is favored by the presence of the parietal lesions described above.

The newer histological findings thus confirm our previously expressed opinion[1,4] that local parenchymatous lesions play a more important part in the causation of epilepsy in angioma than do hemodynamic disorders. Sclerosis with intimal proliferation and histiocytic deposits superimposed on astrogliosis is an important contributory factor. The iron deposits found in areas other than those involved in recent known hemorrhages serve as evidence of small sub-clinical hemorrhages in the past and add to the epileptogenic activity of the irritant tissue lesions. The neurons are also hampered by anoxia due to escape of blood via arterio-venous shunts.

The parietal lesions in question were mainly found in small sized angiomas derived from subjects, almost all of whom suffered from epilepsy. It would therefore appear that the widely held view that small angiomas mainly manifest themselves clinically by the effects of rupture, and large ones by epileptic attacks, is thus undermined. In fact the explanation is provided by the changes in the wall which, on their appearance, affect the progress of small angiomas in such a way that they act as epileptogenic foci without, however, eliminating the risk of hemorrhage; attacks of apoplexy marked the onset in only 2 of our 9 cases of small angiomas.

CONCLUSIONS

The role of local and systemic atherosclerosis in the progress of cerebral arterio-venous angiomas was investigated in a series of 77 cases by histological examination of malformations removed at operation and comparison of the findings with the clinical facts.

1. Sclerosis of the vascular walls is an almost constant finding. It is not diffuse (71 cases), and for this reason is not thought to be responsible for any particular symptom.

2. In 17 cases more special lesions were noted. They were akin to atheroma but differed from it by the constant absence of porridge-like material and fatty acids. They consisted of conglomerates of histiocytes near areas of endothelial proliferation (pads of Conti) in 5 cases, of calcifications in the wall of the vessels in 6 cases, and of iron deposits other than those left by a known recent hemorrhage in 5 cases. The distribution of these 16 cases in the series classified into Streeter's 3 stages was as follows: type 1 — (6 cases, vascular stage of blastema) — no sclerotic lesions; type 2 — vessels recognizable but not differentiated into arteries and veins — 52 cases; 9 showed histiocytic masses, 4 showed calcifications and 5 — iron deposits; type 3 (a total of 19 cases with predominant arterial, venous and capillary differentiation in 14, 2 and 3 cases respectively) — 2 cases of calcification. It would therefore seem that neither immature angiomas nor highly differentiated ones tend to show major parietal lesions.

The latter seem to be more or less confined to small angiomas (7 out of 9 cases), their development being dependent on hemodynamic disorders (jet lesions).

3. No systemic atheroma was demonstrated in any of the 16 patients with the special parietal lesions which were the subject of this study; the latter must therefore be considered to be purely local tissue lesions. Furthermore, there was no really significant difference between the average age of the patients with special lesion-bearing angiomas and other patients with angiomas.

4. The incidence of migraine among the patients with the special type of lesion is particularly high, being 24% as against 7.5% in other patients.

5. Similarly, the incidence of epilepsy is very high in patients with special lesions (13 out of 17 cases, or 84% as against 40% for other patients). All 5 calcified angiomas were epileptogenic, and in one of these cases iron deposits were also demonstrated.

The local parenchymatous lesions, parietal and interstitial, therefore play a dominant role in the causation of epilepsy. Anoxia due to arteriovenous shunt plays an essential role in the histogenesis of the local lesions but only a secondary one in the pathogenesis of epilepsy. This explains the apparent discrepancy between the greater frequency of the incidents of rupture in small angiomas and the paradoxical predominance of epilepsy in small angiomas bearing the parietal changes in question.

REFERENCES

1 BONNAL, J., BERARD-BADIER, M., WINNIGER, J. AND PAILLAS, J. E. (1963) Epilepsy in subtentorial arterio-venous angiomas. Anatomo-electro-radio-clinical correlations. *Neuro-chirurgie*, **9**, 427–433.
2 HOUDART, R. AND LE BESNERAIS, Y. (1963) Arterio-venous aneurysms of cerebral hemispheres (Report presented at the French Language Congress of Neurosurgery, 1963), Vol. 1, Masson, Paris, 197.
3 PAILLAS, J. E., BERARD, M. AND SERRATRICE, G. (1957) An attempt at classification of arterio-venous angiomas (cirsoid aneurysms) of the brain on the basis of 25 cases including histological examination. *Rev. neurol.*, **96**, 146–148.
4 PAILLAS, J. E., BONNAL, J. AND LEGRE, J. (1960) A study of anatomo-electro-radio-clinical correlations in arterio-venous angiomas complicated by epilepsy. A discussion of 'epilepsy in vascular malformations of the brain' by K. DECKER AND J. KUGLER, in *X-rays, Radio-isotopes and E.E.G. in epilepsy* (7th Marseille Colloquium (1958) of the International Federation of Electroencephalography and Clinical Neurophysiology), Masson, Paris, 155–160.
5 PAILLAS, J. E., BONNAL, J., SERRATRICE, G., BERARD-BADIER, M. AND WINNIGER, J. (1959) Arterio-venous angiomas of the brain. A study of 70 cases of subtentorial angiomas. *Presse méd.*, **59**, 2215–2218.
6 PERRET, G. AND HIRO NISHIOKA (1966) Arterio-venous malformations. An analysis of 545 cases of craniocerebral arterio-venous malformations and fistulae reported to the cooperative study. *J. Neurosurg.*, **4**, 467–489.

Brain Angiomata and Intracerebral Haematoma

N. O. AMELI

Professor of Neurosurgery, University of Tehran (Iran)

In the last 18 years we have seen 76 cases of brain angiomata, of which only 3 were in the posterior fossa. In 16 cases the first indication of any abnormality had been an intracerebral haematoma. There were 9 males and 7 females. Except for a man of 48 the others were all young (6–23 years). In one case the haematoma was intracerebellar and the remainder were intracerebral.

The cases are divided into the spontaneous and post-traumatic groups.

SPONTANEOUS GROUP

In this group of 11 cases two distinct syndromes were encountered.

Syndrome 1

In 6 cases (7–17 years old) the picture was that of a rapidly growing intracranial mass. The length of history varied from two weeks to three months. Apart from headache and papilloedema which were present in all cases, presence of slight neck rigidity in 3 patients was noteworthy.

In a girl of 7 with presence of headache, slight fever and later neck stiffness, diagnosis of typhoid fever and then TB meningitis had been considered, by her physician, until papilloedema appeared and the patient was referred to the Neurosurgical Service. This patient had a large right temporal haematoma with a small angioma.

In two cases haematomata were in the parietal lobe and one in the frontal, one in occipital and two in the temporal lobes. On removal of the clots, angiomata could be seen presenting in the wall of the cavity which were easily dealt with.

Syndrome 2

In 5 cases of rather older age group (19–20–21–23–48) the picture was completely different. In every case there had been a sudden onset of severe headache, vomiting and loss of consciousness of short duration. In 3 cases that had lumbar puncture CSF was blood stained. All the patients had slight to severe hemiparesis, and one patient also had complete loss of vision when he regained consciousness a week later. Hemiparesis in all patients gradually improved. Two patients also had dysphasia. Except in one case the others were referred to us not earlier than one month after the haemorrhage. Angiography in each case demonstrated a small angioma with displacement of main arterial tree suggestive of an intracerebral mass. In two patients there was also an aneurysmal dilatation in the angioma. One patient, after recovering from an attack of haemorrhage 12 months previously had repeated temporal epilepsies. Angiography demonstrated an angioma plus an aneurysm. At operation there was a cavity filled with yellow fluid and the aneurysm presented into this cavity as a round white mass. The angioma was completely removed. Pateint has been free of attacks in the last 5 years with small doses of phenobarbital in the first 2 years.

In a man aged 23 who had two attacks of intracerebral haemorrhage with hemiplegia, angiography demonstrated a small haematoma with aneurysm in the parasagittal parietal region. At operation exactly the same picture was seen as in the previous case. Another patient aged 48 had persistent headache and dysphasia after recovering from haemorrhage. Angiography demonstrated an angioma with two large feeding arteries and much displacement (Fig. 4). At operation a large cavity with a slightly coloured fluid was found with the angioma on its posterior wall.

A case seen recently (a boy of 19) had sudden attack of headache, loss of consciousness, neck rigidity and left hemiplegia. CSF was markedly blood stained. Patient was treated conservatively. Patient's hemiplegia gradually recovered without

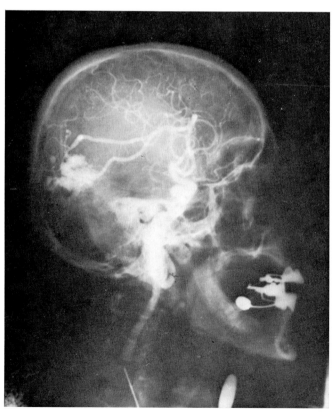

Fig. 1. Small angioma presenting in the wall of a large intracerebral cavity.

operation. But as headache persisted two months after the haemorrhage, it was decided to explore. In this case there was no cavity and angioma was very deeply situated and it was decided not to remove the lesion. Although we had no success with radiotherapy in the past, as this patient's angioma consisted mostly of small vessels, 3,800 r was given. Angiogram three months later showed that the angioma had disappeared.

POST-TRAUMATIC GROUP

5 cases all young (6–23 years) had delayed intracerebral haematoma after slight head injuries. 4 were intracerebral and one intracerebellar. This last patient was interesting as his haematoma appeared after a fist fight but was not referred until a month later, when he had signs of raised intracranial pressure and cerebellar signs on the right side. There was a large congenital angioma of the right half of his tongue (Fig. 2).

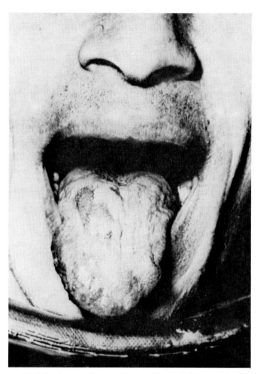

Fig. 2. Angioma of right half of the tongue in a patient with post-traumatic right cerebellar haematoma

In one case a child of 6. patient developed haematoma after a slight injury when playing with other children. At autopsy frontal haematoma was seen and on carefully washing away the blood clot a small angioma was discovered.

In another case a boy of 12, whilst swimming, hit his head against the wall of the swimming pool. When seen the next day he was semicomatose with hemiparesis.

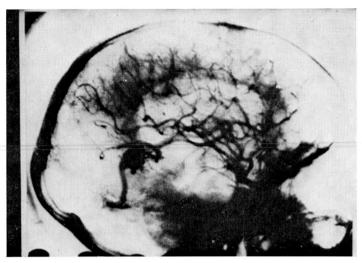

Fig. 3. A small angioma, a cause of post-traumatic intracerebral haematoma.

With the diagnosis of extradural haematoma a burr hole was made under local anaesthesia; as this proved negative a canula was introduced into the temporal lobe and 40 ml of dark blood aspirated. Later an angiogram demonstrated the angioma (Fig. 3). Further operation for removal of the angioma was refused. Patient is alive and well 18 years later.

Another patient (a boy of 12) who developed haemorrhage after falling off his bicycle; angiography showed a small angioma in the left parietal region. Operation was refused. Patient is well with slight right hemiparesis 7 years later.

Of the 16 cases under discussion, in 10 the angiomata were removed. In 5 other cases with large angiomata the malformation has been completely removed. There has been no mortality in this series.

DISCUSSION

Haemorrhage is an important complication of congenital arteriovenous malformations of the brain. This complication seems to occur with small angiomata and in young people. A number of cases of intracerebral haematoma from small angiomata and microangiomas have been reported (Ameli, 1956, 1957, 1964; Crawford and Russel, 1956; Krayenbuhl and Siebenmann, 1964).

In many cases the haemorrhage is spontaneous but in some patients it occurs after a slight head injury (Ameli, 1957). In post-traumatic group patients are usually children and young adults; and therefore in a child with post-traumatic intracerebral haematoma the presence of a congenital angioma should be kept in mind.

The haemorrhage can occur slowly, and mimic a brain tumour or it may come on suddenly with symptoms of a cerebro-vascular catastrophe. In the latter case the haemorrhage may cease spontaneously and the resultant haematoma is absorbed, leaving a cavity filled with a xanthochromic fluid. In the wall of this cavity part of the angioma may protrude as an aneurysm. Repeated haemorrhages may occur in this cavity. On the whole brain angiomata compared to aneurysms are benign lesions. Many patients after one haemorrhage lead a normal life and second haemorrhage may never occur.

It is suggested that operation for removal of angiomata should be considered in the following circumstances:

1. In the course of evacuation of a haematoma.
2. More than one attacks of haemorrhage.
3. Progressive deterioration in patients symptoms, *e.g.* hemiparesis or dysphasia.
4. Uncontrollable epilepsy.

As the operative mortality with modern facilities is negligible, in presence of one of the above indications the size of haematoma even on the dominant hemisphere should not deter the surgeon.

REFERENCES

AMELI, N. O., (1956); *Act. Med. Iranica.*, **1**, 53–68.
—, (1957); *Act. Med. Iranica.*, **1**, 267–291.
—, (1964); *Act. Med. Iranica.*, **7**, 10–18.
CRAWFORD, J. V., AND RUSSEL, D. S., (1956) *J. Neurol., Neurosurg. Psych.*, **19**, 1–11.
KRAYENBUHL, H., AND SIEBENMANN, R., (1965); *J. Neurosurg.*, **22**, 7-20.

Angiomatous and Fistulous Arteriovenous Aneurysm in Children

With comments on the opportunity and results of treatment in 27 cases

RAUL CARREA AND J. MARTIN GIRADO

Centro de Investigaciones Neurológicas and Servicio de Neurocirugía, Hospital de Niños, Buenos Aires (Argentina)

It is the purpose of this communication to offer some comments on the type, location and surgical results in 27 arteriovenous aneurysms admitted to the Buenos Aires Children's Hospital during the last 10 years.

In constrast to adult material (MacKenzie, 1953; Potter, 1955; Gould *et al.*, 1955; Olivecrona and Ladenheim, 1957; Pool, 1962; French *et al.*, 1964), this type of vascular lesion has in children three distinctive features: (a) more than one fourth of the malformations are arteriovenous fistulae, (b) midline encephalic structures are involved in one half of the angiomatous arteriovenous aneurysms, and (c) about one fourth of acute cerebrovascular accidents due to the rupture of cirsoid aneurysms require radical surgery within the first twelve hours.

Our material is summarized on Table I. Angiomatous lesions involved midline

TABLE I

ARTERIOVENOUS ANEURYSMS IN CHILDREN AND ADULTS

	Children	27
ANGIOMATOUS		
Not involving midline structures	9	
Involving midline structures	11	
		20
FISTULOUS		
Posterior cerebral - vein of Galen	2	
Middle cerebral - lateral sinus	1	
Carotid - cavernous sinus	1	
Middle meningeal - dural sinus	1	
Occipital - lateral sinus	1	
Vertebral - supraclavicular vein	1	
		7
	Adults	7
ANGIOMATOUS		
Not involving midline structures	6	
Involving midline structures	1	
FISTULOUS	*none*	

structures in eleven cases whereas they did not in 9 out of 20 patients. There were seven congenital arteriovenous fistulae of various types as listed in the Table. Of the seven adult cases operated during the same period and shown here only as a control, only one lesion involved midline structures.

Figs. 1 to 3 illustrate what we mean by involvement of midline structures. The case whose cerebral angiographies are shown in Figs. 1 and 2 was treated by intra-cranial occlusion of the main afferent vessels and subsequently by ventriculocister-nostomy and the patient is alive and well. The patient illustrated on Fig. 3, an infant, with severe hydrocephalus, died 24 h following a ventriculocaval shunt.

There were in this series two cases of the well known fistulae of the posterior cere-bral artery into the vein of Galen (Alpers and Foerster, 1945; Boldrey and Miller, 1949; French and Peyton, 1954). Intracranial ligation of the posterior cerebral artery was carried out in one of these with success but the child died of an intercurrent disease one year later. In the second case, both posterior cerebral arteries entered into the grossly dilated vein of Galen and there was a severe progressive hydro-cephalus. This improved following a ventriculocisternal shunt and the patient will be subjected to artificial embolization in the near future.

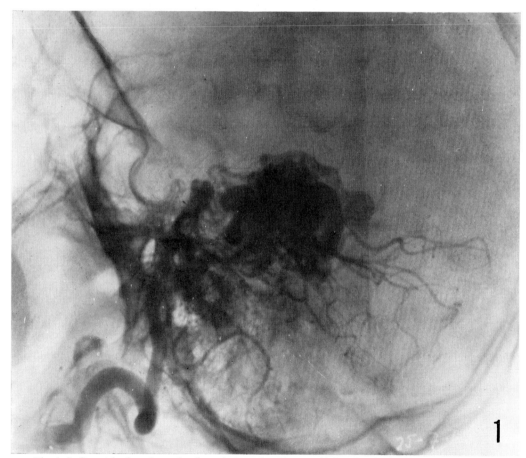

Fig. 1. Left vertebral angiography, lateral view of a 13 year old female who had headaches, a right hemiplegia, left IIIrd nerve palsy, cerebellar signs, papilledema and a cephalic bruit. Intracranial ligation of the main afferent vessels was carried out with success. Two years later progressive hydro-cephalus was controlled with a ventriculocisternal shunt.

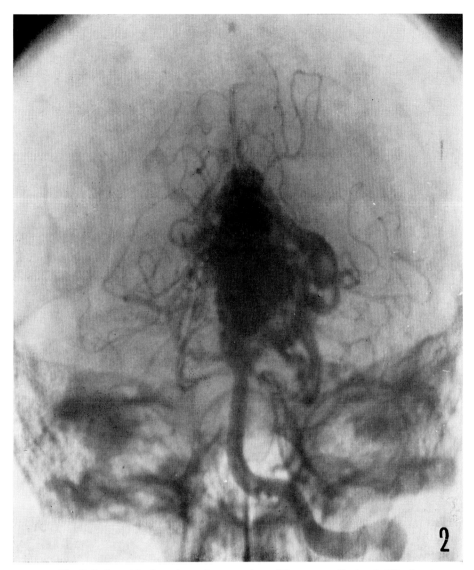

Fig. 2. Left vertebral angiography, a.p. view of the same patient as in Fig. 1.

A 10 month old infant had a fistula of an enlarged branch of the left middle cerebral artery into the lateral sinus. This child had severe cardiac failure and recovered following intracranial occlusion of the fistula.

Table II shows the fate of the nine children with cirsoid aneurysms who were good candidates for radical excision. Two children died shortly after admission before arteriography could be carried out, three and a half and six and a half hours following the onset of symptoms, the lesion being verified at autopsy. Radical removal was carried out in the remaining seven cases with no deaths but three patients had to be operated within 12 h of the onset of symptoms. Similar good results were ob-

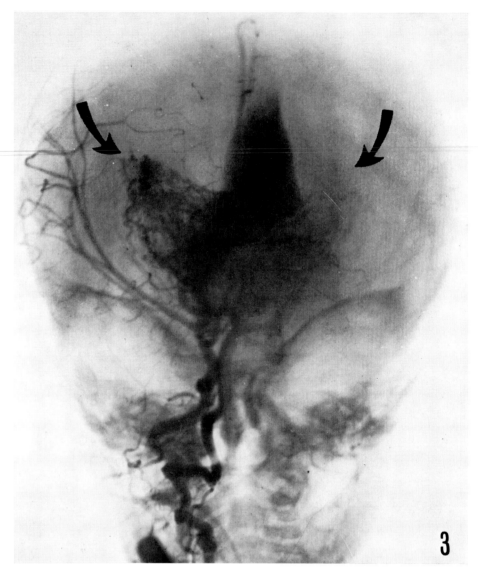

Fig.3. Right brachial angiography in a 3 month old child with progressive hydrocephalus. The lesion involved both thalami (as verified by autopsy). The child died with acute intracranial bleeding following ventriculocaval shunt.

tained in the adult control series but no emergency operation was required in these.

Emphasis should be placed upon the frequency of cases with early deepening coma and decerebrate rigidity. There were six cases of this type in this series. Two cases, as mentioned above, could not receive the benefit of surgery. In three patients, surgery began six, seven and nine and a half hours, respectively, following the initial symptoms and successful radical excision could be performed. In one of these, an 11 year old child, the arteriography was carried out two hours after the onset of symptoms. The 3.5 cm diameter cirsoid aneurysm ruptured directly into the lateral ventricle

TABLE II

ANGIOMATOUS ARTERIOVENOUS ANEURYSMS NOT INVOLVING MIDLINE STRUCTURES

CHILDREN	dead	alive	total
Died before angiography could be carried out (3½, 6½ h)	2	0	2
Operated within 12 h	0	3	3
Operated between 4 and 63 days	0	4	4
Total	2	7	9
ADULTS			
Operated on 2nd week or later	0	6	6

and this is why no midline shift was observed in the a.p. arteriographies. It was radically excised, intraventricular clots were aspirated from both lateral ventricles, by opening the septum pellucidum, and from the third ventricle, and a ventricular drainage was left in place for 48 hours. The child fully recovered following a somewhat difficult postoperative course. The sixth patient, a two month old infant, was such a poor surgical risk that the operation was deferred but a large frontal clot and the lesion could be successfully removed on the fourth day.

TABLE III

ANGIOMATOUS ARTERIOVENOUS ANEURYSMS INVOLVING MIDLINE STRUCTURES

CHILDREN	dead	alive	total
Intracranial occlusion of afferent arteries	0	2	2
Idem plus Torkildsen	0	1	1
Ventriculo-caval shunt	2*	0	2
Unoperated	2	4	6
Total	4	7	11

* One late death

Table III summarizes what was done in the eleven cases in which radical excision could not be attempted. Intracranial ligation of the main afferent vessels to the lesion was carried out in three cases with no ill effects and gave some benefit. A ventriculo-cisternal shunt was carried out in addition in one of these cases who had severe headaches and increasing papilledema as a result of hydrocephalus due to aqueduct stenosis (Figs. 1 and 2). The situation was similar in two other cases where we had, at a previous date, performed a ventriculo-caval shunt: one died on the first postoperative day with intracranial bleeding (Fig. 3) while the other showed progressive signs of brain stem involvement, lapsed gradually into coma and died four weeks later. Such procedure seems, therefore, highly contraindicated.

Of the six unoperated cases, four are alive and well although one had recurrent subarachnoid bleeding. This agrees with other observations in adults (Svien et al., 1956).

Ligation of the afferent artery in fistulous arteriovenous aneurysms is a rather simple and successful procedure. Occlusion of the afferent artery was carried out successfully in six out of seven cases, intracranially in two, extracranially in four. A Torkildsen procedure was employed as already mentioned in one case with a bilateral fistula of the posterior cerebral arteries into the vein of Galen. There were no operative deaths and only one patient died of an intercurrent disease one year following surgery.

Finally, Table IV shows that twenty of these twenty-seven cases are alive and fairly

TABLE IV

ARTERIOVENOUS ANEURYSMS IN CHILDREN. MANAGEMENT AND RESULTS

ANGIOMATOUS	early deaths	late deaths	total deaths	alive	total
Radical operations	0	0	0	7	7
Palliative operations	1	1	2	3	5
Not operated	2	2	4	4	8
Subtotal	*3*	*3*	*6*	*14*	*20*
FISTULOUS					
Radical operations	0	1	1	5	6
Palliative operations	0	0	0	1	1
Subtotal	*0*	*1*	*1*	*6*	*7*
TOTAL	3	4	7	20	27

well one month to ten years following their initial symptoms. Although the table is self-explanatory, it should be pointed out that: (a) out of the 12 operated angiomatous arteriovenous aneurysms the only two deaths were the result of ill-advised palliative ventriculocaval shunts, (b) there was no mortality following radical surgery (7 cases) or after intracranial ligation of afferent vessels or Torkildsen procedure (3 cases), (c) one half of unoperated cases died, and (d) the only late death following the treatment of a fistulous lesion was due to an unrelated cause.

CONCLUSIONS

1. Fistulous arteriovenous aneurysms are much more frequent in children than in adults and can be easily and successfully treated by ligation of afferent arteries.

2. Only one half of the angiomatous arteriovenous aneurysms in children are amenable to radical surgical removal.

3. Intracranial bleeding due to cirsoid aneurysms with early deepening coma and decerebrate rigidity requires extremely urgent arteriography and surgical treatment. The results of radical surgery within the first 12 h are in such cases highly rewarding.

4. Hydrocephalus due to aqueduct stenosis in lesions involving the brain stem can improve with ventriculocisternostomy. Ventriculovenous shunts are contraindicated in these cases.

REFERENCES

ALPERS, B. J. AND FORSTER, F. M. (1945) Arteriovenous aneurysm of great cerebral vein of Galen and arteries of Circle of Willis. *Arch. Neurol. Psychiat., Chicago*, **54**, 181–185.

BOLDREY, E. AND MILLER, E. R. (1949) Arteriovenous fistula (aneurysm) of the great vein (of Galen) and the Circle of Willis. Report of two cases treated by ligation. *Arch. Neurol. Psychiat., Chicago*, **62**, 778–783.

FRENCH, L. A., CHOU, S. N. AND STONY, J. L. (1964) Cerebrovascular malformations. *Congr. Neurol. Surgeons*, **11**, 171–182.

FRENCH, L. A. AND PEYTON, W. T. (1954) Vascular malformations in the region of the great vein of Galen. *J. Neurosurg.*, **11**, 488–498.

GOULD, P. L., PEYTON, W. T. AND FRENCH, L. A. (1955) Arteriovenous malformations of the brain. *Bull. Univ. Minn. Hosp.*, **26**, 611–622.

MACKENZIE, I. (1953) The clinical presentation of the cerebral angioma. A review of 50 cases. *Brain*, **76**, 184–214.

OLIVECRONA, H. AND LADENHEIM, J. (1957) *Congenital arteriovenous aneurysms of the carotid and verebral arterial systems*. Berlin, Springer, 91 pp.

POOL, J. L. (1962) Treatment of arteriovenous malformations of the cerebral hemisphere. *J. Neurosurg.* **19**, 136–141.

POTTER, J. M. (1955) Angiomatous malformations of the brain. Their nature and prognosis. *Ann. Roy. Coll. Surg.*, **16**, 227–243.

SVIEN, H. J., OLIVE, I. AND ANGULO RIVERO, P. (1956) The fate of patients who have cerebral arteriovenous anomalies without definitive surgical treatments. *J. Neurosurg.*, **8**, 381–387.

Surgical Treatment of Carotid-Cavernous Fistulas

A. I. ARUTIUNOV, F. A. SERBINENKO AND A. A. SHLYKOV

*The N. N. Burdenko Research Institute of Neurosurgery, Academy of Medical Sciences, Moscow
(U.S.S.R.)*

Carotid-cavernous fistulas are rather frequent and take a typical clinical course. Their incidence rate takes the second place, after the arterial aneurysms of the brain.

Functionally, a carotid-cavernous fistula is an arterio-venous aneurysm, while from a structural-anatomical point of view a fistula and an aneurysm are completely different pathological forms.

This fact determines the following most important postulation: in cases of fistulas, in contrast to arterio-venous aneurysms, it is impossible to restore the separate arterial and venous circulation, since surgical intervention is impossible within the fistula itself. This, in its turn, puts forward the operative task of the distant occlusion of the afferent arteries, or of an intravascular closure of the defect in the carotid artery.

Our experience comprises 200 cases of carotid-cavernous fistulas; 142 patients were operated by different methods. This permits to make certain generalized conclusions, which in a summarized form prove that:

1. After ligation of the common carotid artery the carotid-cavernous fistula continues to carry out its draining function, being supplied from the ipsilateral external carotid artery and the circle of Willis. Consequently, the therapeutic effect achieved with this operation is insignificant.

2. Ligation of the internal carotid artery in the neck, being a comparatively more

TABLE 1

No.	Type of operation	No. of operations	Recovery	Cerebral complications		
				transient hemi-plegia	persistent hemi-plegia	died
1	Ligation of the common carotid artery	24	—	—	2	—
2	Ligation of the internal carotid artery	29	10	3	2	—
3	Occlusion of flow in the internal and external carotid arteries	16	2	—	1	2
	Total	69	12	3	5	2

TABLE 2

No.	Type of operation	No. of operations	Intracranial clipping of the carotid artery	Recovery
1	Ligation of the common carotid artery	24	8	—
2	Ligation of the internal carotid artery	29	10	5
3	Occlusion of the internal and external carotid arteries	16	9	6
	Total	69	27	11

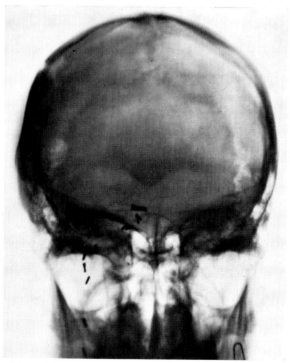

Fig. 1. Plane film of skull after one-stage occlusion of the carotid artery intracranially and in the neck and tamponage of the internal carotid artery with marked muscular pieces (temporary clip on the carotid artery).

TABLE 3

One-stage intracranial occlusion of the internal carotid artery in the neck with muscular tamponage of the fistula	Occlusion of the ophthalmic artery	Recovery (on the basis of clinical and angiographic data)	Died
60	32	56	1

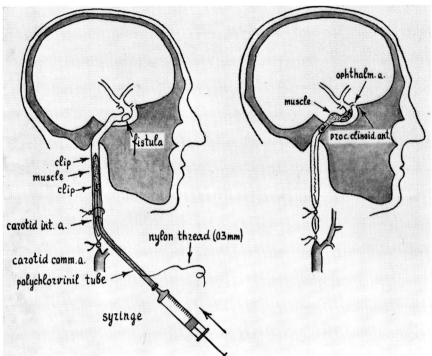

Fig. 2. Scheme of tamponage of the intracavernous part of the shunted carotid artery with marked
pieces of muscle.

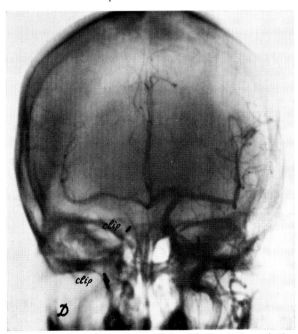

Fig. 3. Angiographic view of collateral circulation of the right hemisphere via the anterior communicating artery after muscular tamponage of the intracavernous part of the right carotid artery; clips
on the cranial and caudal ends of the muscular embolus.

effective operation than ligation of the common carotid artery, also gives results that are hardly satisfactory.

3. Simultaneous ligation of the external and internal carotid arteries in the neck increases the flow from the circle of Willis to the cavernous sinus and depresses the blood supply to the middle cerebral arterial region. Hence, the unfavourable results (Table 1).

4. Intracranial clipping of the carotid artery, after its ligation in the neck, is performed to block the blood supply to the carotid-cavernous fistula via the anterior, ipsilateral posterior communicating and ophthalmic arteries. As a rule, however, the fistula continues to function because of the reverse flow via the external carotid artery, ophthalmic artery and the pituitary and meningeal collaterals.

Intracranial clipping of the carotid artery was performed in 27 of the 69 operated patients. The results of their treatment are presented in Table 2 illustrating the poor effect of the surgical methods mentioned.

The next 60 patients were operated by means of simultaneous intracranial occlusion of the carotid artery with tamponage of the cavernous part of the carotid artery with a piece of muscle marked with a silver clip and ligation of the internal carotid artery in the neck. This operation permits avoiding all cerebral complications and prevents blood supply to the fistula, thus providing full success of the operation. In all these cases the muscular embolus was transported to the fistula hydraulically through the plastic tube inserted into the internal carotid artery. This group of patients is presented in Table 3.

One of the 60 operated patients died. The fatal outcome was caused by the incision of a pre-operatively not recognized traumatic pseudo-aneurysm at the supraclinoidal part of the carotid artery.

Finally, the last group: intravascular tamponage of the fistula. This operation can be performed with the help of any plastic material, but in our opinion, muscle is the best one. The original Brooks operation has one important drawback: the muscular embolus is not controlled and may embolize the middle cerebral artery. In our modification of this operation, we use a piece of muscle, 4–5 cm long, marked with a silver clip. This piece is hydraulically transported through a plastic tube under TV-control to the intracavernous part of the carotid artery and tamponades the fistula. The distal end of the muscle piece is fixed to a thin Capron thread and its position may be corrected and the muscle may be drawn back, if necessary.

13 patients were successfully operated with this method.

A New Surgical Method for Treatment of Pulsating Exophthalmus

T. RIECHERT

Neurosurgical Clinic,* University of Freiburg i. Br. (Germany)

Intracranial injuries to the internal carotid in the region of its passage through the cavernous sinus are becoming more and more important by the increase in traffic accidents. Spontaneous healing occurs, as we know, only in a low percentage of the cases and is mostly a consequence of thrombosis. Surgical therapy does not possess an absolutely reliable method. There are limitations to the possibility of ligation of vessels because disturbances of brain circulation may easily be caused. On the other hand a ligature often remains uneffective if the collateral circulation is strongly developed. In recent times Dwight Parkinson has shown the difficulties prohibiting a definitive improvement by ligation of arteries.

A further method of operative management is the introduction of a small embolus of muscle after Brooks. This method is only possible in those cases in which the fistula is large enough to let the muscular tissue pass through the opening of the cavernous carotid. Things being as they are, the most promising method would be a direct approach to the fistula in the cavernous sinus. Such a procedure has so far been declined by all authors even in progressive cases, principally because of the serious hemorrhages to be expected during such an intervention. Parkinson recently treated a case of progressive exophthalmus by direct approach. He performed ligatures around the carotid, incised it and packed it with muscle. The artery was then clipped and ligated. Because of the hemorrhage to be expected the operation was conducted under hypothermia with the heart exposed and simultaneous occlusion of the great vessels from the arch of the aorta. A cardiac arrest was additionally provided after incision of the sinus. The operation had a good effect and there was no evidence of a neurological deficit, although the patient died on the third postoperative day from a cardio-pulmonary complication.

In the patient operated on by us we also planned a direct approach because the typical operations had remained unsuccessful and there was a deterioration of symptoms. We attempted a primary occlusion of the fistula with subsequent thrombosis in the region of the cavernous sinus. For this purpose we tried to fix a tantalum plate in the region of the base of skull above the cavernous sinus in such a way that a firm

---

* Director: Prof. Dr. T. RIECHERT

References p. 448–449

compression of the fistula and subsequent thrombosis was attained. In order to avoid vascular injuries due to the pressure of the tantalum, we interposed several layers of dura mater and of nylon gauze between the metal and the sinus. For obtaining a lasting and efficient compression it was necessary to fix the tantalum immovably on the base of skull. For this purpose we used steel tacks which were inserted into the base of skull with the help of a special instrument developed by myself. This instrument has proved useful in numerous operations for liquorrhea. Even in large defects of the base of skull we were able to fix the fascia lata by means of these tacks above the defect so that we reached a water-tight occlusion.

The patient operated on by us was an 8-year-old boy who had suffered a blunt head injury. Within a few days a pulsating exophthalmus developed with chemosis and a bruit. The presence of an aneurysm was first suggested by the finding of the Ophthalmological Clinic (Director: Prof. Dr. Wegner) of the University of Freiburg i. Br.

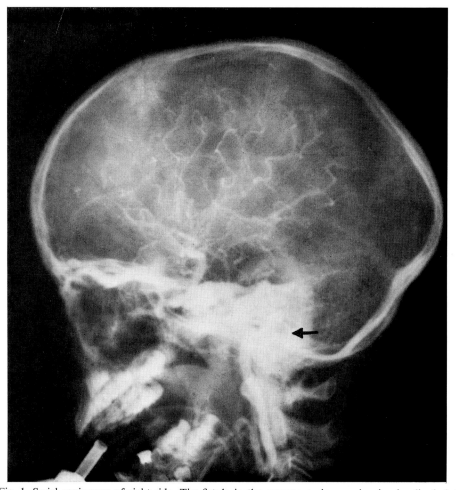

Fig. 1. Serial angiogram of right side. The fistula in the cavernous sinus region is visualized. (←)

The angiogram sequence of the right side visualized a typical fistula of the carotid in the region of the cavernous sinus (Fig. 1). The normal brain vessels were also filled, a sign that the fistula was relatively small and not suitable for a treatment by muscle embolism after Brooks. The angiogram of the left (healthy) side demonstrated a complete double filling.

Therapy: The right common carotid was ligated in stages with a Selverstone carotid artery clamp. As the symptoms, particularly the bruit, did not improve, a ligation of the right internal carotid was performed 8 days later. This intervention also remained without success, so that, after experimental dissection of the cavernous carotid on autopsy specimens, the operation mentioned above had to be undertaken*.

Report of operation: Right-sided frontal trephination and exposure of chiasma, intracranial carotid and posterior communicating artery, ligation of ophthalmic artery. The access is made difficult by enlargement and tension of the cavernous sinus and by adhesions. The ophthalmic and then the internal carotid arteries are ligated and dissected. Puncture of the cavernous sinus causes a large arterial hemorrhage, a sign that, in accordance with Parkinson's description, the collateral blood supply to the fistula has not yet been blocked. Thereupon the 3rd cranial nerve is exposed and isolated in order to avoid injury to this nerve. A tantalum plate is adapted to the size of the free space above the dilated cavernous sinus. Drillings are performed in the metal for the fixation of this plate on the base of skull with steel tacks. In order to reach a more effective compression by the tantalum plate and to avoid, on the other hand, a damage to the vessels by this metal, a layer of Spongioprot (R) (enveloped by a dacron net) and dura mater is interposed between the plate and the cavernous sinus. Under temporary compression of the left carotid in the neck, the plate is impressed on the cavernous sinus and the first steel tack is inserted. This causes a profuse arterial bleeding. Only after the second steel tack has been fixed and the pressure of the plate has increased, the bleeding stops and the previously tightly filled vessels of the base of skull collapse (Fig. 2). There were no postoperative complications in this case. Objectively and subjectively the bruit had completely disappeared immediately after the operation, the other symptoms showed progressive improvement. There was an incomplete postoperative paresis of the third cranial nerve and partial hemianopsia. The oculomotor paresis disappeared nearly completely within a few weeks.

DISCUSSION

After failure of the typical operations, a traumatic fistula of the cavernous carotid was approached directly by intracranial exposure. Thrombosis was for the first time caused by pressure on the cavernous sinus with a small tantalum plate and the patient

---

* We are obliged to Prof. Dr. STAUBESAND, Director of the Anatomical Institute of Freiburg University for his aid.

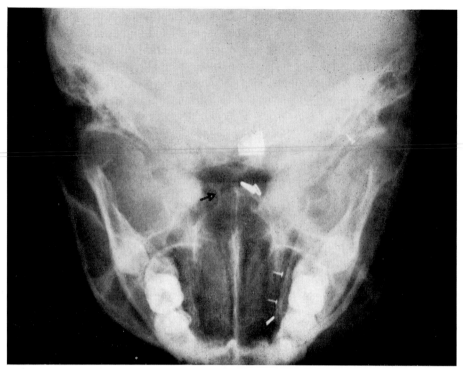

Fig. 2. Occlusion of the fistula with a tantalum plate. (→)

was cured. The described method had already been successfully used by the author in a previous case of inoperable aneurysm of the internal carotid at the base of skull. The method was also employed in basal meningiomas in which the bleeding could not be managed by the typical interventions. By a modification of the technique an exact fixation of the tantalum plate can be reached even in cases with pathologic erosion of the base of skull.

SUMMARY

A case of pulsating exophthalmus is described in which after failure of the typical surgical methods the fistula in the cavernous sinus was directly approached.

Thrombosis was induced by compression of the cavernous sinus with a tantalum plate.

REFERENCES

BROOKS, B., (1930); Treatment of traumatic arteriovenous fistula. *Sth. med. J. (Bgham, Ala.)*, **23**, 100–106.

HAMBY, W. B., (1964); Carotid-Cavernosus Fistula. Report of 32 Surgically Treated Cases and Suggestions for Definitive Operation. *J. Neurosurg.*, 859–866.

ISFORT, A., AND ESCH, R., (1965); Ist die Muskelembolie nach BROOKS bei den traumatischen Carotis-Sinus cavernosus-Fisteln heute noch zweckmässig? *Neurochir.*, **8**, 11–19.

KAUTZKY, R., (1953); Fehlerquellen bei der Durchführung des operativen intrakranialen Karotis-verschlusses. *Zbl. Neurochir.*, **18**, 65–71.

PARKINSON, D., (1964); Collateral circulation of cavernous carotid artery: anatomy. *Canad. J. Surg.*, **7**, 251–268.

—, (1965); A Surgical Approach to the Cavernous Portion of the Carotid Artery. *J. Neurosurg.*, 474–483.

—, AND RAMSAY, R. M., (1963); Carotid cavernous fistula with pulsating exophthalmus: a fortuitous cure. *Canad. J. Surg.*, **6**, 191–194.

RIECHERT, T., (1964); Klinik und operative Therapie der intrakraniellen infektiösen Erkrankungen. *Archiv Ohren-, Nasen- und Kehlkopfheilk.*, **183**, 147–164. (Kongressbericht, 1964; Bad Reichenhall, Teil II)

—, (1967); *Fortschritte in der Behandlung von Aneurysmen und Gefässtumoren des Hirns.* Jubiläums-heft der Wissenschaftlichen Zeitschrift der Humboldt-Universität Berlin.

—, AND GABRIEL, E., (1967); Eine neue chirurgische Methode zur Ausschaltung von biologischem Gewebe durch induktive Erwärmung (Indukoagulation). *Dtsch. med. Wschr.*, **92**, 513–516.

SUNDER-PLASSMANN, P., AND TIWISINA, Th., (1952); Die Behandlung der Aneurysmen im Sinus cavernosus (Exophthalmus pulsans). *Chirurg*, **23**, 376–382.

WALTER, W., AND BISCHOF, W., (1966); Die Durchblutungsstörung des Gehirns bei Sinus-Cavernosus-Aneurysmen. *Zbl. Neurochir.*, **27**, 139–155.

WOLFF, H., AND SCHMID, B., (1939); Das Arteriogramm des pulsierenden Exophthalmus. *Zbl. Neurochir.*, **4**, 241–319.

Discussion on Aneurysm

P. RÖTTGEN

53 Bonn-V., Heinr.-Fritsch-Str. 16, Germany

Until April 1967 we observed 726 cases of spontaneous cerebral hemorrhage (Fig. 1).

The great number of cerebral hemorrhages of unknown origin is striking although the 4 main cerebral arteries were arteriographically demonstrated and in some cases the angiography was even repeated later.

Fig. 2 shows the results of 233 berry aneurysms whose necks were intradurally clipped. I prefer this method (occasionally the ligation of the aneurysm's neck by a thread, too) since the aneurysm has to be prepared anyway and the coating of the aneurysm with plastic materials offers no advantage. In the beginning younger neurosurgeons generally prepare the aneurysms not exactly enough fearing a rupture (magnifying glasses, micro-instruments). A hypotension from 30 to 70 mm Hg is necessary. The preparation of the carotid arteries in the neck for a temporary ligation is unnecessary in our opinion. The digital compression of the carotid arteries is sufficient. We think that the temporary compression of the anterior cerebral arteries in cases of aneurysms of the anterior communicating artery is noxious because of endangering the hypothalamic vessels. The hypothermia from 28 to 30°C prevents hypotension injuring the brain and permits the compression of both carotid arteries for 10 minutes if necessary.

From 15 comatose patients operated upon in the time of acute cerebral hemorrhage 12 died. Therefore an operation during this phase seems to be unreasonable. A patient not overcoming the comatose state usually shows a perforation into the ventricle and has an unfavorable prognosis.

ANEURYSMEN, ANGIOME UND UNKLARE CEREBRALE
BLUTUNGEN

Aneurysmen	324
Angiome	185
Spontane Subarachnoidealblutungen unklarer Genese	184
Spontane intracerebrale Blutungen unkl. Genese	33
	726

Abb. 1

OP.-RESULTATE (intradurales Verklippen) BEI 233 ANEURYSMEN

Sitz	*Zahl*	*Op. i. Blut. stadium*	†	*Op. i. Intervall*	†
Com. ant.	91	8	7	83	11 (13%)
Supraclin.	80	1	—	79	7 8,8%)
Media	35	5	5	30	3
Gabel	12	1	—	11	1
Com. post.	7			7	1
Sonstige	8			8	—
	233	15	12	218	23 (10,5%)

Abb. 2

The high mortality of aneurysms of the anterior communicating artery seems not only to depend on the difficulty of this operation. There we find especially marked defects caused by secondary ischemia in both hemispheres. The greater part of our patients is even more than 50 years old. The total mortality naturally contains the first experiences of operating such cases. The occlusion (by clipping or ligating) of the aneurysms without injuring the artery is according to our experience the method of choice.

Pathogenesis of Hypertensive Intracerebral Hemorrhage: A Hypothesis with Supporting Data[*]

GEORGE MARGOLIS, JACOB ABRAHAM, AYKUT ERBENGI, JOHN O'LOUGHLIN AND W. C. MACCARTY, JR.

Department of Pathology, Dartmouth Medical School, and the Departments of Neurosurgery and Radiology, Mary Hitchcock Memorial Hospital, Hanover, New Hampshire 03755 (U.S.A.)

Hypertensive intracerebral hemorrhage is a unique pathological phenomenon, a comparable process occurring in no other organ system. Evidence indicates that this lesion results from a necrotizing arteriopathy in the cerebral vascular bed, the onset and progression of which precedes similar changes in the systemic vasculature. During a period of intensive study of the dynamics of cerebrovascular disease a hypothesis of the pathogenesis of this process has been constructed[**]. This hypothesis is based upon two premises, namely;

(1) It is not elevated blood pressure per se, but rather the tonic reaction of vessels to this stress, which is responsible for the widespread vascular injury occurring in hypertension.

(2) The cerebral vascular bed is peculiarly susceptible to injury in hypertension because of structural and physiologic differences between it and the systemic vasculature which place it at a disadvantage in withstanding the sustained load of perfusion by an elevated pressure head.

This hypothesis is, admittedly, speculative and difficult to prove. Succinctly, it demands the demonstration of a strong superiority of the extra-neural over the neural vascular beds in reactivity to baroreceptor, chemoreceptor and neurogenic influences. Such supporting evidence, provided from our own studies and from the literature, is cited herein.

Physiologic studies of structure and stresses in vessels[2,3] furnish cogent arguments against vascular injury in hypertension solely on the basis of increased intravascular pressure. The physical equilibrium of the vascular wall is the resultant of the two opposing forces, luminal pressure and wall tension. Luminal pressure, tending to stretch the wall, is resisted by tension in the wall, according to the formula[3]

$$\text{wall tension} = \text{distending pressure} \, \frac{\text{vessel radius}}{\text{wall thickness}} \, .$$

Tension has two components. One, *elastic tension*, is the passive resistance to stretch

* Supported by Grant NB-05160 from the National Institute of Neurological Diseases and Blindness, and Grant GM-10210 from the National Institute of General Medical Sciences.
** Historical aspects of the development of prevailing concepts of the genesis of hypertensive apoplexy, histopathologic features of salient vascular lesions, and a discussion of physical principles underlying these changes have been presented elsewhere[1].

References p. 461–462

of the physiologically inert vascular elastic tissue. The other, *active tension*, is dependent upon vasomotor tone, to which the sole contributor is smooth muscle. Only the action of this latter component requires the expenditure of energy. Changes in wall tension are of great magnitude because of the dependence upon radial dimensions. Hence the fall in wall tension between aorta and capillary is of a far larger order than the 4-fold drop in blood pressure in this portion of the vascular bed. Considering that at the arteriolar level — the order of vascular size involved most extensively in hypertension — the factor of wall tension is of small magnitude *at any pressure level*, it is difficult to conceive of small vessels being injured or ruptured simply because of increased tangential forces applied to their walls *unless* they respond by a myogenic reaction of excessive degree and/or uncontrolled duration. An exaggerated myogenic reflex to abrupt or severe elevations of pressure could lead to vascular necrosis through ischemia, anoxia, and/or exhaustion of available substrates as a consequence of energy utilization during prolonged vasospasm.

A striking demonstration of the differential reactivity of neural and extraneural vascular beds has been encountered by us in studies of the pathogenesis and therapeutics of neurotoxic effects of roentgen contrast agents[4,5]. These studies are based on the observation that radiopaque media used in clinical angiography are capable of producing a necrotizing lesion if they reach target organs in high concentrations. In an experimental model of retrograde aortography in the dog the spinal cord is the majo

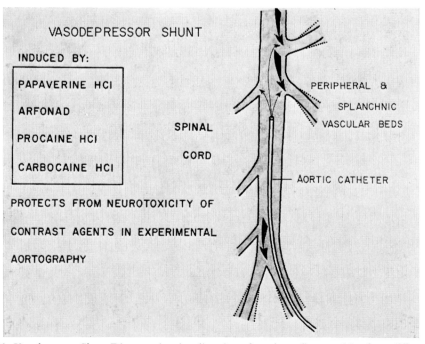

Fig. 1. *Vasodepressor Shunt*. Diagram showing diversion of aortic outflow resulting from differential action of vasodepressor agents upon resistance vessels of neural and extraneural vascular beds. This directional shunting was deduced from studies with a model of experimental retrograde aortography in the dog, exemplified by Fig. 2, and confirmed by flow studies.

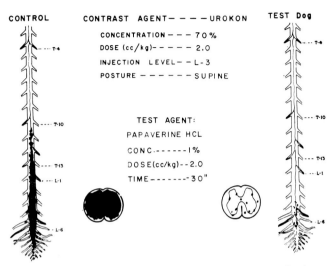

PROPHYLAXIS OF CONTRAST MEDIUM INJURY

CONTROL   CONTRAST AGENT — — — UROKON   TEST Dog

CONCENTRATION — — — 7 0 %
DOSE (cc/kg) — — — — 2.0
INJECTION LEVEL — — L-3
POSTURE — — — — — SUPINE

TEST AGENT:
PAPAVERINE HCL
CONC.------1%
DOSE(cc/kg)--2.0
TIME-------30"

Fig. 2. Protective action against neurotoxic effect of a noxious intraaortic injection mass induced by the vasodepressor shunt depicted in Fig. 1. Urokon[R], the contrast agent used in this study (now no longer available except on an investigative basis) is severely histotoxic at dosage and concentration levels far below those employed here, thereby rendering this study a most rigorous test of prophylactic action of the therapeutic agent.

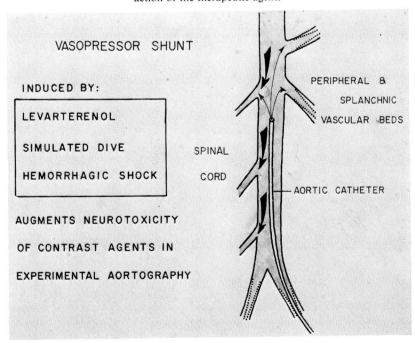

VASOPRESSOR SHUNT

INDUCED BY:

LEVARTERENOL

SIMULATED DIVE

HEMORRHAGIC SHOCK

AUGMENTS NEUROTOXICITY

OF CONTRAST AGENTS IN

EXPERIMENTAL AORTOGRAPHY

PERIPHERAL &
SPLANCHNIC
VASCULAR BEDS

SPINAL
CORD

AORTIC CATHETER

Fig. 3. *Vasopressor Shunt.* Diagram showing diversion of aortic outflow resulting from differential action of vasoconstrictor influences upon resistance vessels of neural and extraneural vascular beds. This directional shunting was deduced from studies with a model of experimental retrograde aortography in the dog exemplified by Fig. 4, and confirmed by flow studies.

AUGMENTATION OF CONTRAST MEDIUM INJURY

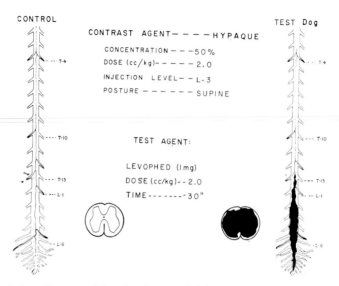

CONTROL   TEST Dog

CONTRAST AGENT— — — —HYPAQUE

CONCENTRATION — — —50%

DOSE (cc/kg)— — — — —2.0

INJECTION LEVEL— —L-3

POSTURE — — — — —SUPINE

TEST AGENT:

LEVOPHED (1mg)

DOSE (cc/kg)— -2.0

TIME— — — — — —30"

Fig. 4. Augmentation of neurotoxicity of an intraaortic injection mass produced by the vasopressor shunt depicted in Fig. 3. Hypaque[R], the contrast agent used in this study, is otherwise innocuous at this dosage and concentration, but is severely histotoxic when shunted toward the vascular bed of the spinal cord without significant dilution.

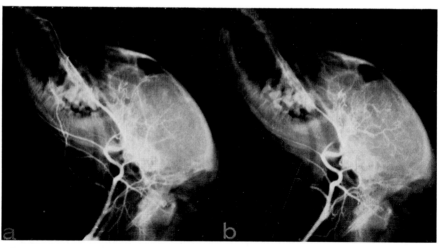

Fig. 5. *Vasopressor Shunt*. Diagram showing redistribution of flow of common carotid injection mass induced by differential action of a vasoconstrictor agent upon the cerebral and extracerebral vasculature of the dog. (a) In the control angiogram the flow is distributed to both the external and internal carotid systems, with the former being dominant. (b) After the intracarotid injection of levarterenol. constriction of the extracerebral vessels, closure of anastamoses, and dominance of the intracerebral angiogram are demonstrated.

target area for this destructive action. Since this necrotizing effect is a concentration dependent action the degree of injury to the spinal cord may be used as a semi-quantitative index of direction of outflow of the intra-aortic injection mass. By pharmacologic induction of altered tonus of the vascular system it is possible to demonstrate a 10-fold or greater difference in the neurotoxic action of these media. At one hand extreme vaso-inhibitor agents (procaine HCl, papaverine HCl and Arfonad [trimethapan camphorsulfonate]), by inducing a shunt away from the spinal cord, exert a protective effect (Figs. 1 and 2). On the other hand, the vasoconstrictor agent, levarterenol, by inducing a shunt toward the cord, greatly potentiates the neurotoxic action of contrast media (Figs. 3 and 4). Clearly, these studies indicate a strong dominance of extraneural over neural vascular beds in response to vasoactive drugs.

Studies of these same influences using electromagnetic flow meters and cineaortography to measure blood flow confirm these findings[6]. Under the influence of levarterenol the major outflow routes from the aorta close down, leaving the paired lumbar arteries as the major means of forward flow of the injection mass, with selective diversion of flow to the essentially passive vascular bed of the spinal cord via anterior and posterior radicular arteries. Conversely, the changes induced in vascular tonus by the vasodepressor, papaverine HCl, result in a great lowering of peripheral resistance in the splanchnic and somatic vascular beds, an increased speed of aortic outflow, a dilution of the injection mass, and a shunting away from the spinal cord.

The subordinate status of the neural vasculature is even more clearly manifest in studies of the cerebral circulation in the dog[7]. In this animal there are rich anastomoses between the cerebral and extracerebral arterial trees, which facilitate the observation of modifying influences of pharmacologic agents. In a state of normal vascular tonus an injection of contrast medium into the common carotid artery will be distributed to both external and internal carotid systems, with the former being dominant. Under a vasoconstrictor stimulus, radiographic studies of flow demonstrate a constriction of the extracerebral vessels, a shutting down of anastomotic channels, and a dominance of the intracerebral angiogram (Fig. 5). The converse picture is produced by a state of vasodilator induced hypotonus (Fig. 6). These same directional diversions of flow are seen in angiographic studies when injections are made selectively into either the external or the internal carotid artery. These findings are corroborated by electromagnetic flow meter studies of these two arterial trees.

Another set of studies has demonstrated a striking difference in reactivity of the retinal and cerebral circulations to respiratory gases[8,9]. Oxygen at high concentrations and pressures is a potent cell toxin. The vascular system responds to an excess of oxygen by a generalized constrictor action, a reaction interpreted as a homeostatic protective mechanism preventing the tissues from being flooded with oxygen. Under conditions of hyperbaric oxygenation the vascular bed of the canine retina overreacts to such a degree that microscopic foci of ischemic necrosis develop. This retinal ischemic lesion can be prevented by the addition of carbon dioxide to the respiratory gas. As a result of the vasodilating action of carbon dioxide, however, the direct toxic action of oxygen on the brain is augmented and convulsive responses, paralysis, neuronal necrosis and death are accelerated in onset and increased in incidence.

References p. 461–462

A recent study by Harper[10] demonstrates that with hypercapnia the autoregulatory capacity of the cerebral vascular bed is lost, thereby explaining the increased toxicity of oxygen for the brain in the presence of CO_2. The investigations of Balentine shed further light on this phenomenon. By repeatedly exposing rats to oxygen at high pres-

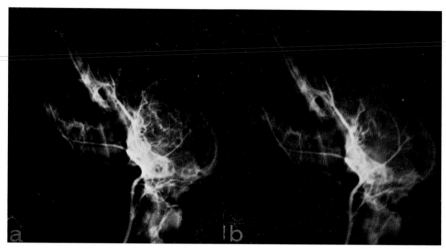

Fig. 6. *Vasodepressor Shunt*. Diagram showing redistribution of flow of an intracarotid injection mass induced by differential action of a vasoinhibitor agent upon the cerebral and extracerebral vasculature of the dog. (a) In the control angiogram, flow is distributed to both the external and internal carotid systems, with the latter being unusually well shown. (b) After the intracarotid injection of papaverine the external carotid and its major branches are dilated and readily seen, but there is virtually no demonstrable filling of the distal internal carotid tree.

sure, he has been able to produce regularly bilateral symmetrical necrotic lesions in the substantia nigra[11]. But with unilateral ligation of the carotid artery, a procedure that renders the ipsilateral cerebral cortex vulnerable to anoxia, he has been able to protect the ipsilateral deep nuclei from toxic effects of hybaroxia[12]. We conclude from his study that the cerebral vasculature, in contrast to the retinal vessels, does not overrespond to hybaroxia to the point of inducing a paradoxical ischemia. Further, its protective constrictor response against excess oxygen is easily overcome by the vasodilating influence of hypercapnia. In Balentine's studies the protective effect of carotid ligation against excess perfusion by hyperoxygenated blood is comparable to the effect of this procedure against cerebral vascular injury in experimental hypertension[13].

Although the relative inertness, or resistance to change of the cerebral circulation is a well established phenomenon[14], the magnitude of the difference in reactivity between the neural and extraneural beds has not been strongly emphasized. However, the remarkable circulatory adjustments observed in diving mammals furnish data comparable to ours[15,16]. During simulated dives a widespread peripheral vasoconstriction has been demonstrated, with a sharp drop in intravascular pressure and a virtually complete cessation of blood flow in muscles, extremities, renal and mesenteric arteries. At the same time blood flow to the brain remains constant or may even increase. That this same reflex mechanism with strong shunting of circulation toward the central nervous system, exists in terrestrial animals, has recently been demonstrated in these laboratories. Using the model of experimental aortography described above, Mills *et al.*[17] have demonstrated that during simulated dives otherwise innocuous doses of contrast agents become noxious for the dog as a result of this differential shunting, just as with the use of vasopressor agents.

Despite the relatively passive status of the cerebral vasculature an increase in cerebrovascular resistance paralleling blood pressure rise is a recognized phenomenon in hypertension both in man[18] and animals[10]. Further, animal studies, including observations through plastic skulls and cranial windows and measurements of cerebral blood flow and oxygen tension, have clearly demonstrated an angiospastic mechanism of cerebral vascular injury in hypertension[19,20]. An elevation of pressure head, particularly an abrupt rise, has been observed to induce an excessive and prolonged vasoconstriction, to the point of producing a reduction in flow and oxygen tension, focal permeability breaks, microinfarcts, and vascular necrosis. On the other hand it has been shown by Robert[13] that with unilateral or bilateral ligation of the common carotid arteries in rats with DOCA-hypertension, protection of one or both cerebral hemispheres from edema and hemorrhage may be attained. Similarly, Robert and Nezamis[21] has protected the vascular bed of the eye in hypertensive rats.

Support for the concept that a structurally weaker vascular bed is more susceptible than a stronger system to injury in hypertension is provided by further observations, both in animals and in man. Byrom[22], in rats made chronically hypertensive by unilateral renal artery constriction, observed a striking medial hypertrophy in arteries of the intact kidney and, despite an eventual revascularization, a relative disuse atrophy in the arteries of the restricted kidney. Upon injection of the pressor agent, angiotensin, into rats with chronic unilateral renal hypertension an acute necrotizing lesion was produced in the arteries of the restricted kidney only. He interpreted this finding as the result of the vulnerability of the relatively atrophic arteries to "the double stress of overstimulation and excessive filling tension", stresses which the hypertrophied vessels would be better able to withstand. In man the congenital narrowing, or coarctation, of the thoracic aorta results in a comparable disparity in growth and development of the vasculature. As a compensatory response to the restricted flow in the kidneys a moderate systolic hypertension occurs. But below the site of aortic stenosis the pulse pressure is strikingly reduced, and a relative hypoplasia of the arterial bed results. When this constriction is surgically corrected an acute paradoxical hypertension may develop[23]. This reaction has been explained as an overresponse of the poststenotic portion of the vascular bed upon being abruptly subjected to an unaccustomed distending force. In some instances acute focal arterial necrosis develops, restricted to the hypoplastic vascular bed distal to the site of corrected constriction[23,24]. Giese[25] in his admirable study of the pathogenesis of hypertensive vascular disease, observed that permeability changes, infiltration of fibrin, and necrosis developed in weaker, dilated portions of arterial walls, rather than in constricted zones. It could be queried, however, whether these stages of the vascular lesion had not been preceded by an intense vasoconstrictive response at the maximally affected areas, now no longer capable of

References p. 461–462

reacting against an elevated pressure head; i.e., that the incipient phase of aneurysm formation already existed at the time of these observations.

There are few studies exploring the basis of the structural difference between cerebral and systemic arterial beds. Hassler[26] produced large cranial bone defects in young rabbits and observed that medial hypertrophy and hyperplasia of cerebral arteries occurred in these operated animals. This finding suggested that the damping effect of the closed cranial cavity is a critical factor in creating these differences. Naeye[27,28], studying the postnatal development of the vascular system in man, has observed that in young hypertensives a hypertrophy and hyperplasia of the muscular coat of systemic arteries occurred. These reactive changes exhibited a broad spectrum of severity. Surprisingly, the arterial bed of the brain manifested a greater degree of hyperplasia and hypertrophy than found in any other site. Another significant finding was the inverse correlation between changes displayed by arteries of supply and their terminal beds. For example, the mesenteric arteries, supplying the bowel, were most severely altered. Yet, the intrinsic arteries and arterioles of the gastrointestinal tract were unaltered. These unanticipated findings are readily explained by our thesis. A vasotonic reaction of proximal regions of an arterial tree would protect distal zones, and at the same time determine the localization of the major reactive changes and injurious effects invoked by an elevated pressure head. Further, Selye[29] using rats and Brownlee *et al.*[30] with dogs have demonstrated that surgical constriction of a proximal mesenteric vessel during the developmental stages of experimental hypertension will protect the distal beds from arteriolonecrotic lesions. This reciprocal relationship between proximal vasotonic response, site of vascular injury, and protection of the distal vascular bed is exemplified by the hypertensive kidney. Here the delicate glomerular capillary network remains uninjured, being protected by the afferent arteriole, the locus both of vasospasm and of arteriolosclerosis.

Finally, the deep, rather than surface localization of hypertensive intracerebral hemorrhage must be explained. Particularly germane to these considerations is the study of Hughes[31] concerning the pathogenesis of "lacunes", the small foci of cavitation and softening in the basal ganglia which constitute the most frequent of all cerebrovascular lesions. He places emphasis upon the unique anatomical arrangement of the paramedian arteries, small hair-like vessels which arise from surface arteries and almost immediately penetrate the brain. The steep gradient in caliber between the main arterial trunk and the paramedian arteries, unmatched elsewhere in the vascular system, exposes these frail vessels to an inordinately high pulsatile pressure. Clearly, this anatomic feature adds to the stresses which must be withstood by a vascular bed whose homeostatic mechanisms are already overtaxed. We postulate that in hypertension the superior reactivity of extraneural vascular beds tends to drive blood into the brain in increasing quantities, to the point of overcoming its autoregulatory mechanisms[10]. The brain, with a capillary pool in gray matter[32] amounting to but 1% of wet tissue mass, has little ability to accommodate an increased blood volume. Further, the penetrating arteries supply a system of end arteries, in contrast to the rich anastomotic network of the cortical vessels. Manifestly, the vasotonic response to an increased pressure head would require greater work in a terminal vascular bed than in a system with abundant collaterals which would accommodate a large runoff, thereby attenuating the perfusion load.

SUMMARY

A hypothesis is advanced explaining the vulnerability of the cerebral vasculature in hypertension and the pathogenesis of hypertensive intracerebral hemorrhage. This postulate is based upon two premises: (1) It is not elevated blood pressure per se, but rather the tonic reaction of vessels to this stress, which causes the widespread vascular injury occurring in hypertension. (2) Structural and functional properties of the cerebral vasculature place it at a disadvantage in withstanding an elevated pressure head, rendering it particularly susceptible to injury in hypertension. This hypothesis has been tested by studies comparing differential reactivity of neural and extraneural vascular beds to vasoactive agents at two sites, namely: (1) The internal versus the external carotid arterial flow distributions. (2) Aortic outflow into the vascular bed of the spinal cord versus splanchnic and somatic vasculature. Electromagnetic flow meters, thermistors, serial and cineangiograms, and neurotoxic effects of roentgen contrast media have been used as indicators of blood flow. While the extraneural vasculature responded strongly to vasoactive agents, responses of the neural vasculature were essentially passive, their primary reactions being overriden by stronger responses of extraneural vessels. Consequently, vasoconstrictor agents induced a strong centripetal shunt, diverting flow toward the central nervous system. Conversely, vasoinhibitor agents induced a strong centrifugal shunt, diverting flow toward splanchnic and somatic vascular beds. The striking superiority of extraneural over neural vascular beds in reactivity to a broad spectrum of vasoactive agents provides strong supporting evidence for the proposed hypothesis. Pertinent supporting evidence from the literature is also cited.

REFERENCES

1 MARGOLIS, G. (1966) *The vascular changes and pathogenesis of hypertensive intracerebral hemorrhage.* Chapter IV in *Cerebrovascular Disease,* Association for Research in Nervous and Mental Diseases, Vol. **41,** 73–91. Williams & Wilkins Co., Baltimore.

2 BURTON, A. C. (1965) *Physiology and Biophysics of the Circulation.* Chicago, The Year Book Medical Publishers.

3 PETERSON, L. H. (1962) Properties and behavior of living vascular wall. In Proceedings of a Symposium on Vascular Smooth Muscle. *Physiol. Rev.,* **42,** *Suppl.,* 5, 309.

4 MARGOLIS, G. AND YERASIMIDES, T. G. (1966) Vasopressor potentiation of neurotoxicy in experimental aortography. Implications regarding the pathogenesis of contrast medium injury. *Acta Radiol.* (Diagnosis) 5, 388–412.

5 YERASIMIDES, T. G., MARGOLIS, G. AND PONTON, H. J. (1963) Prophylaxis of experimental contrast medium injury to the spinal cord by vasodepressor drugs. *Angiology,* **14,** 394.

6 ABRAHAM, J., MARGOLIS, G., O'LOUGHLIN, J. C. AND MACCARTY, W. C., JR. (1966) Differential reactivity of the neural and extraneural vasculature. I. Role in the pathogenesis of neurotoxic effects of contrast media. *J. Neurosurg.,* **25,** 257–269.

7 MARGOLIS, G., ABRAHAM, J., ERBENGI, A. AND MACCARTY, W. C., JR. (1967) Differential reactivity of the neural and extraneural vasculature. II. Contribution to the dynamics of cerebrovascular disease. In preparation.

8 MARGOLIS, G. AND BROWN, I. W., JR. (1966) Hyperbaric oxygenation: The eye as the critical limiting factor. *Science*, **151**, 466.

9 MOOR, G., FUSON, R. L., BROWN, I. W., JR., MARGOLIS, G. AND SMITH, W. W. (1966) An evaluation of the protective effect of hyperbaric oxygenation on the central nervous system during circulatory arrest. *J. Thoracic and Cardiovascular Surg.*, **52**, 618–628.

10 HARPER, A. M. (1966) Autoregulation of cerebral blood flow: Influence of the arterial blood pressure on the blood flow through the cerebral cortex. *J. Neurol. Neurosurg. Psychiat.*, **29**, 398.

11 BALENTINE, J. D. AND GUTSCHE, B. B. (1966) Central nervous system lesions in rats exposed to oxygen at high pressure. *Amer. J. Pathol.*, **48**, 107.

12 BALENTINE, J. D. (1967) *Pathogenesis of central nervous system lesions induced by exposure to hyperbaric oxygen. Amer. J. Pathol.*, **50**, 12a.

13 ROBERT, A. (1956) Complete prevention of cerebral accidents in malignant hypertension. *Circ. Res.*, **4**, 527–532.

14 SOKOLOFF, L. (1959) The action of drugs on the cerebral circulation. *Pharmacol. Rev.*, **11**, 1.

15 BRON, K. M., MURDAUGH, H. V., JR., MILLEN, J. E., RASKIN, P. AND ROBIN, E. D. (1966) Arterial constrictor response in a diving mammal. *Science*, **142**, 540.

16 ANDERSEN, H. T. (1966) Physiological adaptations in diving vertebrates. *Physiol. Rev.*, **46**, 212.

17 MILLS, L. R., MARGOLIS, G. AND NAITOVE, A. M. (1968) *Augmentation of neurotoxic effects of experimental aortography by the vascular reflexes induced during simulated diving.* In preparation.

18 LASSEN, N. A. (1959) Cerebral blood flow and oxygen consumption in man. *Physiol. Rev.*, **39**, 183.

19 MEYER, J. S., WALTZ, A. G. AND GOTOH, F. (1960) Pathogenesis of cerebral vasospasm in hypertensive encephalopathy. I. Effects of acute increases in intraluminal blood pressure on pial blood flow. *Neurology*, **10**, 735.

20 BYROM, F. B. (1959) *The significance of hypertensive encephalopathy.* In Lectures on the Scientific Basis of Medicine, Vol. 8. London, Athlone Press, 1958–59, p. 256.

21 ROBERT, A. AND NEZAMIS, J. E. (1957) Hypertensive eye lesions in the rat. Effect of carotid ligation. *Experientia (Basel)*, **13**, 457–459.

22 BYROM, F. B. (1964) Angiotensin and renal vascular damage. *Brit. J. Exptl. Pathol.*, **45**, 7.

23 SROUJI, M. N. AND TRUSLER, G. A. (1965) Paradoxical hypertension and the abdominal pain syndrome following resection of coarctation of the aorta. *Canad. Med. Ass. J.*, **92**, 412.

24 BENSON, W. R. AND SEALY, W. C. (1956) Arterial necrosis following resection of coarctation of aorta. *Lab. Invest.*, **5**, 359.

25 GIESE, J. (1966) *The Pathogenesis of Hypertensive Vascular Disease.* Munksgaard, Copenhagen, 177 pages.

26 HASSLER, O. (1961) Morphological studies on the large cerebral arteries with reference to the aetiology of subarachnoid haemorrhage. *Acta Psychiat. Neurol. Scand.*, **36**, Suppl. 154, 145 pp.

27 NAEYE, R. (1967) Development of systemic and pulmonary arteries from birth through early childhood. *Biol. Neonatorum*, **10**, 8.

28 NAEYE, R. (1967) Arteriolar abnormalities with chronic systemic hypertension: A quantitative study. *Circulation*, **35**, 662.

29 SELYE, H. AND HEUSER, G. (1954) *Fourth Annual Report on Stress.* Montreal, p. 47.

30 BROWNLEE, G. V., HOPKINS, E. L., JASON, R. S. AND HAWTHORNE, E. W. (1959) Arterial pressure level and the pathogenesis of arteriolonecrosis in dogs with experimental malignant hypertension. *Med. Ann. D.C.*, **28**, 121–124.

31 HUGHES, W. (1965) Hypothesis: Origin of lacunes. *Lancet*, **2**, 19.

32 SOKOLOFF, L. (1961) *Local circulation at rest and during altered cerebral activity induced by anesthesia or visual stimulation.* Regional Neurochemistry. New York, Pergamon, p. 107.

The Diagnosis and Treatment of Intraventricular Haemorrhages

H. W. PIA

Director of the Neurosurgical Clinic of the University of Giessen/Lahn, Germany

Since Sanders[5] in 1881 first published a description of intraventricular haemorrhage, there have been numerous reports, mostly morphological and clinical case histories, in which attention has been drawn to the various forms of haemorrhage and abnormal clinical symptoms and courses, to spontaneous recoveries and to cases subjected successfully to operation, but so far in the neurosurgical literature there have been no systematic examinations. A review of our personal case material (Table 1) has recently been undertaken and shows the principal causes and distribution of the haemorrhages. Out of 145 cases of spontaneous intracerebral haematoma, approx. half were due to cerebral vascular diseases, mostly as a consequence of hypertension, while the other half were due to cerebral vascular malformations. With a numerically equal distribution of the haemorrhages, aneurysms are involved less frequently than angiomata: 20% and 45% respectively. 43 per cent of the mass haemorrhages were associated with an intraventricular haemorrhage, the frequency being 6% for aneurysms but 30% for aneurysmal haematomata, 24% for angiomata and 50% for angiomatous haematomata, and 44% for haematomata of a different origin.

TABLE 1

INTRACEREBRAL AND INTRAVENTRICULAR HAEMORRHAGE

Etiology	Number of cases	Intracerebr. haematomas		Intraventricul. haemorrhage	
		Number	%	Number	%
Aneurysms	156	33	21	10	6
Angiomas	63	29	46	15	24
Intracerebral haematomas of other etiology		73	—	29	40
		135	40	54	

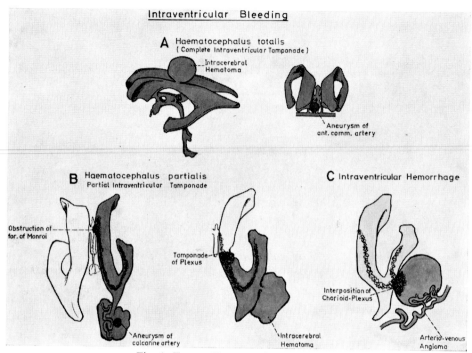

Fig. 1. Types of intraventricular bleeding.

MORPHOLOGY

Morphologically, we have been able to distinguish 3 typical forms of ventricular haemorrhage: (Fig. 1): Total haematocephaly presents the picture of a ventricular effusion with a clot or haematoma of the entire ventricular system. In partial haemato-cephaly, blood masses fill circumscribed portions of the ventricular system, usually a lateral ventricle, only rarely both lateral ventricles. We have observed haematomata in circumscribed areas of one lateral ventricle only in the posterior horn and in the inferior horn, at times extending to the trigonum. Other types often encountered in autopsy cases are a clot of the 3rd ventricle, aqueduct and 4th ventricle or of isolated areas. In the third group, that of intraventricular haemorrhage, the ventricular CSF contains variable amounts of fresh blood without showing any signs of a haematoma.

The causes and the pathogenic mechanism of these typical forms of intraventricular haemorrhages have so far hardly been discussed. According to our personal ex-perience, the ventricular bottlenecks: the foramen of Monro and the outlet of the 4th ventricle, and especially the choroid plexus are of the greatest importance in the formation of localized ventricular haematomata and for the closure of ventricular ruptures. Out of 9 cases with a complete clot of a lateral ventricle, the plexus had shifted the foramen of Monro in 2 proved cases. In one case of haematoma of the inferior horn, the plexus at the level of the compressed trigonum prevented a further advance of the haemorrhage. Out of 27 cases of ventricular haemorrhage there were 9 in which portions of the plexus bulged into the haematoma cavity and the rupture had

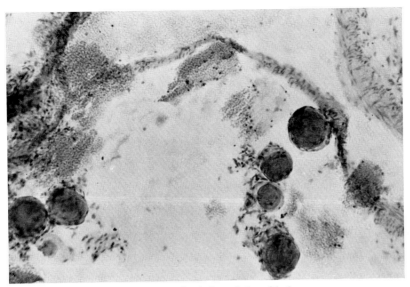

Fig. 2. Compressive lesion of choroid plexus.

been closed by this prolapse. The effective closure of the rupture by the plexus is proved by the histological findings in a postmortem case of plexus prolapse (Fig. 2). The plexus presents severe degenerative changes with cyst formation and thrombotic occlusions of the widely dilated stromal vessels, in other words a picture of compression damage. A further protective mechanism which may be mentioned is the local and general mass shifts with narrowing or displacement of the ventricular lumen.

AETIOLOGY

In our personal material there were 16 cases of total haematocephaly, 19 cases of partial haematocephaly and 27 cases of ventricular haemorrhage. Cases of hypertension appear to be divided equally over all forms, aneurysms show a tendency to the severest forms of haemorrhage and angiomata a tendency to ventricular haemorrhage (Table 2). The causes of this distribution pattern, which is not fortuitous, are

TABLE 2

MORPHOLOGY AND ETIOLOGY OF INTRAVENTRICULAR BLEEDING

Etiology	Number of cases	Haematoceph. totalis	Haematoceph. partialis	Intraventricul. haemorrhage
Hypertension	29	11	8	10
Aneurysms	10	5	4	1
Angiomas	15	—	4	11
	54	16	16	22

outside the scope of the present communication. It must be pointed out that neither
the localization of the haemorrhage nor the age of the patient afford reliable indications
with regard to the aetiology. This is true in particular of the concept that it is only the
capsular haemorrhage which shows a special tendency to ventricular eruption. In
our personal material, 10 haemorrhages had a frontal localization, 37 had a temporo-
parieto-occipital localization and only 13 were in medial structures. Diffuse haematomata were observed in 2 cases.

DIAGNOSIS (Table 3)

The clinical diagnosis of ventricular haemorrhage can be made with a good degree
of probability in the majority of the cases of total haematocephaly and in partial
haematocephaly with involvement of the 3rd or 4th ventricle. These cases show the
classical picture described by Sanders[5] and McDonald[3]: persistent coma of acute
onset, focal losses of function in the early stages, symptoms of mesencephalic
herniation, developing in the case of longer survival into decerebration, meningism
and central regulation disorders that are extremely severe from the beginning. As a
rule, death ensues within 24 hours as a result of respiratory paralysis.

Partial haematocephaly of the lateral ventricle and especially ventricular haemorrhage are frequently not diagnosed clinically or cannot be proved in the case of a
subacute onset, absence of coma, of meningism and of a local syndrome determined
by the site of the haemorrhage, or in the case of rapid spontaneous remission. The
principal diagnostic information consists in the following triad of symptoms:
(1) apoplectic onset, (2) focal losses of function combined with signs of an acute
increase in the intracranial pressure and (3) the demonstration of blood in the CSF.

TABLE 3

SYMPTOMATOLOGY OF INTRAVENTRICULAR BLEEDING

Clinical signs	Haematoceph. totalis	Haematoceph. partialis	Haemorrhagia intraventricularis
Onset	acute	acute	acute and subacute
Coma	+++	+++	++
No coma	ø	seldom	40%
Meningism	+ and ø	+ and ø	+ and ø
CSF	bloody	bloody	bloody
Local symptoms	+	+	+
Symptoms of mesencephalic herniation	+	50%	50%
Decerebration	60%	25%	25%
Central dysregulation	+++	++−+++	+−+++
Spontaneous outcome	Death	Remission possible	Remission in 50%

TABLE 4

ECHOENCEPHALOGRAPHY IN 19 CASES OF INTRACEREBRAL HAEMATOMAS

Number of cases	Normal midline echo	Displacement of midline echo		Echos of haematoma
		3–5 mm	5 mm	
19	1	15	3	7

Withdrawal of a *sample of CSF* is always indicated, because meningism is usually present although the presence of meningism is not evidence of the presence of a haemorrhage. In all the 39 early cases that were examined, the CSF was bloody. *Echo-encephalography* has proved to be a valuable addition to the diagnostic arsenal (Table 4). The shift of the median echo is often only very slight or may be completely absent in cases of intracerebral haemorrhage. We have observed shifts of more than 5 mm. only in children. An observation of decisive importance is that of a pulsating haematoma echo which yields information concerning the localization and extension of the mass haemorrhage (Fig. 3). Since our own 7 cases have been observed only in the last year, I believe that with sufficient experience it will be possible in the future practically always to diagnose correctly the nature and localization of the lesion.

Cerebral angiography is indispensable for the elucidation of the aetiology and for the demonstration of mass haemorrhages. The difficulties of diagnosis in cases of mass haemorrhage are well known and need not be further expounded here. With

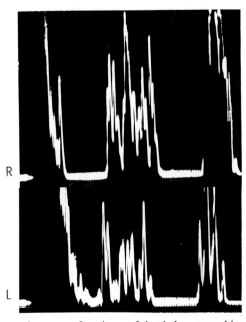

Fig. 3. Echoencephalogram in a case of angioma of the thalamus combined with intracerebral and intraventricular haematomas.

References p. 470

the exception of one case reported by Larson *et al.*[2], so far no ventricular haemorrhages have been diagnosed angiographically, through the demonstration of a still bleeding intraventricular a-v angioma. Two recently treated cases of a-v angioma with intra-cerebral and intraventricular haematoma and involvement of a lateral ventricle presented a uniform shift syndrome: lateral shift of all the extremely stretched insular arteries, caudal shift of the venous angle, with the intraventricular veins stretched, shifted in a caudal direction and forced apart. In none of the other cases could the ventricular haemorrhage be recognized in the angiograms.

VENTRICULOGRAPHY

Guillaume *et al.*[1] have pointed out the possibility of the diagnostic elucidation of intraventricular haemorrhage by ventricular puncture and the possibility of deter-mining the degree of extension by subsequent air filling. Individual cases have been reported in which the correct diagnosis was made with ventriculography or encephalo-graphy, while the primary diagnosis in most of these cases had been that of an intra-ventricular tumour; among these reports there is one by Ojemann and New[4], of a particularly interesting observation with spontaneous reabsorption. With the exception of the subacute and chronic cases, surgical evacuation of the intracerebral and intra-ventricular haematoma must take priority to save the patient's life, so that ventriculo-graphy must be omitted.

PROGNOSIS (Table 5)

The prognosis of total and of partial haematocephaly with involvement of the 3rd ventricle, the aqueduct and the 4th ventricle is unfavourable. All patients died, those not subjected to operation, with one exception, within 24 hours, and those few operated on, during the first week. In the group of partial haematocephaly with involvement of the lateral ventricle, it was possible to save 8 out of 19 patients, and in the group of ventricular haemorrhages, 23 out of 27 patients. As regards the causes of death, in the former group, 5 patients had an intrapontine haemorrhage, and such a

TABLE 5

PROGNOSIS OF INTRAVENTRICULAR BLEEDING

Type of bleeding	Number	(+)	Survived	Operation	(+)	No operation	(+)
Haematocephalus totalis	16	16	—	6	6	10	10
Haematocephalus partialis	16	9	7	13	6	3	3
Intraventricular haemorrhage	22	3	19	22	3	—	—
	54	28	26	41	15	13	13

TABLE 6

PROGNOSIS OF INTRAVENTRICULAR BLEEDING AND ETIOLOGY

	Number	Hypertension (+)		Aneurysms (+)		Angiomas (+)	
Haematocephal. totalis	16	11	11	5	5	—	—
Haematocephal. partialis	16	8	5*	4	3*	4	1*
Intraventricular haemorrhage	22	10	2	1	—	11	1*
	54	29	18	10	8	11	2

* Intrapontine haemorrhage.

haemorrhage was present in 1 of the 3 patients who died in the ventricular haemorrhage group (Table 6).

Compared with the prognostic significance of the nature and cause of the haemorrhage, the factor of age plays a part of some importance only in the senile age group. Even though spontaneous remissions occur among cases of partial haematocephaly, and even in approx. half the number of cases of ventricular haemorrhage, and though this auto-remission leads to partial enclosure of the intracerebral haemorrhage, the constantly demonstrable space-occupying character of the haemorrhage in our cases left very little doubt with regard to the life-saving effect of the surgical treatment. Of the 16 patients in these two groups, 9 were operated on on the day of the haemorrhage and 7 on the next day. Eight patients survived, and 6 of these became symptom-free. With two exceptions it proved possible in 5 patients with aneurysms and 16 with angiomata not only to remove the intracerebral and intraventricular haemorrhage, but also to eliminate the aneurysm or to resect the a-v angioma in its entirety.

INDICATIONS AND SURGICAL TREATMENT

With the exception of extreme cases with very severe central regulation disorders, surgery is always indicated in the treatment of intracerebral and intraventricular haemorrhages with a progressive symptomatology or in the absence of remission. In hyperacute cases, any delay is contraindicated, just as in epidural haematoma. Even though the indications and the optimal moment for the operation are matters of dispute in cases showing an immediate spontaneous remission, our personal experience is that in this category, also, active therapeutic management is to be preferred.

We shall not go into technical details. The principal measures are: incision of the cortex and removal of the intracerebral haemorrhage with a large spoon followed by rinsing, finding of the ventricular perforation and suppression of the ventricular haemorrhage in the same way. If left a few days, the ventricular haematoma will usually be so firm that a more extensive denudation is necessary for its withdrawal. Intracerebral drainage for 24 to 48 hours. In extreme cases we limit ourselves to puncturing the haematoma and the ventricle and rinsing out the haematoma, followed by drainage for a few days.

EXAMPLE

A man aged 20 years old, showed on the day of admission: hemiplegia on the right side, of acute onset in 20 minutes, starting in the leg, together with complete aphasia. After 30 minutes, coma. During the next few hours also: rigidity of the neck, conjugate deviation to the left, blood in the CSF, echo-EG: 3 mm right shift of the median echo. Angiography: a-v angioma in the left parietal region, massive haemorrhage in the parieto-occipital region and left lateral ventricle. Immediate operation: massive haemorrhage of 150 ml in the centre of the angioma, rupture of the posterior horn with ventricular clot. Removal of the blood masses, total extirpation of the angioma. Uneventful course. Patient responsive after 2 days. Regression of the losses of function.

SUMMARY

Owing to the fact that neurosurgeons are being increasingly confronted with cases of vascular diseases of the brain, the clinical and specific diagnostics and the treatment of intracerebral mass haemorrhages and of the frequently associated intraventricular haemorrhages have so much improved in recent years that nowadays half these patients can be saved if operation is performed immediately. A policy of waiting or even resignation is no longer justified; instead, every case of apoplexy with blood in the CSF must be diagnosed as rapidly as possible, and mass haemorrhages of whatever origin must be treated by operation.

REFERENCES

1 GUILLAUME, J., G. MAZARS, R. ROGE AND A. PANSINI (1957) Les accidents circulatoires du cerveau. Presses universitaires de France, Paris.
2 LARSEN, S. J., L. LOVE AND A. MITTELPUNKT (1964) Unilateral intracranial hematoma without shift of the anterior cerebral artery. Am. J. Roentgenol., 92, 786–791.
3 MC DONALD, J. V. (1962) Midline hematomas simulating tumors of the third ventricle. Neurol., 12, 805–809.
4 OJEMANN, R. G. AND P. F. J. NEW (1963) Spontaneous resolution of an intraventricular hematoma. J. Neurosurg., 20, 899–902.
5 SANDERS, E. (1881) A study of primary, immediate or direct hemorrhage into the ventricles of the brain. Am. J. Med. Sci. (N. Ser.), 82, 85–128.

Epicerebral Angiography by Fluorescein during Craniotomy [*]

WILLIAM FEINDEL, CHARLES P. HODGE AND Y. LUCAS YAMAMOTO

Cone Laboratory for Neurosurgical Research, Montreal Neurological Institute and McGill University, Montreal (Canada)

In previous reports we have described the use of radio-active isotopes and Coomassie Blue dye injected by internal carotid catheter for analysis of the regional blood flow in the epicerebral circulation (the pial arteries and veins and the cortical capillary bed) during craniotomy[1]. This method allows for the comparison of quantitative radio-isotopic blood flow curves directly with the anatomical pattern of the normal and abnormal vasculature on the surgically exposed brain. This approach has provided information on changes in blood flow in angiomas and adjacent cortex before and after obliteration of arterial feeders, or after arterial manipulation during clipping of aneurysms, and on abnormal flow rates in tumours with arterio-venous shunts[2]. With Coomassie Blue, a highly coloured non-toxic dye (sodium anazolene) and rapid serial stroboscopic colour photography the anatomical patterns of flow in pial arteries and veins and in the cortical capillary bed can be displayed and analysed. It should be emphasized that this direct comparison of the anatomy and rheology of the cerebral circulation directly from the surface of the brain offers many advantages over the technique of external monitoring by radio-isotopes of cerebral blood flow, where the details of the cerebral microcirculation have not been available.

We now wish to describe the technique of fluorescein angiography as an additional means of examining the surface of the brain during operation.

Details of the method were developed during a study of experimental cerebral ischaemia in cat and monkey brains[3,4]. In the operating room 2 ml of 1 % sodium fluorescein are rapidly injected into an internal carotid catheter. The passage of the dye through the vasculature of the exposed brain is recorded on serial photographs taken at intervals of 0.40 sec by a Nikon camera with motor-driven film changer. The shutter is synchronized with the discharge of a rapid re-charging stroboscopic light. A Wratten 47 colour filter was used over the light and a Wratten 58 over the camera lens for Tri-X film to obtain black and white photographs. Using high-speed Ektachrome film (daylight), the camera filter was changed to Wratten 29 with a 2-B ultra-violet absorbing filter and the film processed as Ektacolor to give an enhanced contrast and a speed of ASA 1200.

The timing of the interval between photographs was measured to within 0.02 sec

---

[*] This work was supported by the Cone Memorial Fund and the Medical Research Council of Canada.

by recording from a cadmium photo-cell placed near the strobe light. Thus the velocity of flow in individual vessels could be calculated from the serial photographs.

The most important feature of fluorescence angiography is the display of the small pial arteries and veins and the cortical capillary bed, all of which appear in high contrast and in great detail. These are vessels of a size which are not visible on standard X-ray angiography, and the additional vasculature seen on the fluorescence photographs and on direct observation of the brain is often remarkable. The arterial and venous vessels stand out distinctly during their separate phases. Because of the dense filling of the capillary bed of the cortex the "water-shed" of the major arterial territories is clearly defined. The dynamics of central and mural laminar flow appear in detail, particularly in larger veins. In cerebral tumours, the fine blood vessels in the tumour bed show up earlier than the normal vascular bed and remain filled later than the normal venous phase, so that the tumour stands out with considerable prominence from the surrounding normal tissue. Shunting of the fluorescein from arteries to veins is readily seen in some tumours, and the velocity of flow in different draining veins can be distinguished. Areas of ischaemia are well demarcated by absence of fluorescence, while areas of damage may retain the dye beyond the normal circulation time. Such areas may escape detection on X-ray angiography.

Two examples of fluorescein epicerebral angiograms in brain tumours taken from our series will serve to illustrate some of these points.

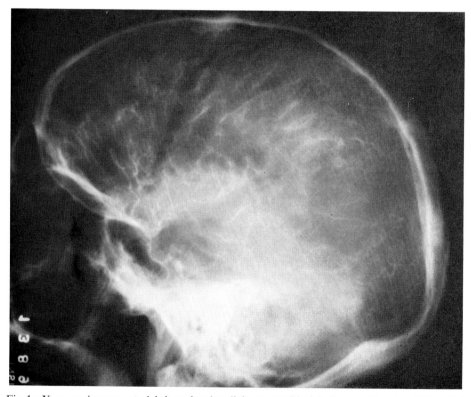

Fig. 1a. X-ray angiogram, arterial phase showing slight tumour blush in the parietal region. Patient J. J.

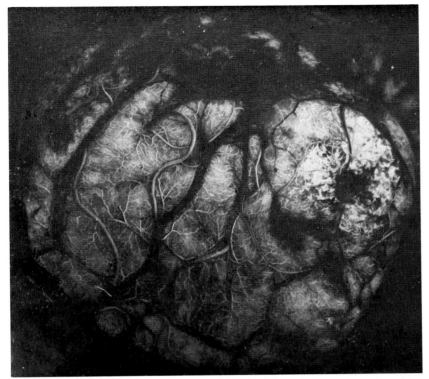

Fig. 1b. Fluorescein angiogram, arterial phase from exposed brain. Note intensity of tumour blush and filling of small arterial vessels. Patient J. J.

In the first example, a patient with carcinoma of the colon who began to have dysphasia, the X-ray film in the arterial phase showed a definite though scanty tumour blush in the left parietal region (Fig. 1a) which persisted in the venous phase (Fig. 2a). In two frames from a 36-frame fluorescein series and on direct observation, the tumour blush of fine vessels was quite obvious. In the venous phase especially the tumour is clearly demarcated from the normal brain (Figs. 1b and 2b). The arteries and the capillary bed appear pale grey or white (Fig. 1b). The veins at this stage are dark, since they are not yet filled with fluorescein. During the venous phase, rather complex laminar flow patterns of alternating dark and light can be seen in the pial veins. The tumour as defined by fluorescence of its vascular bed was excised carefully but radically. The patient recovered a great deal of his speech function and a clearing of his confusion and was discharged home.

The second example, a patient with an intrinsic brain tumour, presented clinically with a sudden onset of dysphasia. X-ray angiography showed a well defined highly vascular tumour in the posterior sylvian area with an arterio-venous shunt. Exploration was carried out. The superior detail of the fluorescein angiogram is depicted in Figs. 3a and 3b, comparing the X-ray arterial phase with the fluorescein arterial phase. Note especially the dense filling of the cortical capillary bed, the large pair of veins which were filled early with arterialized blood, and the central area of tumour

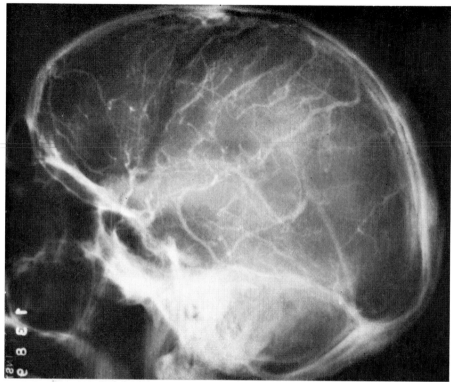

Fig. 2a. Venous phase, X-ray angiogram. Patient J. J.

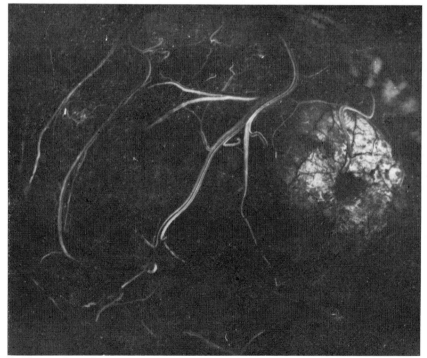

Fig. 2b. Venous phase, fluorescein angiogram. Note high contrast from fluorescein retained in tumour.

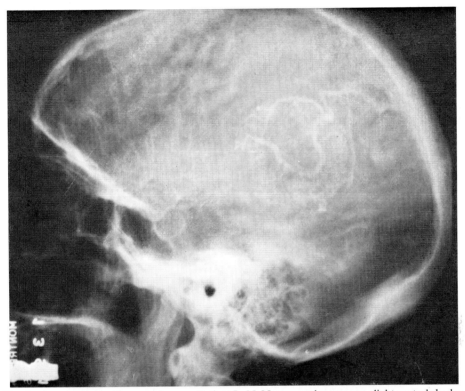

Fig. 3a. Arterial phase, X-ray angiogram. Patient L. N. Note vascular tumour, slight central shadow of lesser vascularity in centre of the tumour and the early filling veins.

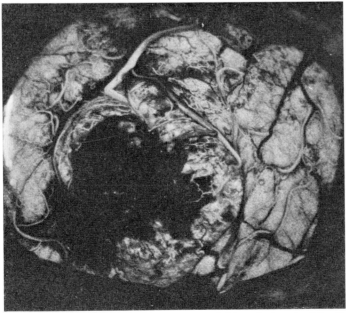

Fig. 3b. Arterial phase, fluorescein angiogram. Patient L. N. Note the increased detail and contrast especially of the microvascular bed as compared to X-ray angiogram. Patient L. N.

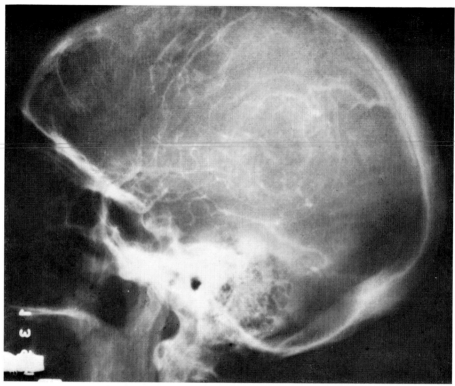

Fig. 4a. Venous phase, X-ray angiogram. Patient L. N.

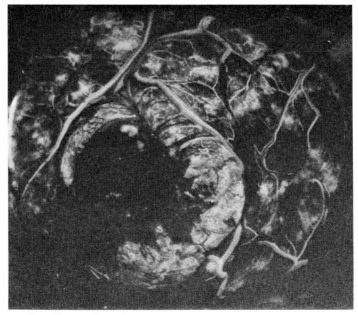

Fig. 4b. Venous phase, fluorescein angiogram. Patient L. N. Note retention of fluorescein in the margin of the tumour marking it out clearly from the surrounding brain.

which fails to show fluorescence. In this part of the tumour, small thrombosed veins were found and this was considered to be evidence of a vascular occlusive phenomenon which went on within the neoplasm and gave an explanation for the onset of symptoms simulating a stroke. This area of avascularity was not as clear on the X-ray films in either the arterial or venous phases, being obscured by the dense subcortical vascular bed of the tumour which was on biopsy a malignant glioma (Figs. 4a and 4b).

In summary, a new method of fluorescein angiography for demonstration of the epicerebral circulation during craniotomy provides for rapid sequential recording of the flow in the pial and cortical vessels. The advantages of the method include the display of the small vessels of the brain not seen on X-ray angiography so that examination of the cerebral microcirculation *in vivo* now becomes possible. Secondly, it allows the neurosurgeon to study the anatomical pattern of the epicerebral vessels in man under a wide variety of abnormal conditions.

Thirdly, though techniques for external measurement of cerebral blood flow by radioactive Xenon or Krypton have been of value, it has not been possible to correlate the many data from these techniques with the anatomical picture of the cerebral microcirculation. This now becomes possible with fluorescein angiography when combined with intracarotid radio-isotopic tracers[5]. The use of fluorescein angiography therefore, has a wide application for examination of the cerebral circulation under neurosurgical conditions. We consider that it will help to explain many of the features of local cerebral blood flow which have not so far been understandable by using only the external radio-isotopic measurement techniques.

REFERENCES

1. FEINDEL, W., GARRETSON, H., YAMAMOTO, Y. L., PEROT, P. AND RUMIN, N. (1965) Blood flow patterns in the cerebral vessels and cortex in man studied by intracarotid injection of radioisotopes and Coomassie Blue dye. *J. Neurosurg.*, **23**, 12–22.
2. FEINDEL, W. (1963) Scandinavian symposium on cerebral circulation. *Canad. Med. Ass. J.*, **88**, 951–952.
3. FEINDEL, W., YAMAMOTO, Y. L. AND HODGE, C. P. (1967) The human microcirculation studied by intra-arterial radio-active tracers, Coomassie Blue and fluorescein dyes. *Proc. 4th European Conference on Microcirculation*, Cambridge, England, June, 1966. *Bibl. Anat.*, fasc. **9**, 220–224.
4. FEINDEL, W., YAMAMOTO, Y. L. AND HODGE, C. P. (1967) Intracarotid fluorescein angiography: A new method for examination of the epicerebral circulation in man. *Canad. Med. Ass. J.*, **96**, 1–7.
5. FEINDEL, W. AND YAMAMOTO, Y. L. (1967); Luxury-Perfusion Syndrome. *Lancet*, **i**, 48–49.

The Protective Effect of Hyperbaric Oxygenation in Experimentally Produced Cerebral Edema and Compression

SIDNEY A. HOLLIN, MICHAEL H. SUKOFF AND JULIUS H. JACOBSON II

Department of Neurosurgery, and the Department of Surgery, The Mount Sinai Hospital, Ner York, U.S.A.

Recent studies indicate that hyperbaric oxygenation may be beneficial in the management of ischemic disorders of the brain[12,14,15,17,43,44,51]. Other reports have appeared suggesting that hyperbaric oxygenation has a protective effect in cerebral trauma[8,11]. The cerebral vasoconstriction caused by hyperbaric oxygenation[13,19,20,31,32] in combination with increased available oxygen[1,2,4,23,26,30,31,45,46,51] are factors which might be of value in the treatment of cerebral edema.

The purpose of the present study has been to evaluate the effect of hyperbaric oxygenation on cerebral edema and compression produced by acutely and slowly expanding intracranial space-occupying lesions.

METHODS

Two methods have been used for the experimental production of cerebral edema. A gradually expanding intracerebral mass has been produced by psyllium seeds, a hygroscopic material which gradually expands approximately ten-fold after insertion into the brain[47]. The second method has been the placement of an extradural balloon which could be inflated at any time subsequently[18].

Psyllium seed technique: Adult mongrel dogs weighing between 15 and 20 kg were used. Operations were performed with sterile technique under intravenous surital anesthesia.

An 8 mm burr hole was made 3 cm anterior to the external occipital protuberance and 2 cm lateral to the midline. Through small dural and cortical incisions a 4 mm diameter ventricular cannula was inserted into the subcortical white matter for a depth of 7 mm. One ml of dry sterilized psyllium seed was gently packed into the white matter with a stylette. The bone button was replaced and the incision closed. Dogs not surviving through the first postoperative day were excluded from the study.

Extradural balloon techniques: Operative conditions were similar to the psyllium seed group. An 8 mm bone button was removed from the left parietal region. The dura was separated anteriorly from the overlying calvarium and a modification of the Jacobson catheter[21] was inserted. This consisted of a collapsed balloon attached to a connecting catheter which, in turn, led to a self-sealing rubber diaphragm (Fig. 1).

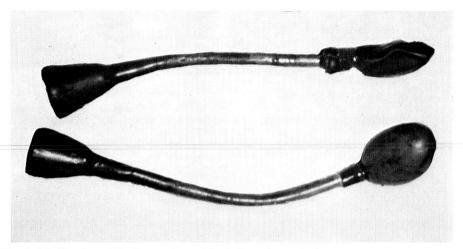

Fig. 1. Modification of Jacobson catheter. The balloon is attached to a catheter which ends in a self-sealing rubber diaphragm.

The balloon was placed extradurally overlying the left frontoparietal cortex. The trephine opening was slightly enlarged anteriorly to accommodate the catheter and the bone button replaced. The self-seeling rubber diaphragm was placed in the sub-cutaneous tissue of the dorsal neck where it could be easily palpated for subsequent insertion of a needle to inflate the balloon (Fig. 2).

Animals were observed during a one-week recovery period and those showing neurologic or systemic deficits were excluded from the study. On the eighth post-operative day a #20 hypodermic needle was inserted percutaneously into the self-

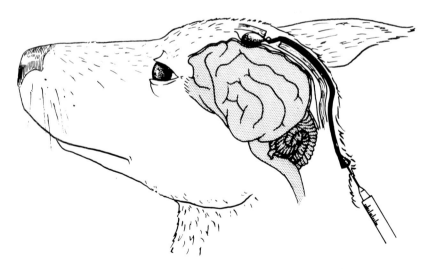

Fig. 2. Extradural placement of the balloon which may be inflated by subcutaneous injection of the self-sealing rubber diaphragm.

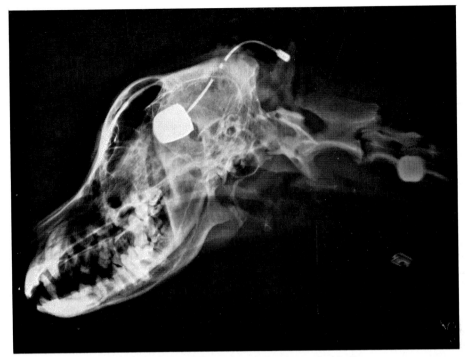

Fig. 3. X-ray visualization of the inflated extradual balloon.

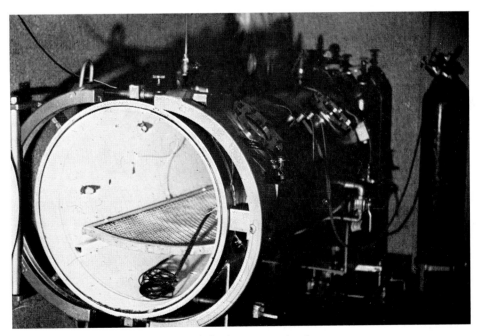

Fig. 4. Animal treatment chamber.

sealing catheter tip. This was, in turn, attached to a length of plastic tubing and syringe. Balloons were inflated with 5 ml of 50% Hypaque solution to permit x-ray visualisation and exclude possible leakage (Fig. 3). Injection of the contrast material was carried out with the syringe in a micrometer vise to assure uniformity of inflation. The time utilized for balloon inflation was 2 min in one group and 10 min in another. Balloons were inflated at ambient pressure or under hyperbaric conditions.

Hyperbaric oxygenation treatment: Hyperbaric oxygenation at 3 atmospheres absolute (30 p.s.i.g.) was used in the treatment groups of all experiments. The animal treatment chamber (Fig. 4) measures 3 feet in diameter and 8 feet in length. Oxygen flushing was initially accomplished so that the concentration of oxygen in the chamber was always above 95% at 3 atmospheres absolute. Compression was carried out at 2 to 3 lbs/min.

When balloons were inflated under hyperbaric conditions the animals were pressurized in our walk-in hyperbaric chamber[24]. Inasmuch as this chamber is compressed with air, the dogs were placed in a plexiglass box which reached the same percentage levels of oxygen as the animal chamber. In the box and the animal chamber oxygen flow was sufficient to keep the CO_2 environmental levels normal. Periodic samples of the inspired air were tested to assure that the O_2 concentration was above 95% and that the CO_2 was not elevated[22].

Treatment periods under hyperbaric oxygenation were for 45 min. Treatment was instituted 24 h after the completion of surgery in the psyllium seed experiment or at the time of, or immediately following, balloon inflation. Hyperbaric therapy was continued at 8-h intervals unless obvious clinical improvement occurred, in which case treatments were given only twice or once a day. Two control animals from both psyllium seed and balloon groups were exposed to 100% oxygen at ambient pressures for similar durations.

Postoperative hydration was maintained parenterally as necessary. In representative animals, cisternal pressures were measured just prior to therapy and immediately thereafter.

Pathological evaluation: Gross pathological examination of all brains was carried out as close to the time of death or sacrifice as possible. All surviving dogs were sacrificed on the eighth postoperative day by perfusion of intracardiac formaldehyde.

In an equal number of control and treatment specimens in the seed group, the brain was transected and the hemispheres weighed separately. A cross-section through the level of the anterior commissure was made and the distance from the septum pellucidum to the cortical surface on both sides was measured. After formalin fixation, sections of white matter were taken from identical areas of the left frontal region and stained with hematoxylin and eosin for light microscopic examination. The amount of cerebral edema was graded by a neuropathologist. He was not informed if the specimen came from control or treatment groups.

RESULTS

Psyllium seeds: (see Table 1) There were 32 dogs in this group. Seventeen served as controls and the remainder were treated by hyperbaric oxygenation. On the first

TABLE 1

ILLUSTRATING RESULTS IN PSYLLIUM SEED EXPERIMENT. ATA REPRESENTS ATMOSPHERES ABSOLUTE

		Psyllium seeds Number of animals	Deaths	Mortality rate
Controls	Ambient Air	15	12	83%
	Ambient 100% O_2	2	2	
Treatment-100% O_2 — 3 ATA		15	4	27%

postoperative day all animals were only minimally sluggish. Beginning on the second day all control animals showed a progressive downhill course characterized by hemiparesis and extreme lethargy. Death occurred in 83% (14 out of 17 animals) by the fifth day. This includes the two controls given 100% oxygen at ambient pressures.

In the hyperbaric oxygen group the progressive neurological deterioration was interrupted. Improvement was apparent immediately after treatment in most animals. In others, the maximum degree of improvement occurred 2 or 3 h after hyperbaric oxygen exposure. At the onset, improvement was temporary in all treated animals and regression was seen after 4 or 5 h. By the fourth or fifth day, however, improvement was progressive in all but the 4 treatment failures. By the eighth day surviving treated animals were neurologically normal except for mild contralateral weakness. The mortality rate in these treated animals was 27% (4 out of 15 animals).

Extradural balloon: Inflation at ambient pressure (see Table 2): Inflation of the extradural balloon was carried out at ambient pressure over a 10-min period in 22 dogs, 12 to be controls and 10 to be hyperbarically treated. Two of the 12 control animals were given 100% oxygen at normal ambient pressure after balloon inflation. In all animals, progressive deterioration of level of consciousness with contralateral hemiparesis and ipsilateral pupillary dilatation was observed by the time balloon expansion was completed.

Although some degree of spontaneous clinical improvement was noted initially in the 12 controls, the mortality in this group was 100% by the fourth postinflation day.

TABLE 2

ILLUSTRATING RESULTS IN GRADUAL BALLOON INFLATION. ATA REPRESENTS ATMOSPHERES ABSOLUTE

		Extradural balloons — Inflation over ten-minute period Number of animals	Deaths	Mortality rate
Controls	Ambient Air	10	10	100%
	Ambient 100% O_2	2	2	
Treatment — 100% O_2 — 3 ATA		10	5	50%

References p. 487–489

In 10 animals treated by intermittent exposure to hyperbaric oxygenation immediately after balloon inflation, the mortality rate was 50%. Surviving animals were neurologically normal by the sixth postinflation day. Their course was similar to the treated psyllium seed dogs (see above).

Extradural balloon: Acute effects of rapid inflation: Four control animals had their balloons inflated over a 2-min period. They became rapidly comatose and decerebrate. All died from within 30 min to 12 h later.

In another 4 animals, balloons were inflated over the same 2-min period while the animals were breathing 100% oxygen at 3 atmospheres absolute. Only evidence of discomfort during balloon inflation and mild contralateral weakness were seen. All remained stable until sacrifice 12 h later.

In an additional 2 animals, balloons were inflated as above under hyperbaric oxygenation. The response again was slight discomfort during balloon inflation and mild weakness of the contralateral extremities. After 15 min of observation, the balloons were deflated. The dogs were observed for the next 2 days. During this time, they remained neurologically normal. Inflation was then carried out again, but this time while breathing air at ambient pressure. In all animals immediate coma developed followed by decerebration, death occurring within 12 h.

Pathological findings: All brains showed gross evidence of cerebral edema (Fig. 5). There was widening of the sulci and flattening of the gyri, most marked in the non-treated dogs in both groups. No intracranial hemorrhage was present. In the seed experiment treated brains weighed less on the average. They had a smaller individual difference between hemispheric weights. The cross-sectional hemispheric difference between each brain was greater in the controls (see Discussion).

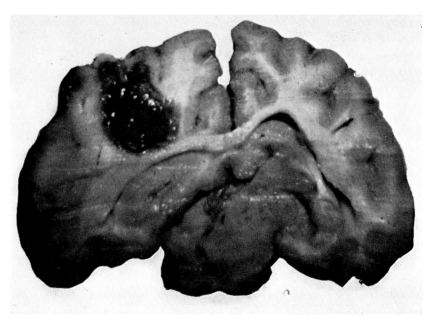

Fig. 5. Cross-section of brain demonstrating psyllium seed lesion and cerebral edema.

Microscopic studies: Histological evaluation demonstrated less severe edema in the control groups as compared to the treatment groups (see Discussion).

DISCUSSION

These experiments indicate that hyperbaric oxygenation has a protective effect against experimental cerebral edema and compression. The morbidity and mortality of all groups treated by hyperbaric oxygenation were decreased. Protection against an acutely expanding mass afforded by hyperbaric oxygenation was dramatic. In place of rapid coma and decerebration only excitation and mild contralateral weakness occurred.

In all animals tested, cisternal pressures were reduced after treatment. The shortcomings of this method in determining intracranial pressure have been discussed[7,37,29]. Clinical observations, demonstrating a decrease in cerebral spinal fluid pressure during hyperbaric oxygenation, lend validity to the experimental observations.

The decreased mortality and morbidity in the animal experiments were reflected by the pathological findings. Treated brains appeared less edematous. The average weights of the treated brains and, more significantly, the difference between the weights of the separate hemispheres in the treated animals were less. In addition, the difference between the cross-sectional measurements of the two cerebral hemispheres was less in the treated groups. This suggests a reduction in the amount of swelling of the edematous brain afforded by the hyperbaric oxygen treatment[27]. Light microscopic studies demonstrated less severe edema in the treated animals. Absence of precise quantitative criteria and other difficulties[6] exist in this method of evaluating cerebral edema. Similarly, because the control animals survived only 2 to 4 days and the treatment dogs usually were sacrificed on the eighth day, further refinements of our quantitative measurements of cerebral edema are warranted.

The production of cerebral edema by intracerebral insertion of psyllium seeds and inflation of an extradural balloon are wellestablished procedures. In addition, the extradural balloon may be expanded rapidly, causing acute changes in intracranial dynamics. The balloon technique used in the present experiment is similar to that employed by others[16,35,36,40], but has the advantage of allowing the animal to recover from surgery prior to balloon inflation and reduces the risk of infection in the chronic preparation. Balloon inflation can be carried out in the awake animal and neurological examinations can be performed during the acute or chronic phases of the experiment.

The psyllium seed technique is a modification of Sperl's method[47] and has been previously used to illustrate the effectiveness of steroids in the treatment of cerebral edema[37,38]. In the present experiments, a larger quantity of seeds was introduced in order to produce a greater mortality rate.

Because animals were treated in the awake state and the main intent was to evaluate neurological status and mortality rates, routine determination of blood gases, pH levels and cerebral blood flow was not performed. As a result, physiological measurements have been limited and the work must still be considered preliminary regarding the clarification of the reasons for the protection afforded. However, other experiments in our laboratory have shown consistent arterial pO_2 levels between 1000–1500 mmHg in dogs treated under similar conditions. Hyperbaric oxygenation, as used in this study, increases the amount of oxygen dissolved in the plasma 15 to 20 times[30]. Volume of oxygen which can be supplied per unit of blood, in terms of arteriovenous extraction ratios, is approximately doubled. The physiological effect of this oxygen at high pressure is much greater, however, as attested to by the relatively rapid onset of oxygen toxicity at increased ambient pressures[31].

The effects of hyperbaric oxygenation on the cerebral blood flow have been well studied. It has been demonstrated that in response to hyperbaric oxygenation cerebral blood flow is decreased because of cerebral vasoconstriction[13,19,28,49]. Debate exists as to whether the vasoconstriction is a result of high blood oxygen per se or a secondary change in carbon dioxide[48]. Even in the presence of cerebral vasoconstriction, the total amount of oxygen available to the brain is believed to be increased[4,12,14,29,46,50,51]. However, it can be argued that the relief of cerebral anoxia may be completely negated by the decrease in blood flow[5,20]. In quantitative terms, Lambertsen[31] and Jacobson[19] have shown that blood flow is decreased by approximately 25%. At 3 atmospheres absolute the additional oxygen dissolved in the plasma is increased by 100% in terms of normal arteriovenous oxygen extractions, thereby increasing available oxygen[25,26].

In the present study, the working hypothesis has been that the protective effect of intermittent hyperbaric oxygenation is the production of cerebral vasoconstriction and decreased blood flow in the presence of adequate or increased oxygenation of the brain. Both cerebral anoxia[3] and increased cerebral blood flow[33,36,39,42,45] are factors which aggravate cerebral edema. Evidence[34,35] has recently been offered supporting the view that expansion of an intracranial balloon institutes a cycle of vasodilatation, probably caused by anoxia, and increased cerebral blood flow. The increased blood flow causes further rise in intracranial pressure, additional anoxia and eventual vasomotor paralysis. Hyperbaric oxygenation serves to break this cycle presumably by combatting the anoxia while, at the same time, decreasing cerebral blood flow by vasoconstriction.

The mechanisms of the protective effect against a rapidly expanding mass are not clearly understood. They may be related to the ability of hyperbaric oxygenation to protect against the acute ischemic phenomenon caused by the rapidly expanding balloon[16] and/or to afford protection by decreasing brain volume.

In a recent report[9] the reduction in mortality of dogs with experimental head trauma was similar after treatment with either hyperbaric oxygenation or 97% oxygen at ambient pressure. The authors concluded that additional benefit from hyperbaric oxygen over ambient oxygen was not manifested because of cerebral vasoconstriction. However, in their studies, animals received only a single 2-h treatment.

In the present study, duration of treatments and atmospheric pressures used were arbitrarily chosen to avoid oxygen toxicity. It seems likely that a superior treatment schedule can be developed[1,2].

Further experience is necessary before any definitive statements can be made regarding the effectiveness of hyperbaric oxygenation in the clinical management of cerebral edema. Current methods of treating cerebral edema are not entirely satis-factory[10,41]. It has recently been stated that "the therapy of brain swelling secondary to cerebral vascular dilatation should be directed towards reduction of brain blood volume and not water content"[35]. Hyperbaric oxygenation, in addition to combatting anoxia, may accomplish this.

SUMMARY

(1) Hyperbaric oxygenation appears to decrease the mortality of experimentally produced cerebral edema and compression.

(2) Mechanisms involved may be related to the dual effect of hyperbaric oxygenation in increasing available oxygen while decreasing cerebral blood flow by vasoconstriction.

REFERENCES

1 ACKERMAN, N. B. AND BRINKLEY, F. B. (1966) Development of cyclic intermittent hyperbaric oxygenation as a method for prolonging survival during chronic hyperbaric exposure. *Surgery*, **60**, 20.

2 ACKERMAN, N. B. AND BRINKLEY, F. B. (1966) Cyclic intermittent hyperbaric oxygenation: a method for prolonging survival in hyperbaric oxygen. In I. W. Brown, Jr., and B. G. Cox (Eds.), Proceedings of the Third International Conference on Hyperbaric Medicine, Duke University, Durham, North Carolina, November 17–20, 1965. Washington, D. C.: *Natl. Acad. Sci.-Natl. Res. Council Publication No. 1404*, 796 pp. (See p. 200).

3 BAKAY, L. AND LEE, J. C. (1965) *Cerebral edema*. Springfield, Illinois: Charles C. Thomas, 200 pp. (See p. 78).

4 BERGOFSKY, E. H., WANG, M. C. H., YAMAKI, T. AND JACOBSON, J. H. II (1964) Tissue oxygen and carbon dioxide tensions during hyperbaric oxygenation. *J. Amer. Med. Assoc.*, **189**, 841.

5 BERGOFSKY, E. H. AND BERTUN, P. (1966) Response of regional circulations to hyperoxia. *J. Appl. Physiol.*, **21**, 567.

6 BLINDERMAN, E. E., GRAF, C. J. AND FITZPATRICK, T. (1962) Basic studies in cerebral edema: its control by a corticosteroid (Solu-Medrol). *J. Neurosurg.*, **19**, 319.

7 BULLOCK, L. T., GREGERSEN, M. I. AND KINNEY, R. (1935) The use of hypertonic sucrose solution intravenously to reduce cerebrospinal fluid pressure without secondary rise. *Am. J. Physiol.*, **112**, 82.

8 COE, J. E. AND HAYES, T. M. (1966) Treatment of experimental brain injury by hyperbaric oxygenation: a preliminary report. *Amer. Surg.*, **32**, 493.

9 DUNN, J. E., II AND CONNOLLY, J. M. (1966) Effects of hypobaric and hyperbaric oxygen on experimental brain injury. In I. W. Brown, Jr., and B. G. Cox, (Eds.), Proceedings of the Third International Conference on Hyperbaric Medicine, Duke University, Durham, North Carolina, November 17–20, 1965. Washington, D. C.: *Natl. Acad. Sci.-Natl. Res. Council Publication No. 1404*, 796 pp. (See p. 447).

10 EINSPRUCH, B. C., AND KEMP, C. (1965) Further studies on the effectiveness of agents used to lower intracranial pressure. *J. Neurosurg.*, **23**, 45.

11 FASANO, V. A., BROGGI, G., URCIUOLI, R., DeNUNNO, T. AND LOMBARD, G. F. (1966) Clinical applications of hyperbaric oxygen in traumatic coma. In *Proceedings of the Third International Congress of Neurological Surgery, Copenhagen, Denmark*, August 23–27, 1965. New York: Excerpta Medica. (See p. 502).

12 FUSON, R. L., MOOR, G. F., SMITH, W. W., AND BROWN, F. W. (1965) Hyperbaric oxygenation in experimental cerebral ischemia. *Surg. Forum*, **16**, 416.

13 HARPER, A. M., JACOBSON, I. AND McDOWALL, D. G. (1965) The effect of hyperbaric oxygen on the blood flow through the cerebral cortex. In *Proceedings of the Second International Congress. Baltimore*: Williams & Wilkins Co. (See p. 185).

14 HEYMAN, A., SALTZMAN, H. A. AND WHALEN, R. E. (1966) The use of hyperbaric oxygenation in treatment of cerebral ischemia and infarction. *Circulation*, **33**, 20.

15 HEYMAN, A., WHALEN, R. E. AND SALTZMAN, H. A. (1964) The protective effect of hyperbaric oxygenation in cerebral hypoxia. *Trans. Amer. Neurol. Ass.*, **89**, 59.

16 HUNT, W. E., MEAGHER, J. N., FRIEMAMS, A. AND ROSSEL, C. W. (1962) Angiographic studies of experimental intracranial hypertension. *J. Neurosurg.*, **19**, 1023.

17 INGVAR, D. H. AND LASSEN, N. A. (1965) Treatment of focal cerebral ischemia with hyperbaric oxygenation. Report of four cases. *Acta Neurol. Scand.*, **41**, 92.

18 ISCHII, S., HAYNER, R., KELLY, W. A. AND EVANS, J. P. (1959) Studies of cerebral swelling. II. Experimental cerebral swelling produced by supratentorial extradural compression. *J. Neurosurg.*, **16**, 152.

19 JACOBSON, I., HARPER, A. M. AND McDOWALL, D. G. (1963) The effects of oxygen under pressure on cerebral blood flow and cerebral venous oxygen tensions. *Lancet*, **2**, 549.

20 JACOBSON, I. AND LAWSON, D. D. (1963) The effect of hyperbaric oxygen on experimental cerebral infarction in the dog. *J. Neurosurg.*, **20**, 849.

21 JACOBSON, I. AND McALLISTER, F. F. (1957) A method for the controlled occlusion of larger blood vessels. *Ann. Surg.*, **145**, 334.

22 JACOBSON, J. H., II, MORSCH, J. H. C., RENDELL-BAKER, L. (1965) The historical perspective of hyperbaric therapy. *Ann. N. Y. Acad. Sci.*, **117**, 651.

23 JACOBSON, J. H., II, WANG, M. C. H., FREEDMAN, P., REICH, T., CHEZAR, J. AND RENDELL-BAKER, L. (1966) Hyperbaric oxygenation as an aid to the surgery of abdominal aortic aneurysm. In I. W. BROWN, JR. AND B. G. COX (Eds.), Proceedings of the Third International Conference on Hyperbaric Medicine, Duke University, Durham, North Carolina, November 17–20, 1965. Washington, D.C.: *Natl. Acad. Sci.-Natl. Res. Council Publication No. 1404*, 796 pp. (See p. 463).

24 JACOBSON, J. H., II (1964) The large chamber for hyperbaric oxygenation: instrumentation and monitoring problems. *Trans. New York Acad. Sci.*, **26**, 474.

25 JACOBSON, J. H., II, WANG, M. C. H., YAMAKI, T., KLINE, H. J., KARK, A. E., AND KUHN, L. A. (1964) Hyperbaric oxygenation in diffuse myocardial infarction. *Arch. Surg.*, **89**, 905.

26 JACOBSON, J. H., II, WANG, M. C. H. AND REICH, T. (1967) *The role of hyperbaric oxygenation in the treatment of cardiovascular disease.* New York, Meredith Publishing Co. (See p. 166).

27 JAVID, N., GILBOE, D. AND CESARIO, T. (1964) The rebound phenomenon and hypertonic solutions. *J. Neurosurg.*, **21**, 1059.

28 KETY, S. S. AND SCHMIDT, C. F. (1948) The effects of altered arterial tensions of carbon dioxide and oxygen on cerebral blood flow and cerebral oxygen consumption of normal young men. *J. Clin. Invest.*, **27**, 484.

29 KOCH, A. AND VERMEULEN-CRANCH, D. M. (1962) The use of hyperbaric oxygen following cardiac arrest. *Brit. J. Anesth.*, **34**, 738.

30 KUHN, L. A., KLINE, H. J., WANG, M. C. H., YAMAKI, T. AND JACOBSON, J. H., II (1965) Hemodynamic effects of hyperbaric oxygenation in experimental acute myocardial infarction. *Cir. Res.*, **16**, 499.

31 LAMBERTSEN, C. J. (1965) Effects of oxygen at high partial pressure. In W. O. FENN AND H. RAHN (Eds.), *Handbook of Physiology, section 3, vol. 2 (Respiration)*. Washington, D.C.: *Amer. Physiol. Soc.* (See p. 1027).

32 LAMBERTSEN, C. J., KOUGH, R. H., COOPER, D. Y., EMMEL, G. L., LOSSCHCKE, H. H. AND SCHMIDT, C. F. (1953) Oxygen toxicity. Effects in man of oxygen inhalation at 1 and 3.5 atmospheres upon blood gas transport, cerebral circulation and cerebral metabolism. *J. Appl. Physiol.*, **5**, 471.

33 LANGFITT, T. W. AND KASSELL, N. F. (1966) Acute brain swelling in neurosurgical patients. *J. Neurosurg.*, **24**, 975.

34 LANGFITT, T. W., TANNENBAUM, H. M. AND KASSELL, N. F. (1966) The etiology of acute brain swelling following experimental head injury. *J. Neurosurg.*, **24**, 47.

35 LANGFITT, T. W., WEINSTEIN, J. D. AND KASSELL, N. F. (1965) Cerebral vasomotor paralysis produced by intracranial hypertension. *Neurology*, **15**, 622.

36 LANGFITT, T. W., KASSELL, N. F. AND WEINSTEIN, J. D. (1965) Cerebral blood flow with intracranial hypertension. *Neurology*, **15**, 761.

37 LIPPERT, R. G., SVIEN, H. J., GRINDLAY, J. H., GOLDSTEIN, N. P. AND GASTINEA, C. F. (1960) The effect of cortisone on experimental cerebral edema. *J. Neurosurg.*, **17**, 583.

38 LONG, D. N., HARTMANN, J. H. AND FRENCH, L. A. (1966) The response of experimental cerebral edema to glucosteroid administration. *J. Neurosurg.*, **24**, 843.

39 LUNDBERG, N. (1960) Continuous recording and control of ventricular fluid pressure in neuro-surgical practice. *Acta Psychiat. Scand.*, **36**, 193.

40 McQUEEN, J. D. AND JEANES, L. D. (1962) Influence of hypothermia on intracranial hypertension. *J. Neurosurg.*, **19**, 277.

41 MANDELL, S., TAYLOR, J. M., KOTSILIMBES, D. G. AND SCHEINBERG, L. (1966) The effect of glycerol on cerebral edema induced by triethyltin sulphate in rabbits. *J. Neurosurg.*, **24**, 984.

42 PILCHER, C. (1937) Experimental cerebral trauma. The fluid content of the brain after trauma to the head. *Arch. Surg.*, **35**, 512.

43 SALTZMAN, H. A., SMITH, W. W., FUSON, R. L., SIEKER, H. O. AND BROWN, I. W. (1965) Hyperbaric oxygenation. *Monogr. Surg. Sci.*, **2**, 1.

44 SALTZMAN, H. A., ANDERSON, B., JR., WHALEN, R. E., HEYMAN, A. AND SIEKER, H. O. (1966) Hyperbaric oxygen therapy of acute cerebral vascular insufficiency. In I. W. BROWN, JR. AND B. G. COX (Eds.), Proceedings of the Third International Conference on Hyperbaric Medicine, Duke University, Durham, North-Carolina, November 17–20, 1965. Washington, D.C.: *Natl. Acad. Sci.-Natl. Res. Council Publication No. 1404*, 796 pp. (See p. 440).

45 SHAPIRO, P. AND JACKSON, H. (1939) Swelling of the brain in cases of injury to the head. *Arch. Surg.*, **38**, 443.

46 SMITH, G., LAWSON, D. D., RENFREW, S., LEDINGHAM, I. McA. AND SHARP, G. R. (1961) Preservation of cerebral cortical activity by breathing oxygen at two atmospheres of pressure during cerebral ischemia. *Surg. Gynec. Obstet.*, **113**, 13.

47 SPERL, M. P. JR., SVIEN, H. J., GOLDSTEIN, N. P., KERNOHAN, I. W. AND GRINDLAY, J. H. (1957) Experimental production of local cerebral edema by an expending intracerebral mass. *Proc. Mayo Cl.*, **32**, 744.

48 TINDALL, G. T., WILKINS, R. H., ODOM, G. L. (1965) Effect of hyperbaric oxygenation on cerebral blood flow. *Surg. Forum*, **16**, 414.

49 TINDALL, G. T., WILKINS, R. H. AND ODOM, G. L. (1966) Effect of hyperbaric oxygenation on blood flow in the internal carotid artery of the baboon. In I. W. BROWN, JR. AND B. G. COX (Eds.), Proceedings of the Third International Conference on Hyperbaric Medicine, Duke University, Durham, North Carolina, November 17–20, 1965. Washington, D.C.: *Natl. Acad. Sci.-Natl. Res. Council Publication No. 1404*, 796 pp. (See p. 236).

50 WANG, M. C. H., REICH, T., LESKO, W. S. AND JACOBSON, J. H., II (1966) Hyperbaric oxygenation: oxygen exchange in an acutely ischemic vascular bed. *Surg.*, **59**, 94.

51 WHALEN, R. E., HEYMAN, A., AND SALTZMAN, H. (1966) The protective effect of hyperbaric oxygenation in cerebral anoxia. *Arch. Neurol.*, **14**, 15.

Some Concluding Remarks

F. LOEW

Universitätsklinik, 665 Homburg/Saar, Germany

While walking along the shore of the ocean, St. Augustine puzzled over a problem. This was to describe and recognize the mystery and power of God. Suddenly he came upon a young boy who was attempting an impossible feat — that of emptying the ocean with a seashell. He realized that he, too, had attempted the impossible. I find myself in a position similar to that of St. Augustine, though I cannot call myself a saint and also show few other similarities to St. Augustine. It is absolutely impossible to give a general discussion of this congress, at which more than 200 reports and other papers were given, without boring you to death with a terribly long speech. Therefore, I ask your patience and understanding. I cannot touch upon every paper — not even each theme — but can only spotlight a few areas at random.

A large part of the congress dealt with the basis of cerebral circulation; not only normal and pathological anatomy, but especially physiology and patho-physiology. New methods, such as isotope clearance or dilution methods and measuring with heat-clearance-probes, have given us the possibility of replacing the hypotheses with positive knowledge. Physiology textbooks show that the brain blood flow is self-regulated and relatively independent of the condition and disturbances of the general circulation. It must be emphasized that this self-regulating system deals only with the normal brain; this system is abolished by diseases, trauma, and brain operations. That is, without a doubt, one of the most important results of research in the past few years, which has been reflected in the papers of the congress. As we neurosurgeons deal in most cases with a non-healthy brain, it is of utmost importance that we recognize this fact. The circulation in the damaged areas is passively dependent upon the heart output and the blood pressure. The increase of the intra-cranial pressure disturbs the circulation more markedly and earlier in the damaged brain than in the normal brain. At the beginning of a brain edema, carbohydrate utilization is disturbed, even before the cerebral blood flow is diminished. This disturbance of carbohydrate utilization may well be responsible for the consequential barrier disturbances with the resulting electrolyte and water imbalance of the brain tissue.

The experienced neurosurgeon has long been aware of and taken into consideration the increased vulnerability of damaged brain tissue to oxygen deficiency, decrease of blood pressure, and increase of intracranial pressure. We now have a more exact basis for further improvement of therapy. I am convinced that in the near future especially important advancements in this field will be made.

The papers have given the impression that the indication and technique of operating on aneurysms and angiomes are internationally uniform. Results are also correspondingly similar. The initial enthusiasm for the deep hypothermia, isolated brain cooling and circulatory arrest has been replaced by critical research and strong indication. As this is quite common with new methods, this should not limit its further development.

The leading word "cold" makes one think of the interesting research in Cryosurgery, the possibilities and limits of which have still not been established. The same holds true for hyperbaric oxygenation, which shows much promise in the future.

With regards to operative techniques, you may remember the use of the operation microscope, the neurosurgical microsurgery, and the possibility of nerve-root transplantion, for example in cases with neurogenic bladder.

In reflecting upon the diagnostic methods, the brain scanning is finding its place next to the time-proven angiography. The papers of this congress indicate the possibility that in the future the diagnosis of the pathology of a lesion could be made, in addition to its localization; for example, by the simultaneous application of different isotopes and through the notation of the time differences of the concentration in the focus.

In reviewing the congress, it becomes rather clear to me that the greatest advances have taken place between the field of neurosurgery and its neighboring specialties. Occasionally such fruitful areas of contact are found in a single person; for example, the contacts with anatomy in our friends and colleagues Lazorthes and Van den Bergh. We, the remaining, more simple structured neurosurgeons, who have no such ideal combination of more then one specialty combined within us, must promote cooperation with our neighboring specialist and profit from their methods. This is possible by teamwork with physiologists, biochemists, physicists, neurologists, and so on. It is important that we look past the boundaries of our highly specialized area. At the same time, it is also important to promote increased contact between the neurosurgeons of different nations. The international contact that we have experienced here in Madrid, has been highly successful. We enjoyed the pleasant atmosphere, beautiful surroundings, gracious hospitality and cultural stimulation. For this and much more, we are indebted to the organizers of this Congress.

Rheoencephalography

Supplementary Information in Tables, Compiled for the Participants of the IIIrd
Europ. Congr. of Neurosurgery

F. L. JENKNER

Fichtnergasse 22, Vienna, Austria

The following tables concerning Rheoencephalography contain in concise (but not
complete) form essentials on (a) apparatus available for the purpose (tables 1 and 2);
(b) attempts at evaluation (tables 3 and 4); and criteria in use (table 5) for evaluation;
(c) a compilation of those diagnoses amenable to the technique as regarded by various
investigators (table 6) and already in routine use in several countries. From these
tables everyone may derive some idea on REG. Further information on details such
as *e.g.* names (if desired addresses) of investigators will be gladly supplied by your
reviewer. A bibliography of REG has not been published as yet. Whatever information
is available will also be provided to interested neurosurgeons.

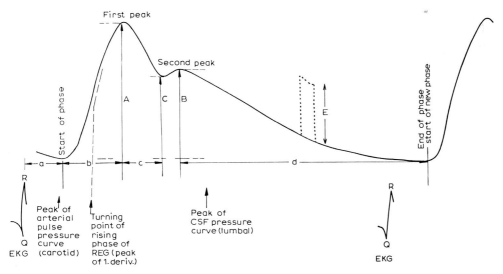

Fig. 1.

TABLE 1

INSTRUMENTS AVAILABLE COMMERCIALLY FOR RHEOENCEPHALOGRAPHIC USE. SEPARATE RECORDING DEVICES REQUIRED IN ALL INSTANCES (OF ECG AMPLIFICATION QUALITY). SIMULTANEOUS RECORDINGS OF OTHER PARAMETERS POSSIBLE WITH ALL UNITS BUT FROM IDENTICAL ELECTRODES ONLY WITH SOME UNITS. SPECIFICATIONS OBTAINABLE FROM MOST MANUFACTURERS.

Country	Model and data (type, frequency etc.) available
AUSTRIA	RHEOGRAPH (Dr. Schuhfried) Models with separate power supply Type I (single channel), Type II (2 channels). Self contained units (power supply in housing, use off mains): Type III (two channels) and type IV (4 channels) Frequencies from 20 to 60 kc, depending on model. 2 (4) channel models have 2 (4) frequencies. Circuitry supplied with all models. Bridge type. Medium size. Calibration: 0.05, 0.1, 0.5 and 1.0 ohm.
CSSR	L2-1 VUT PODEBRADY (Podebrady). Single channel model, rather large. Frequency, circuitry obtainable in CSSR only. Bridge.
FRANCE	ALVAR (Montreuil sous Bois) Bridge type, no other information.
ITALY	GALILEO (OTE Firence) Single channel model. Latest model is transistorized plug-in module, fairly small. Bridge type.
HUNGARY	ORION EG1–01, Type 4551 (METRIMPEX, Budapest) Model has 4 parts (large and heavy): electronic unit, power supply, push cart frame and carrying case. Single channel model, 30 kc (variable from 0.5 to 70 kc). Circuitry available with all data on the parts. Bridge type.
USA	BIOCOM Inc. Universal transistorized transducer. Smallest & most compact model on market. No bridge. 50 kc. Excellent for use also in physiology (adapter for recording EEG/ECG from same electrodes simult. available). Battery powered. E. and M. Instr. Co. Universal transducer, 2-channel model, 75/85 kc, battery powered, no cross talk, medium size; circuit available on request. Recording other parameters from same electrodes possible (ECG, EEG etc). Also for physiological use. HEWLETT PACKARD (former PI/Florida model) Bridge type unit, battery powered, medium size. (Is being improved). LEAR-SEAGLER, PARKS ELECTR., REFLECTONE ELECTR., SPACELABS Inc. are also producing models, no information obtained so-far.
USSR	BIOFIZPRIBOR produces one model, reported bridge type, no data available.

TABLE 2

PILOT MODELS OF INDIVIDUAL OR INSTITUTIONAL DESIGN, FOR RESEARCH AND CLINICAL ROUTINE USE OF RHEOENCEPHALOGRAPHIC INVESTIGATIONS. NO ATTEMPT MADE TO OBTAIN COMPLETE INFORMATION FROM ALL INSTITUTIONS USING THESE TECHNIQUES SINCE THE NUMBER OF INSTITUTES IS FAR TOO LARGE. THIS TABLE REPRESENTS SMALL SURVEY ONLY.

Country	Model	Remarks
AUSTRIA		RODLER pilot model, no bridge, multichannel model. Tracing does not change on clamping of internal carotid artery. Only block diagram published. One frequency (9 kc) with all channels.
CHECHOSLOVAKIA		LOSENICKY (electrotechnical university model) pilot model, no data available.
FRANCE		GOUGEROT pilot model one frequency, no bridge multichannel model. Block diagram published. Significance for evaluation of intracranial hemodynamics under investigation. No other data.
ROUMANIA		SOTIRESCU type I model (bridge) and type II model (no bridge), no other data. Simple circuit given.
USA		LIFSHITZ pilot models of various types (bridge and no bridge) for research, automatic evaluation.
		THE MAYO CLINIC and other institutions (*e.g.* Stanford Research Institute and many others) have pilot models for institutional use only. Research on special problems and basic research. On these apparatus no data available so far.
USSR		ARNAUTOV private model for routine use. Reported to be best Soviet design. Data given in USSR scientific journal. No other data available.
		FEDOROVSKIY private model, frequency 60–80 kc, reportedly automatic without controls. All other data available.
		YARULLIN institutional model for routine use. Bridge type 4-channel model using one frequency for all channels. (between 100 and 150 kc). No other data available.
		MOSKALENKO institutional model, transistorized, smallest model known to reviewer. Experimental use and basic research only. No other data.

496

TABLE 3

ATTEMPTS AT QUANTITATIVE EVALUATION

Name	Year	Formula
A. A. KEDROW	1948	$\Delta V = \dfrac{\Delta R}{R} \cdot G(g/cm^3)$
BONJER	1950	$\Delta V = \dfrac{\Delta R}{R} \cdot rho \cdot \dfrac{l^2}{r}$
J. NYBOER	1950	$\Delta R = \dfrac{R_s \cdot R_d}{\Delta R}\quad (R = R_d - R_s)$
A. I. NAUMENKO W. W. SKOTNIKOW	1954	$\Delta V = rho \cdot l^2 \cdot \dfrac{\Delta R_o}{R_o}$
K. POLZER F. KAINDL KUNERT F. SCHUHFRIED	1958	$\Delta V = \dfrac{\Delta R}{R} \cdot \dfrac{1}{T}\quad (T = \dfrac{60}{P})$
JANTSCH	1948	$\Delta V = \dfrac{\Delta R}{R}$
BIRZIS TACHIBANA	1962	Experimental comparison of imp. changes and flow rate in a diagram (linear quantitative correlation).

TABLE 4

ATTEMPTS AT QUALITATIVE EVALUATION (SYMBOLS A, B, C, D, A, B, C + E TAKEN FROM FIG. 1 DIAGRAMMATIC PRESENTATION OF CURVE PHASE)

Term	Symbol	Formula	Author
Celerita	C		Gentili
Komplex	K	$\dfrac{b}{b + c + d}$	Poilici
Quotient	Δt_2		Kunert
Quotient	ΔR	A/E	Kunert, Zouhar
Quotient	Δt_1	$\dfrac{a + b}{b + c + d}$	Kunert
Verzögerungszeit		$\Delta t_1 - \Delta t_2$	Kunert
Quotient	h/alpha	A/b	Hadjiev
Herzhirnzeit	t	a + b	Jenkner
		QR + a + b	Kunert
		"Cardiac period to 1. peak	Angelino
Index	I	A/B	Komrska
Index		A/C	Fedorowskij
Circulation rate		QR + a	Hadjiev

TABLE 5

SURVEY ON SOME CRITERIA IN USE FOR EVALUATION OF REG-TRACINGS

From this, it is evident, that standardisation is imperative!

Term/Symbol		Authors	Normal values	Mode of calculation (quotient of time intervals)	Remarks
CELERITA	C	GENTILI DOMONTOVITSCH			
KOMPLEX	K	POILICI, SOTIRESCU, NAS	0.10-0.18		
QUOTIENT	Δt_2	KUNERT ZOUHAR, NEVRATAL	3-6a =0.11 15-30a 0.13 45-60a 0.26 6-14a 0.12 20-45a 0.22 60 u.m. 0.28	onset of phase to first peak	in arterioscl.
QUOTIENT		POLZER, SCHUHFRIED	0.10-0.15	onset of phase to end of phase	0.20-0.40
QUOTIENT		FEDOROVSKIJ			
QUOTIENT	ΔR	KUNERT, ZOUHAR NEVRATAL CHRAST	300 (depends on age)	$\dfrac{\text{amplitude of curve}}{\text{height of cal. sign.}} \cdot 0.1\ \text{Ohm}$	signif. in carot. occl. and compr.
QUOTIENT	Δt_1	KUNERT	9-20 a 0.155) 0.16 60-70 · 0.31 20-30 a 0.165) 70-80 · 0.31 40-50 a 0.26 80-90 · 0.35 30-40 a 0.24 }0.26 or 50-60 a 0.26 60-90 · 0.3-0.35	$\dfrac{Q_{EKG}\ \text{to}\ Max_{REG}}{\text{length of phase}}$	arteriosclerosis (10 cases) 0.23-0.47
RETARDATION TIME		KUNERT	no change with age	$\Delta t_1 - \Delta t_2$	
INDEX	I	KOMRSKA	til 40 a : 0.50, over 40 a : 1.50	$\dfrac{\text{ampl. of first peak}}{\text{ampl. of second peak}}$	
QUOTIENT RHEOGR. QUOT.	A/C RQ	FEDOROWSKIJ JANTSCH + others	depending on vascular tone no change with age	ampl. in 1st peak/absc. of dip $\Delta R/R$	
RELATIVE PULSE (WAVE) VOLUME	P_R	KAINDL, POLZER SCHUHFRIED, JENKNER	1-2 ‰, no change with age	$RQ \cdot \dfrac{1}{T},\ T = \dfrac{60}{P}$	changes with funct. e.g.: CVI, ASCL, compr.
HEART BRAIN TIME	t	ANGELINUS KUNERT / JENKNER	to 50 yrs – 0.18 over 50 yrs – 0.22 changes with age changes with age and path.	"total heart period" to REG-peak Q_{EKG} to 1st peak R_{EKG} to 1st peak	changes with shunt, ASCL, occl.
CIRCULATION VELOCITY QUOTIENT	h/alpha	POILICI, NAS, SOTIRESCU HADJIEV, TZENOV	changes with age changes with age	Q_{EKG} to onset of phase ampl. of curve (1st peak)/rise time	

TABLE 6

TABULATION OF DIAGNOSIS FOR WHICH REG IS USED CLINICALLY (IN SOME COUNTRIES ROUTINELY); LAST TWO PARAGRAPHS MAINLY FOR STUDY AND INVESTIGATION

Diagnosis	Authors
Arteriosclerosis	Almay, Angelino, Auinger, Azzolini, Beer, Dobner, Fasano, Fedorovskij, Hadjiev, Garbini, Gentili, Jenkner, Kaindl, Kunert, Minc, Neumaier, Nevratal, Oehninger, Orlandi, Polzer, Ronkin, Schuhfried, Tzenov, Zouhar.
Hematoma (sub-, epidural, intra cerebral, also neonatal)	Almay, Fasano, Jenkner, Sakata, Sato, Semino, Suzuki, Takemoto.
Vascular occlusion (of carotid acute or chronic), compression or ligation (clamping, in human subjects) or stenosis (also of other cerebral vessels)	Almay, Chrast, Geddes, Gentili, Hadjiev, Hall, Hoff, Jarullin, Jenkner, Kottmeyer, Kunert, Lifshitz, Miller, Namon, Nevratal, Nas, Markovich, Poilici, Polzer, Ronkin, Schuhfried, Sotirescu, Tzenov, Zouhar (mostly more than one condition studied).
Arterio-venous shunts	Almay, Angelino, Jarullin, Jenkner.
Headache, migraine	Almay, Garbini, Gentili, DiMarchi, Jenkner, Oehninger, Ratner, Ronkin.
Concussion, contusion, edema	Beer, Evans, Freygang, Fedorovskij, Ischii, Jarullin, Jenkner, Landau, Oehninger, Ronkin.
Cerebral ischemia, cerebro-vascular insufficiency, softening	Almay, Hadjiev, Jarullin, Jenkner, Massmann, Nas, Nevratal, Schaaf, Sotirescu, Poilici, Zouhar.
Orthostatic stress, coma	Ascione, Dobner, Fedorovskij, Jenkner, Ronkin.
Arterial hypertension, coronary disease, myocardial infarction, aortic insufficiency, other	Almay, Beer, Fedorovskij, Garbini and assoc., Oehninger, Poppi, Ronkin.
Varia (lead intoxication, cer. atrophy, collagene disease, cer. tumor-investigational)	Anselino, Ascione, Fasano, Fusco, Jarullin, Jenkner, Komrska, Orlandi, Ronkin, Rossi, Silvestroni. (Only positive evidence of tumors reported by Jarullin)

Author Index

Subject Index